THE BIOCHEMIC SYSTEM OF MEDICINE

COMPRISING OF

THE THOEORY,
PAHTOLOGICAL ACTION,
THERAPEUTICAL APPLICATION,
MATERIA MEDICA & REPERTORY

OF

SCHUESSLER'S
TWELVE BIOCHEMIC REMEDIES

BY

GEORGE W. CAREY, *M.D.*

B. Jain Publishers (P) Ltd.
NEW DELHI-110055

Note from the Publishers

Any information given in this book is not intended to be taken as a replacement for medical advice. Any person with a condition requiring medical attention should consult a qualified practitioner or therapeutist.

Reprint Edition: 2005

Price. Rs. 99.00

Published by Kuldeep Jain for

B. Jain Publishers (P) Ltd.

1921, Street No. 10, Chuna Mandi,
Paharganj, New Delhi 110 055 (INDIA)
Phones: 2358 0800, 2358 1100, 2358 1300, 2358 3100
Fax: 011-2358 0471; *Email:* bjain@vsnl.com
***Website:* www.bjainbooks.com**

Printed in India by

J.J. Offset Printers

522, FIE, Patpar Ganj, Delhi - 110 092

ISBN 81-7021-161-1

BOOK CODE BC-2135

A WORD FROM THE EDITOR

I am extremely glad to have had the opportunity of helping to prepare this new edition of "The Biochemic System of Medicine," because I feel that the practice of supplying cell-salt deficiencies not only affords the most natural and logical method of treating disease, but it also agrees with, and indeed completes, the most modern ideas on internal medicine. I believe that its employment by physicians generally will be followed by a vast increase in the percentage of cures effected in both acute and chronic cases.

Biochemistry does not oppose the simultaneous use of other accepted forms of medication against the germ and bacillus, but while such treatment is being carried on, Biochemistry actually goes to the basic cause of the trouble. It supplies to the affected cells the inorganic salts which they lack, deprives the invading organisms of a breeding place, and restores the tissues to a healthy, normal condition.

Indeed, if proper biochemic treatment is given at the first pathological symptoms present, the trouble may often be aborted, as there will be no breeding place for hostile germs to thrive.

The same thing is true in chronic diseases. Here the cells, through lack of inorganic salts, have established a pathologic condition as practically normal, and it is only by giving them their lacking inorganic constituents that they are enabled to regain their proper composition, and once more function naturally.

In conclusion, I want to thank the many physicians who have co-operated with us by sending clinical reports showing the remarkable therapeutic results accomplished by the Biochemic Remedies. "Experientia docet." This has been a basic truth in medicine since the days of Hippocrates, and nowhere has it proven more resultful than with those who have followed the principles of Biochemistry. Modern medicine has already acknowledged the value of calcium and other cell-salts. The facts of Biochemistry should before long be accepted by all.

Edward L. Perry, M.D.

SAINT LOUIS, MO.
June 15th, 1925.

PREFACE

The following work on Biochemistry is offered to the medical profession as a step in advance in the domain of therapeutics. The simple logic of this theory and the remarkable results that have been obtained in its practical application to the problems of medicinal treatment of the sick must appeal to every intelligent practitioner. Far from refuting what experience in other branches of medical science has taught us, Biochemistry will, on the contrary, clear up many points that have never before been entirely understandable, and fit nicely into those gaps of understanding which have in many places been left in the physician's mind.

It is not claimed that all the matter in this book is original. It is absolutely necessary in preparing a text book on Biochemistry to use, chiefly, the therapeutics and materia medica of Schuessler and the translator, Dr. M. Docetti Walker, of Dundee, Scotland. Many additions have been made, however, founded upon extensive recent experience with the Biochemic Remedies. Hundreds of eminent physicians have given their time and experience to help make this book a complete and modern work on the subject. The theory, in regard to the manner and mode of operation by which the inorganic cell-salts of the human blood unite with organic matter to form the necessary material for carrying on life's processes, has, in this book, been given particular attention in order that the logic and simplicity of application of the Biochemic Theory may be easily understood in the case of each of the several diseases hereinafter mentioned.

Biochemistry is still in its infancy and it is hoped that progressive physicians will investigate, without prejudice, and thereby assist in obtaining a true understanding of the cause and cure of disease.

Introduction

THE process of life, complicated though it may be by countless minor and contributing processes, is in the main a simple one. It is therefore a great relief to find a system equally simple by means of which the ills and accidents to the machinery of life may be understood and overcome.

Nature has intended that all living things shall, for the span of their existence, be strong and healthy to their greatest capacity. Sickness, therefore, is an unnatural condition—one at variance with the intentions of Nature. And nature itself is continually battling against such conditions. Logically, then, man in his endeavor to combat disease, should study nature and in an understanding way help it to overcome its natural enemy, disease.

In the past, however, as a study of medical history will show, man has been groping along the wrong way. Strong drugs, poisons, nauseous chemicals, unnecessary surgery—these were formerly the means employed to overcome disease. But now, after much experiment and investigation, modern laboratory methods have proven that *within the body itself* are to be found the most potent weapons in the battle against disease.

According to the theory of Biochemistry, health is dependent upon the quantity and equalization of the organic and inorganic constituents in the body. The body is merely a collection of cells, each cell being composed of organic and inorganic matter; the former, quantitatively, largely prepondering. But it is the presence of the inorganic matter, which, though in minute quantity, unites with and activates the organic element and causes the cell to function in a normal manner.

Under ordinary conditions, enough of the inorganic cell-salts are supplied by the food to replace those lost in the process of metabolism. But when for any reason the body's power of assimilation fails, as occurs in disease, a lack of inorganic cell-salts results which can only be replaced by introducing them from the outside in assimilable form. A deficiency of one or more of the inorganic constituents will cause a train of symptoms, varying according to the inorganic salt that is lacking, which condition is known as disease.

Such in brief is the simple, natural truth upon which the theory of Biochemistry is founded. It is a logical way of assisting Nature with Nature's own weapons, and as such is bound to impress itself upon the unprejudiced investigator.

In the following pages the author has attempted to set forth in the plainest words the theory and practice of Biochemistry as stated by the famous scientist Dr. W. H. Schuessler, as well as the results of all the important recent developments and discoveries. In every case he has endeavored to trace back the disease to its inception and to show the logical steps in its development and the corresponding biochemic treatment.

It is hoped that this book will find favor wherever it is read and that it may help in creating a fuller understanding of diseases and their cure.

Contents

PART I.

GENERAL SKETCH

OF THE

Biochemic System of Medicine

BIOCHEMISTRY, or biochemic treatment of disease, opens up a new phase of medical science. The treatment of disease, with the inorganic cell-salts is so rational, so in accordance with well-known principles of natural law, that its basic principles need only be presented to the intellect to be understood and adopted.

In 1832 we find the following written in Stapf's *Archiv*: "All the essential component parts of the human body are great remedies." And again, in the same journal, in 1846: "All constituents of the human body act in such organs principally where they have a function."

Later, we find Grauvogl, in his Text-book, taking some notice of those remarks and amplifying them, but it remained for Dr. William H. Schuessler, of Oldenburg, Germany, to develop these suggestions and make the idea foreshadowed in them the basis of a "new system." It was in March, 1873, that he appeared in an article entitled: "Shortened Therapeutics," in which he says: "About a year ago I intended to find out by experiments on the sick if it were not possible to heal them, provided their diseases were curable at all with some substances that are the natural, *i. e.,* physiological function-remedies." Of this very promising communication of Dr. Schuessler no notice seems to have been taken, until some five months later Dr. Lorbacher, of Leipzig, came out in the same journal with some critical considerations. This was followed by a reply from Dr. Schuessler, which ran through seven numbers, giving a more detailed account of his "Abridged System of Therapeutics," the important features of which appear in the following pages.

The original communication by Schuessler to the German journal was translated into English by Dr. H. C. G. Luyties, and soon afterwards appeared a small edition, by Dr. C. Hering, on the Twelve Biochemic Remedies, "recommended for investigation" by this great teacher. Several editions were published in rapid succession, from which this historical sketch is mainly derived, and following these appeared the translation of the twelfth German edition, by J. T. O'Connor, M. D., and one by M. Docetti Walker, of Dundee, considerably enlarged by the addition of an appendix, popularizing the biochemic method.

Later, Doctors Boericke and Dewey, published a book, "The Twelve Tissue Remedies." It was the following words of Professor Moleschott of Rome, in his work on *"Vital Circulation,"* which set Schuessler to thinking that the sick might be healed with *"substances that are natural, i. e., physiological function remedies."* With this object in view he began a system of experiments upon the sick, and fully demonstrated that his ideas, and those of Professor Moleschott, were in full accord with natural law. Professor Moleschott said: "The structure and vitality of the organs depend upon the presence of the necessary quantities of the inorganic constituents."

On this fact is based the high estimation in which of late years, the subject of the relative proportions of the inorganic substances to the individual parts of the body has been held.

In the face of such positive facts, it can no longer be denied that the substances which remain after incineration or combustion of the tissues—the ashes—are as important and essential to the inner composition, and consequently to the "form-giving" and "kind-determining" basis of the tissues, as those substances which are volatilized during combustion.

A glue-furnishing base and bone-earth are essential constituents of bone. Without either there can be no true bone; so also, there can be no cartilage, without cartilage-salt; nor blood without iron, nor salines without potassium chloride.

The word biochemistry is formed from *bios* (the Greek for life) and chemistry. Webster defines chemistry as "that branch of science which treats of the composition of substances and of the changes which they undergo." Therefore, Biochemistry, taken literally, means that branch of science which treats of the composition of living substances, both animal and vegetable, and of the processes of their formation. But usage has given the word a somewhat different signification, and the following is a more accurate definition: That branch of science which treats of the composition of the bodies of animals and vegetables, the processes by which the various fluids and tissues are formed, the nature and causes of the abnormal condition called disease, and the restoration of health by supplying to the body the deficient cell-salts.

The chemical composition of nearly every fluid and tissue in the human body has long been known, but until Biochemistry was introduced, no practical use had been made of this knowledge in the treatment of the sick. Biochemistry is the only system of medicine which answers satisfactorily and fully the question: "What is disease?" It not only does this but it gives a logical reason for every dose of cell-salt prescribed; and describes its action in the system.

Biochemistry is science, not experimentalism. There is no more of mystery and miracle about it than about all natural laws. The food and drink taken into the stomach, and the air breathed into the lungs furnish all the materials of which the body is composed. By the juices of the stomach, pancreas, and liver, the food is digested and the useful particles are taken up by the villi of the small intestines. These are carried by the blood to the various parts of the body where they are needed and where they are absorbed. The blood thus supplies the materials necessarv for forming every tissue and fluid in the body and for carrying forward every process.

An analysis of the blood shows it to contain organic and inorganic matter. The organic constituents are sugar, fats and albuminous substances. The inorganic constituents are water and certain minerals, commonly called cell-salts. Of a living human being, water constitutes over seven-tenths, the cell-salts about one-twentieth, organic matter the remainder.

Not until recently were the inorganic cell-salts understood and appreciated. Being little in quantity, they were thought to be little in importance. But now it is known that the cell-salts are the vital portion of the body, the workers, the builders; that the water and organic substances are simply inert matter used by these salts in building the cells of the body.

Should a deficiency occur in one or more of these workers, of whom there are twelve, some abnormal condition arises. These abnormal conditions are known by the general term disease, and according as they manifest themselves in different ways and in different parts of the body, they have been designated by various names. But these names totally fail to express the real trouble. Every disease which afflicts the human race is due to a lack of one or more of these inorganic workers. Every pain or unpleasant sensation indicates a lack of some inorganic constituent of the blood. Health and strength can be maintained only so long as the system is properly supplied with these cell-salts.

Man, through the medium of plant life, is a product of the soil. All the main elements enter into his composition. Were the soil barren of its constituent matters, plant life would be unknown and man would cease to exist. An equilibrium of the inorganic constituents is as necessary in fertile soil and plant life as in the human organism. It is a law immutable and has existed since the world's creation.

Having learned that disease is not a thing, animate or inanimate, but a condition due to a lack of some inorganic constituent of the system, it follows naturally that the proper method of cure is to supply to the system that which is lacking. While in the treatment of disease, the use of products not constituents of the system may be very necessary and useful, a complete return to health cannot be expected until the missing cell-salts are supplied.

Biochemistry would seek to ascertain what is lacking and supply it in just the form needed. Any disturbance in the molecular motion of these cell-salts in living tissues constituting disease can be rectified and the requisite equilibrium re-established by administering the same mineral salts in small quantities. This is brought about by virtue of the operation of chemical affinity in the domain of histology, and hence this therapeutic procedure is styled by Schuessler the Biochemic Method, and stress is laid on the fact that it is in harmony with well-known facts and laws in physiological chemistry and allied sciences.

It is the blood that contains the material for every tissue of the body, that supplies nutriment to every organ, enabling it to perform its individual function; it is, indeed, a microcosm, able to supply every possible want to the animal economy.

Two kinds of substances are needed in the process of tissue building, and both are found in the blood, namely, the organic and the inorganic constituents.

Among the former are the sugar, fat and albuminous substances of the blood, serving as the physical basis of the tissues; while the water and salts, namely, potash, lime, silica, iron, magnesium and sodium, form the inorganic substances, which determine the peculiar kind of cell to be built up. Other salts may from time to time be found; but these constitute those constantly present. Whenever, then, in the animal organism new cells are to be generated and formed, there must be present, in sufficient quantity and proper relation, both these organic and inorganic substances; by their presence in the blood, all the organs, viscera and tissues in the body are first formed, fixed and made permanent in their functions, and a disturbance here necessitates disturbed function.

The cells are not fed. They feed themselves. Witness Virchow's researches, Lecture 14: "The absorption of matter into the interior of the cells is unquestionably *an act* of the cells themselves, for we are as yet acquainted with no method enabling us to produce this kind of proliferation in the body, by any mode of experimentation, through the medium of the agency primarily affecting either the nerves or the vessels."

Lecture 13, page 306, Virchow says—in relation to white matter in the spinal cord: "Every special function possesses its special elementary cellular organs; every mode of conduction finds paths distinctly traced out for it."

Thus we find the white fibres of the nerve or muscle act as conductors for Magnesia Phos. and indicate a lack of this salt by certain signs or words. (See repertory.) Other groups of fibres are conductors of other salts.

Alfred Binet, a French scientist of note, in his work, "The Psychic Life of Micro-organisms," says: "The micro-organisms do not nourish themselves indiscriminately, nor do they feed blindly upon every substance that chances in their way. Also, when they ingest food through some point or other of their bodies, they understand perfectly how to make a choice of the particles they wish to absorb. This choice is sometimes quite well defined, for there are species which feed exclusively upon particular foods. Thus, there are herbivorous and carnivorous infusoria."

Again—"The following is what occurs when the amœba, in its rampant course, happens to meet a foreign body: In the first place, if the foreign particle is not a nutritive substance, if it be gravel, for instance, the amœba does not ingest it, it thrusts it back with its pseudopodia. This little performance is very significant, for it proves, as we have already said, that this microscopic cellule in some manner or other knows how to choose and distinguish alimentary substances from inert particles of sand."

As the researches of Binet, the French scientist, show that micro-organisms—infusoria—select their own food from the material at hand, so does the German scientist, the great Virchow, clearly demonstrate that the cells which build the human form also select their own nourishment from the material at hand, and that nothing foreign to their constituent parts can be forced upon them, except to produce injury or death. The learned Pomeranian lectures, delivered in Berlin, many years ago, and published as "Virchow's Cellular Pathology," demonstrate the fact that all disease is caused by altered or abnormal cells, but he did not lay down the law of cure. The work of formulating a system of medicine and proclaiming to the world that the basic law of cure was at last discovered, remained for Dr. Schuessler, of Oldenburg, Germany.

The inorganic materials of nerve cells are Magnesia Phos., Kali Phos., Natrum and Ferrum. Muscle cells contain the same, with the addition of Kali Mur. Connective tissue cells have for their specific substance Silicea, while that of the elastic tissue cells is Calcarea Fluor. In bone cells we have Calcarea Fluor. and Magnesia Phos. and a large portion of Calcarea Phos. This latter is found in small quantities in the cells of muscle, nerve, brain and connective tissue. Cartilage and mucous cells have for their specific inorganic material Natrum Mur., which occurs also in all solid and fluid parts of the body. Hair and crystalline lens contain, among other inorganic substances, also Ferrum. The carbonates, as such, are, according to Moleschott, without any influence in the process of cell formation.

They are reserve materials out of which phosphates and sulphates can form themselves. Sulphuric and phosphoric acids unite with the bases of the carbonates and carbonic acid is given off. In this way sulphates and phosphates are produced.

The oxygen of the air, upon reaching the tissues through the blood by means of the respiration, acts upon the organic substances which are to enter into the formation of new cells. The products of this action are the organic materials which form the physical basis of muscle, nerve, connective tissue and mucous substances; each of these substances is the basis of a particular group of cells, to which, by means of chemical affinity, the above mentioned cell-salts are united, and thus new cells are produced. With the production of new cells there occurs at the same time a destruction of the old ones, resulting from the action of oxygen on the organic substances forming the basis of these cells. This oxidation has, as a consequence, a breaking-down effect on the cells themselves.

Urea, uric acid and sulphuric acid are the result of the oxidation of the albuminous substances, while phosphoric acid is produced by the oxidation of lecithine contained in the nervous tissue, brain, spinal cord and blood corpuscles. Lactic acid results from the fermentation of milk-sugar, and finally breaks down into carbonic acid and water. Sulphuric and phosphoric acids unite with the basis of the carbonates, forming sulphates and phosphates, and set free carbonic acid.

Uric acid unites with sodium, forming sodium urate, which, being of no use to the animal economy, is eliminated from the system; while partial failure of this, and its accumulation in the neighborhood of joints, together with albuminous substances, gives rise to gout. Natrum Sulph. removes the water resulting from the oxidation of the organic substances of the body, in which are suspended or dissolved the mineral matters set free in the retrograde cell metamorphosis, as well as the newly-formed organic substances, such as urea, uric acid, etc.

Disturbances of the function of the molecules of Natrum Sulph. may be followed, according to its duration or extent, as well as its location, by a retarded removal of this water of oxidation and its dissolved or suspended matter. This implies a slower tissue change and a consequent liability to diabetes, gout, etc.

It is interesting to note that Natrum Sulph. and Natrum Mur. act in opposite ways; for while the former—the sulphate—removes from the tissues the water, according to the process just described, the muriate—the common salt—enters the tissues dissolved in the water from the blood plasma, in order that the requisite degree of moisture proper for each tissue may be maintained.

By means of the presence of Natrum Phos. in the system, lactic acid is decomposed into carbonic acid and water. This salt has the power of holding carbonic acid in combination, fixing it, and does this in the proportion of two parts of carbonic acid to one of phosphoric acid which it contains. This combination is carried to the lungs, and there, by the action of oxygen from the inhaled air, the carbonic acid is set free from its loose union with Natrum Phos.—is exhaled and exchanged for oxygen.

Thus, of the sodiums, it will be noted that Natrum Phos. creates, Natrum Mur. distributes and Natrum Sulph. eliminates water.

The final products of the oxidation of the organic substances are urea, carbonic acid and water. These, together with salts set free, leave the tissues and thereby give place to less fully oxidized organic bodies, which in turn undergo finally the same metamorphosis.

The products of this retrograde tissue change are conveyed through the lymphatics, the connective tissue and the veins to the gall-bladder, lungs, kidneys, bladder and skin, and are thereby removed from the organism with the excretions, such as the urine, perspiration, feces, etc.

The importance and dignity of the function of the connective tissue has been established, since the researches of Virchow and Von Recklinghausen have led to its close study and proven its fertile activity. That which formerly seemed only intended as a filling-in, or protective covering, appears now as a matrix, in which the minute capillaries carry the plasma from the blood to the tissues and return the same to the blood-vessels, and at the same time serves as one of the most important breeding places for young cells, which are capable of developing out of the embryonic latent forms to the most differentiated structure of the body.

Health may be considered to be the state characterized by normal cell metamorphosis; thus, when by means of digestion of food and drink taken, recompense is made to the blood for the losses it sustained by furnishing nutritive material to the tissues, when this compensation is supplied in requisite quantities and in proper places, and no disturbance of the motion of the molecules occurs, *"Under these conditions alone will the building of new cells and the destruction of old ones proceed normally and the elimination of useless materials be furthered."*

Disease is the result of a loss of the power of union with organic matter by one or more of the inorganic cell-salts, which exhausted salt or salts are then carried out of the system. The cure consists in supplying the proper quantity of active inorganic cell-salts to replace that which has been thrown out of the system, and, by uniting with the organic matter, thus allows the affected cells to function properly.

The blood not being perfectly balanced in all its parts, does not feed and nourish the nerves, muscles and other tissues of the body. Thus a certain condition arises called disease, which, through the medium of the senses sends a call for certain materials which have not been supplied. These calls asking for material with which to carry on the process of life are the symptoms of disease; the names differ accordingly as the point is located in the body, from whence the call, or dispatch for cell-food is sent. The call or symptom is disagreeable or painful in order that we may heed it; for if it were pleasant or made an agreeable impression, we would be pleased and make no effort to prevent its repetition.

It is not the symptom that must be cured, but the underlying cause for which the symptom is only the body's warning that there are deficiencies to be supplied, for example:

A man goes without food for three days and nights, and, consequently, has pains, fever, headache, etc. Obviously he hasn't a disease, but simply lacks food. Obviously, too, he will die if the food is not supplied, but the symptoms or calls for food will not kill him; a lack of food will kill him. You know this and you give him food; but if you did not know it you might proceed to try to cure the pain, fever, headache, etc., arising from his lack of nourishment with some drug or medicine. So it is with the inorganic cell salts; a lack of any of them will set up certain symptoms which are merely Nature's method of indicating that certain of the vital workers of the body are absent and must be supplied.

Virchow defines disease as "a lack of some constituent part of the blood at the part affected."

Each mineral salt has a special work to do. Each has an affinity for certain organic materials used in building up the human frame. Thus, Kali Mur. molecules work with fibrin. If a deficiency occurs in this salt, a portion of the fibrin not having this inorganic salt to unite with becomes a disturbing element and may be thrown out of the vital circulation, through the nasal passages, lungs, kidneys or bowels, producing conditions called catarrhs, colds, coughs, etc.

Virchow's Lecture 7, page 167, "Cellular Pathology," says: "This dissociation of fibrin from the other fluid constituents of the blood is, to a certain extent, of real value, because fibrin, like the blood corpuscles, is quite a peculiar substance, and so exclusively confined to the blood and the most closely allied juices, that it really may be viewed as connected rather with blood corpuscles than with the mere fluids which circulate as serum."

The above gives us an insight into the workings of the molecules of Kali Mur. The reason the fibrin is "more plainly discerned in blood corpuscles than in the serum" is because only the organic material for fibrin is found in the serum. Kali Mur. salt unites with albumen and other substances and forms fibrin, and thus furnishes the corpuscles with the building material for tissue.

Our position is strengthened by a further quotation from same lecture: "Fibrin, which is, first of all, gelatinous, becomes differentiated into a fibrillar mass. It must be borne in mind, that this substance originally existed in a homogenous, amorphous, gelatinous condition and can again be reduced to it." Page 99, same lecture, Virchow says: "I do not think, therefore, that we are entitled to conclude that in a person who has an excess of fibrin in his blood, there is on that account also a greater tendency to fibrinous transudation."

The criticism we offer to the above is this: We claim an excess of fibrin never occurs in the blood, not even in embolus. The fault lies in a deficiency in Kali Mur. molecules—the workers in fibrin—the creators of fibrin. When this salt falls below the standard the fibrin collects in quantities, is not diffused properly through the blood, and might easily mislead the scientific investigator, simply studying the question from the point of organic chemistry.

In Bright's disease we find pure albumen a disturbing element. There is an affinity between lime phosphate and albumen. When the lime molecules fall below the standard, a portion of the albumen becomes non-functional and is thrown off through the kidneys.

Furnish lime phosphate in molecular form to fill the gap, to again establish the continuity in the salt, and the albumen will again be properly distributed through the organism.

If the albuminous substance thus thrown off should reach the skin in quantities too great to be excreted through the pores, it breaks down the tissue of the epidermis, or, in other words, eats a small section of the skin and thus escapes. Such a condition is called eczema, a word derived from a Greek word "to boil out."

When the deficiency is great, of course, more organic material must be disposed of, hence fevers or inflammation. The circulation is increased and the motion being changed to heat, by the law of conservation of energy, causes the symptom called fever. (See article on typhoid fever.)

The circulation is increased: 1. To throw off the waste organic matter or heteroplasm. 2. To try to furnish material to all parts of the system to sustain life. 3. To carry a sufficient amount of oxygen with the limited amount of iron molecules at hand. Of course, when a great lack of iron occurs, the blood must move much faster, for iron molecules are carriers of oxygen, and without that creative element life cannot be sustained.

Any tissue of the body deprived of oxygen dies at once. For the life of the individual cell is very brief, and without oxygen no new cells can be built; neither can they be built without a proper balance of inorganic salts.

Biology shows Biochemistry to be a science. The practical counterpart of the abstract science of Virchow's "Cellular Pathology" is formed by cellular therapeutics, or the system of introducing molecular cell-salts. Biochemic treatment is the outcome of the teachings of biology and those sciences which of late years have disclosed nature's ways and foot-steps by aid of the microscope and spectroscope.

The value of this system of medicine will be found by every medical man or student who tests the inorganic cell-salts in disease in accordance with the rules and practice of Biochemistry.

CELLULAR PATHOLOGY

ALL diseases that are curable, are cured in a *natural manner* through the circulation; the constituent parts of the human organism that are carried by the blood-vessels and transude through the walls of the veins and capillaries into the surrounding tissue, restore normal conditions when the blood contains the proper amount of its inorganic salts, water, sodium, ferrum, potassium, calcium, silica and magnesium.

When a deficiency of one or more of the constituent parts of the blood occurs, a disturbance arises in some part of the organism and a symptom (pain, fever, spasm or some cry of distress) is set up, in order that the intellect may heed and supply the want; or it may be that while the blood contains a proper balance of the vital principles, a disturbance may arise because of a pathological condition in a group of cells, tissue or nerves, and in supplying the cell-salts needed to overcome this condition, the quantity of cell-salts in the blood may fall below normal. In either case, a fine dilution of the salt indicated by the symptoms is needed, either to supply the lack of it in the blood, or to restore the normal condition of the part affected. It will be observed that there is nothing miraculous about this process—it is simply a *natural law;* and in no other way can a normal condition be restored in disease.

No improvement can be made on the human organism in this respect. The constituent parts of our bodies all keep in perfect harmony when rightly understood; and harmony can only be preserved by supplying these elements, the lack of which prevent harmony in the system.

We do not claim for the biochemic remedies magical curative properties, without giving any reason or explanation of the law of cure on which it is based. Let it be borne in mind that there is only one way to be restored to health, and that is the natural way; through the blood, by supplying deficiencies.

It will require just as much time to cure as nature requires, working in a natural way; by supplying the deficiencies. The salt *called for* must be supplied; other medicines may be given to alleviate pain or to overcome certain conditions in order that the Biochemic Remedies may work more accurately, but as they are not constituent parts of the blood found in the human organism, they will not, in themselves, effect a cure.

When a twig is broken from a tree we know a new twig will again grow to the same size if water is supplied to the soil, and the conditions favorable to the tree are kept up.

We realize the twig must be restored in a *natural* manner. The human system can only use its constituent parts. "The cells are *not fed,*" they feed themselves. They *reject* what they do not need; it cannot be forced on them, except to the detriment or death of the body. The vital forces are at once set to work to get rid of anything that does not belong to our organism, or will not assimilate with blood, bone, muscle, tissue, etc.

Dr. Schuessler says: "The inorganic substances in the blood and tissues are sufficient to heal all diseases which are curable at all. The question whether this or that disease is or is not dependent on the existence of fungi, germs or bacilli is of no importance in biochemic treatment because this treatment goes to the basic cause of the trouble, and, by supplying to the cells the cell-salts needed for a normal condition to exist, thereby destroys the breeding place for the fungi, germs, or bacilli. If the remedies are used according to the symptoms, the desired end, that of curing disease, will be gained in the logical natural way. Long-standing, chronic diseases, which have been aggravated by overdosing, excessive use of such medicines as quinine, mercury, etc., can be cured by minute doses of cell-salts."

Professor Liebig says: "It happens that a tissue in disease reaches such a degree of density, becomes so clogged, that the salt solutions of the blood cannot enter to feed and nourish; but, if for therapeutic purposes a solution of the cell-salt be so triturated, and given so diluted that all its molecules are set free, it is presumable that no hindrance will be in the way of these molecules to enter the abnormally condensed part of tissue."

The body is made up of cells. Different kinds of cells build up the different tissues and organs of the body. The difference in the cells is largely determined by the kind of inorganic salts which enter into their composition. If we burn the body, or any tissue of it, we obtain the ashes. These are the inorganic constituents of the body, the salts of iron, magnesia, lime, etc., which build up the tissues.

They are the *tissue-builders,* therefore, and both the structure and vitality of the body depend upon their proper quantity and distribution in every cell.

The biochemic remedies are these inorganic cell-salts, prepared by trituration, and thereby rendered fine enough to be absorbed by the delicate cells wherever needed.

Health is the state of the body when all the various tissues are in a normal condition; and they are kept in this state when they each receive the requisite quantity of needful cell-salt required for the upbuilding of the different tissues. Disease is an *altered state* of the cell, produced by some irregularity in the supply to the cells of one of the inorganic tissue-salts. Imperfect cell-action results, diseased tissues and organs follow, and all the phenomena of disease are developed. Now, the cure consists in restoring the normal cell-growth, by furnishing a minimal dose of that inorganic substance whose power of union with organic matter has been disturbed, which disturbance has caused the diseased action. To do this successfully, it is necessary to know what salts are needed for the upbuilding of the different tissues and for their normal action. This knowledge is derived from physiological chemistry, and hence this treatment of disease by supplying the needed tissue-salts is called the biochemic treatment.

In the following pages are given, under the different names of diseases, the respective Biochemic remedies that will prove curative, based upon the kind of tissue affected by the different diseases. Thus, in catarrhal conditions, for instance, the remedies will be the same, whether the catarrh shows itself in the throat, nose, or other organs, since it is the mucous membrane that is involved, and the mucous cells, therefore, call for a cell-salt that is lacking.

By giving a Biochemic remedy in such a dose as can be assimilated by the growing cells, the most wonderful and speedy restoration to healthy function is brought about in every case of curable disease. All diseases that are at all curable are so by means of the cell-salt properly prepared to the needs of the organism.

This is very important, and on it depends the success of the treatment, just as much as on the correct selection of the particular cell-salt. It seems reasonable that, to make the cell-salts immediately useful, they should be prepared in the same delicate form in which nature uses them, and that if they are absorbed by the microscopic corpuscles, they must themselves be finer than the corpuscles. We know that the mineral or cell-salts are infinitesimally subdivided in the different kinds of food we take, thus are capable of assimilation by the cells.

The cells of each tissue group receive their own special and peculiar cell-salt; for instance, those entering into the promotion of nerve cells are magnesia, potash, soda and iron; of bone cells: lime, magnesia, silica, etc., etc., which are extracted by the body from the food we take.

There are twelve Biochemic remedies—the twelve inorganic salts found in the ashes of the body—all essential to the proper growth and development of every part of the body. They are the.

Phosphates	of Lime, Calcarea Phosphorica. of Iron, Ferrum Phosphoricum. of Potash, Kali Phosphoricum. of Soda, Natrum Phosphoricum. of Magnesia, Magnesia Phosphorica.
Chlorides	of Potash, Kali Muriaticum. of Soda, Natrum Muriaticum.
Sulphates	of Lime, Calcarea Sulphurica. of Soda, Natrum Sulphuricum. of Potash, Kali Sulphuricum.
Fluoride	of Lime, Calcarea Fluorica.
Pure Silica	Silicea

Of these, those entering into the formation of *Nerve Cells,* and hence useful as remedies in diseases of the nervous system, the principal ones are Magnesia Phos. and Kali Phos.

Of *Muscle Cells*—the same and Kali Mur.

Of *Bone Cells*—Calcarea, Silicea.

This method of treating all forms of disease has been eminently successful, and can be confidently recommended to all practitioners of medicine.

The following indications for the use of these remarkable remedies can be relied upon, and have been verified by hundreds of physicians in all parts of the country.

In order to achieve the striking results recorded, it is essential to procure these remedies prepared strictly according to the Biochemic method.

The best preparation of the biochemic remedies is the triturated form. The original salts are triturated according to the Biochemic method with sugar of milk, one part of the salt to nine of sugar of milk, for one hour, which gives the first decimal trituration. The particles of this are still too large to be readily assimilated by the cells, and experience has taught that for general use the third trituration, where each grain contains the one-thousandth part of a grain of the cell-salt, is the most desirable.

Nature works everywhere with immense numbers of infinitely small atoms which can only be perceived by our dull organs of sense when presented to them in finite masses. The smallest image our eye can see is produced by millions of waves of light. A granule of salt which we can scarcely taste, contains millions of groups of atoms which no human eye will ever discern.

One quart of milk is found by analysis to contain about the six-millionth of a grain of iron; a child fed on milk receives each time one milligramme of iron in a half-pint of milk, which is only the fourth part of the above minute fraction of one part of a grain of iron.

Four milligrammes represents the whole quantity of iron in the milk supplied per day for its nourishment and growth, and this is sufficient to feed all the cells that are known to contain iron, and consequently require iron. This being the fact, how small will be the quantity required to equalize the balance of iron molecules in only a limited portion or group of cells, where, for instance, a molecular disturbance has taken place, and iron has to be supplied medicinally? But if milk contains the whole of the twelve inorganic cell-salts, how small must the quantity be when subdivided so that each drop has its own particle of each of the twelve constituents?

The proportion of fluorine in the human organism is still less than that of iron. From analytical facts it may be estimated that the fluorine in the milk is only present in decimilligrammes. One milligramme of Calcarea Fluor. per dose for a remedy would be quite large. A dose of any remedy used for therapeutic purposes should be rather too small than too large; for if too small, a repetition of the dose will bring about the desired effect, while too large a dose may miss its object altogether. Large doses of iron have a bad effect on the stomach, leaving the complaint unaffected. At the temperature of the body, hydrochloric acid, diluted with one-thousandth part of water, readily dissolves the fibrin of meat and the gluten of cereals, and this solvent power is *decreased,* not *increased,* when the acid solution is made stronger. (Professor Liebig's Chemical Letters.)

Spectrum analysis has opened a new field of truth, showing matter to be capable of endless subdivision.

A loss of the power of union with organic matter of any of the inorganic salts of a tissue produces an altered or abnormal condition, which is termed disease. Professor Virchow, the greatest authority on cellular diseases and cancer-cells, clearly states that the definition of all *disease* resolves itself into this: *"An altered or changed state of cell."* To overcome this condition, Dr. Schuessler supplies the same cell-salt, finely triturated, in fresh, active form. This fresh cell-salt then unites with organic matter and the cell is restored to normal condition. Chemical affinity here plays a particular part, each salt, by virtue of that law existing between organic and inorganic substances, finding its way into its particular tissue where it is wanted. Under this law, nature cures; hence it becomes necessary to administer these salts to the minute cells medicinally in minute quantities. Thus refined, they can be taken up by the cells so changed that they are no longer able to absorb the ordinary molecules of salt out of the plasma. Hence it follows that the ordinary preparations of cell-salts given as medicines are too bulky, and Dr. Schuessler has formulated a saccharated trituration of the twelve constituents of the body in such form that they can pass through the minute passages in the capillaries, and are readily assimilated by the cells of the blood and tissues. One illustration explains this: One red-blood corpuscle does not exceed the one-hundred-and-twenty-millionth of a cubic inch. There are over three million such cells in one droplet of blood, and these cells carry the iron in the blood. How necessary, then, to administer the cell-salt iron (*Ferrum Phos.,* which is the remedy for all inflammations of lungs, pleura, throat, eyes, ears, etc.), to diseased cells in the most minute molecular form. Each one of the twelve inorganic substances (in chemistry called salts) of which the human body is built up, has its own sphere of function and curative action, by reason of the part it occupies in the cells, and the part these have to perform in maintaining and restoring health.

TRITURATION

IT MUST be remembered that an attenuation of an inorganic mineral salt does not lose its entity but is always the same substance, however fine it may be pulverized, however many times it may be subdivided or however highly it may be triturated. The component parts of organic matter, *i. e.,* fibrin, sugar, oil, albumen, etc., leaving out the inorganic salts—the workmen which organize them—may be resolved back to their original elements by trituration. The chemical combination or formula that produces a certain organic substance is broken up by the process of trituration, and the oxygen, hydrogen, nitrogen, etc., that enters into the matter is set free again, and, while nothing is destroyed, a disintegration has taken place, and the organized substance only exists in its original elements.

But the cell-salts found in this organized matter, there to hold the materials together, and through the operation of which the whole substance is united as a functioning entity, cannot be disintegrated or changed to other principles. Iron is always iron. Potassium is always potassium. Silica is always silica.

Professor Liebig, in his chemical letters, says: "The smaller the particles of a prescribed medicine, the less physical resistance they meet in their diffusion in the tissues. It may be possible that a tissue can reach such a degree of density (become so clogged) that it is rendered impenetrable to the salt-solutions of the blood. But if, for medicinal purposes, a solution of salt be given so diluted that all molecules of the salt are set free, no hindrance will be in the way of these molecules to enter the abnormally condensed parts of tissue."

Professor Huxley said, in an address before the Medical Congress in London in 1881: "It will, in short, become possible to introduce into the human organism a molecular mechanism which, like a very cunningly contrived torpedo, shall find its way to some particular group of living elements, etc."

And again, Professor Huxley says: "Those who are conversant with the present state of biology, will hardly hesitate to admit that the conception of life of one of the higher animals as the summation of the lives of a *cell* aggregate, brought into harmonious action by a co-ordinative machinery formed by some of these cells, constitutes a permanent acquistion of physiological science.

"Nature works only with atoms, or groups of atoms, termed molecules. The growth of animals and plants is a synthesis process, atoms or groups of atoms joining the already existing mass of molecules. Every biochemic remedy must be diluted, so that the functions of healthy cells are not disturbed, and so that functional disturbances, when present, can be corrected." (*From Schuessler's Therapeutics.*)

In a thousand grammes of blood-cells, the inorganic salts contained are at this rate:

Iron phosphate	0.998
Potassium sulphate	0.132
Potassium chloride	3.079
Potassium phosphate	2.343
Sodium phosphate	0.633
Sodium chloride	0.344
Calcium phosphate	0.094
Magnesium phosphate	0.060

See Burye's "Manual of Physiology and Pathological Chemistry."

DOSE

The Biochemic Remedies are prepared in the form of triturations (powder form) and tablets. The tablets are the most convenient form, and always insure correct dosage. The genuine Biochemic Remedies in the tablet form are prepared by the Luyties Pharmacal Co., St. Louis, Mo., and are known under the name "Celloids."

The usual dose for adults is 5 Celloids (or 5 grains) of the indicated remedy. For children about one-half the quantity. The remedies can be given dry on the tongue or dissolved in water. When two or more remedies are needed, they should be taken in alternation.

In acute conditions give the remedy every one-half hour to two hours, according to the severity of the case, and every three hours after amelioration. If the pains or symptoms are very severe, the quickest results are obtainable by giving the remedy in hot water, until relief is obtained.

In chronic conditions give two or three doses daily in the morning, at noon and at night before retiring.

PART II.

MATERIA MEDICA

OF THE

Twelve Biochemic Remedies

CALCAREA FLUORICA

SYNONYMS.—Calcii Fluoridum, Calcium Fluoride.

PRESENT NAME.—Calcium Fluoride.

COMMON NAME.—Fluor-Spar.

SYMBOL.—CaF_2.

ORIGIN AND PROPERTIES.—It occurs in nature as the mineral fluor-spar, beautifully crystallized, of various colors, in lead-veins, the crystals having commonly the cubic, but sometimes the octohedral form, parallel to the faces of which latter figure they always cleave. Some varieties, when heated, emit a greenish, and some a purple phosphorescent light. The fluoride is quite insoluble in water, but is decomposed by sulphuric acid, generating hydrofluoric acid.

CALCIUM FLUORIDE is found in the surface of the bones, the enamel of the teeth, the elastic fibres, and the cells of the skin. Wherever elastic fibre is found, be it in the epidermis, the connective tissue or the walls of the blood vessels, there Calcium Fluoride may always be found. A loss of its power to unite with organic matter causes a continued dilatation or relaxed condition of the fibres. This is seen in such conditions as varicose veins, hemorrhoidal tumors, relaxation of the abdominal walls, with consequent sagging of the abdominal viscera, uterine hemorrhages, after pains, etc.

This state of relaxation, occurring in the elastic fibres of the blood vessels, connective tissue or lymphatic system, causes an inability to absorb exudations. This results in indurated glands, lumpy exudations on the surface of bone, encysted tumors, hard swellings, etc.

By supplying the lacking Calcium Fluoride the elastic fibres are again restored to their integrity, resume their power of contractility and functionate properly. Exudations are thrown off and absorbed by the lymphatics.

In general, then, the administration of Calcium Fluoride is indicated in all diseases which can be traced, directly or indirectly, to relaxed conditions of the elastic fibres or those ailments having their seat in the substance forming the surface of bone, enamel of the teeth, walls of the blood vessels and in the cells of the epidermis.

CHARACTERISTIC INDICATIONS

HEAD.—Head troubles, when traced to a relaxed condition of the elastic fibres. Tumors on the heads of new-born infants, blood tumors. Bruises on the bones of the head, when they are hard, rough, uneven lumps. Ulcerations on the bone surface.

EYES.—Cataract of the eye. Blurred vision, after straining the eyes, with pain in the eyeball, better when resting the eyes, caused by a relaxation of the walls of the blood-vessels, allowing an engorgement of blood.

EARS.—Diseases of the ear, when the bone or periosteum is affected or when characteristic of this salt.

NOSE.—Stuffy cold in the head, with thick, yellow, lumpy, greenish, discharge. Offensive lumpy discharges, ozæna (*Kali*

Phos., Silicea). Diseases of the nose, when affecting the bones (*Calc. Phos.*).

FACE.—Hard swelling on the cheek, with pain or tooth-ache. Osseous lumps or growths on the jaw or cheek bones. Chaps or cracks of the lips, or nose cold (*Ferrum Phos.*).

MOUTH.—Cracked lips; very hard swellings on the jaw-bones, traceable to a relaxed condition of the muscular fibres.

TEETH.—When the teeth become loose in their sockets, not during dentition, with or without pain. The enamel of the teeth is largely composed of this salt. Enamel rough and thin, or when very brittle. Rapid decay of the teeth, when the enamel is deficient (alternate *Calc. Phos.*). Teeth tender owing to looseness.

TONGUE.—The tongue has a cracked appearance, tongue becomes indurated after inflammation (*Silicea*). Chronic swellings of the tongue.

THROAT.—Relaxed condition of the throat. Elongation of the uvula, causing tickling cough by dropping into the throat (*Natr. Phos.*). Diphtheria, when the disease has gone to the windpipe (alternate *Calc. Phos.*). Enlargement of the throat (*Natr. Mur.*). Relaxation of the blood-vessels of the throat.

GASTRIC SYMPTOMS.—Vomiting of undigested food. *Ferrum Phos.* is the principal remedy, but when this fails, *Calc. Fluor.* should be exhibited,

ABDOMEN AND STOOL.—Hemorrhoids, when bleeding. Protruding and itching piles, blind piles, accompanied with pain in back and constipation. Alternate with remedies indicated by color of stools or blood (also external application). Piles with rush of blood to the head (requires also *Ferrum Phos.*), confined bowels, inability to expel the feces, due to a relaxed condition of the rectum, allowing a too large accumulation of fecal matter. This condition is frequently met with after confinement, when all the pelvic muscles are relaxed. Fissure of anus, sore crack near end of bowel; should also be used locally.

Urinary Organs.—Increased quantity of urine, when traced to a relaxed condition of the muscular fibres of the urinary organs.

Male Sexual Organs.—Dropsy of the testicle. Hardening of the testicles. In syphilis, when the symptoms indicate this remedy.

Female Sexual Organs.—All displacements of the uterus require this remedy (*Calc. Phos., Kali Phos.*). Falling of the womb. Anteversion, retroversion, and the flexions of the uterus require this salt to tone up the contractile muscles. Dragging pains in the groin and in the lower part of the back. Pains extend to the thighs. Menses excessive, flooding, with bearing-down pains. Uterus very relaxed and flabby, or very hard, like stone, owing to a disorganization of the fluoride of lime molecules.

Pregnancy.—After-pains, when too weak. Hemorrhage, if the uterus does not contract. Hard knots and lumps in the breast (*Kali Mur.*).

Respiratory Organs.—Uvula elongated, causing tickling in larynx, with cough. Cough, when tiny lumps of tough, yellow mucus are expectorated. (*Silicea*). In asthma, when the *expectoration* is *difficult* and *consists of small, yellow lumps* (*Kali Phos.*). Patient is relaxed and prostrated.

Circulatory Organs.—*Varicose veins, and also a tendency to this condition.* Veins seem as if they would burst; use also a lotion of the salt. Dilation of the blood-vessels when the elastic fibres of the walls of the vessels have become relaxed; this is the chief remedy to restore their contractility (*Calc. Phos.*). First stage of aneurism (*Ferrum Phos.*). Hypertrophy, or enlargement of the heart (*Kali Mur.*). Irregularities of the heart's action, when due to prolapsus of uterus and other relaxing diseases.

Back and Extremities.—Pain in lower part of back, weak, with dragging pains. Burning pains in the sacrum, with confined bowels. Hard growths or excrescences on the bone surface. Relaxed conditions of the muscles, allowing easy discoloration of the fingers and toes. Hard swellings. Gouty enlargement of the joints (*Magnes. Phos.*). Varicose ulceration of the veins of the limbs; use also a lotion on cotton. Rubber bandages or elastic stockings should also be used Whitton, gathered fingers; use also a local application (*Silicea, Calc. Sulph.*).

Skin.—Chapped hands or lips from cold (*Ferrum Phos.*). Skin hard and horny; use also plenty of soap and water. Cracks in the palms of the hands; mix a quantity of the salt in vaseline, and after washing the hands rub the ointment in thoroughly. Fissure of the anus, fistulous ulcers, when secreting thick, yellow pus (*Silicea, Calc. Sulph.*).

Tissues.—Suppurations of the bones and periosteum; ulcers, felons, etc. "When a fibrinous exudation is not dissolved by suppuration, but has become hardened, *Calc. Fluor.* must be given" (Schuessler). Encysted tumors, *swellings* and *indurated enlargements, hardened glands,* etc., need this salt (*Kali Mur., Silicea*). Relaxed elastic tissues. Bruises on the bone, with uneven hard lumps. Dropsy from heart disease.

Febrile Conditions.—*Fevers, when arising from relaxed conditions;* for the cause of these fevers, alternate with appropriate remedies.

Modalities.—*Hot applications* will generally relieve, especially in hardened conditions; cold is sometimes beneficial when contraction is required.

CALCAREA PHOSPHORICA

SYNONYMS.—Calcii Phosphas Precipitata, Calcis Phosphas, Precipitated Phosphate of Calcium.

PRESENT NAME.—Calcium Phosphate.

COMMON NAME.—Phosphate of Lime.

FORMULA.—$Ca_3 (PO_4)_2$.

MOLECULAR WEIGHT.—306.

PREPARATION.—The one used for the proving was a mixture of the basic and other phosphates of lime, obtained by Dr. Hering (Correspondenzblatt, 1837), by dropping dilute phosphoric acid into lime water, as long as a white precipitate was formed; this precipitate was washed with distilled water and dried on a water bath. It was first proved by Dr. Hering.

PHOSPHATE OF LIME is destined to play a prominent part in the treatment of the sick, when its range is fully understood by medical practitioners. This salt works with albumen, carries it to bone, tissue or to any part of the body where it may be needed. It uses albumen as a cement to build up bone structure.

Bone is fifty-seven per cent. phosphate of lime, the remainder gelatine; an albuminous, gluey substance, carbonate of soda, magnesium phosphate and sodium chloride. Without the lime phosphate no bone can be made.

When, for any reason, the molecules of this salt fall below the proper standard in the blood, some disturbance in life's processes occur. It may be that bone-cells are not rebuilt as fast as they die. In such cases, if the deficiency exists for a great length of time, a condition of anemia prevails, for the bone is the basis, the foundation-stone, of the organism. Should the albumen, not having a sufficient quantity of the lime phosphate to properly take care of it, become a disturbing element and be thrown off by the kidney route, Bright's disease results. If through the nasal passages, the condition is named catarrh. If by the lungs, a cough is produced. If the albumen reaches the skin, pimples, eruptions, freckles, a condition called eczema, or possibly sores.

Calcium phosphate is found in gastric juice, and a lack of the proper balance is frequently the cause of indigestion. Conditions called rheumatism are sometimes due to a deficiency of this cell-salt. It is well known to Biochemists that a proper balance of sodium phosphate is required to prevent an acid condition from prevailing, and under certain conditions, when calcium phosphate for any reason is not present in proper quantities, the affinities draw upon sodium phosphate in an endeavor to supply the lack, and thus a deficiency in the alkaline salts ensue, which allows an acid condition to prevail, *i. e.,* rheumatism. Calcium phosphate is an auxiliary to the therapeutical effects of magnesium phosphate, as it more nearly resembles that salt than any other. When Magnes. Phos. is clearly indicated, and does not restore the normal condition in a reasonable length of time, Calc. Phos., should be given, for it is quite certain that it has been drawn on from the blood to assist the work of Magnes. Phos., hence the deficiency in the lime-salt.

CHARACTERISTIC INDICATIONS

MENTAL SYMPTOMS.—Peevish, fretful children. Poor memory; incapacity for concentrated thought; mind wanders from one subject to another; weak minds in those practicing, or who have practiced, self-abuse (*Kali Phos.*). Dull, stupid; depression of spirits; anxious about the future. Desires solitude after grief, disappointment, pain, etc.

HEAD.—Headache, with cold feeling in the head, and head feels cold to the touch. Headache on top of head and behind the ears. Tight sensation. Headache of girls at puberty, with restlessness and nervousness. *Headache worse from mental exertion, worse near the sutures. Skull is thin and soft. Closure of the fontanelles delayed or re-opening of same.* Vertigo (*Ferrum Phos.*). *Crawlings over the head, with cold sensations.* Ulcers on top of head.

Dropsy of the brain, and to prevent these conditions. Loss of hair; bald spots. Inability to hold up the head, owing to a deficiency of lime phosphate in the system.

EYES.—Sensitive to artificial light. Eyeballs ache; spasm of the eyelids (*Magnes. Phos.*). Squinting. Hot feeling in the lids. Paralysis of the retina, causing dimness and loss of sight (*Kali Phos.*). Neuralgic pain in eyes, when *Magnes. Phos.* fails. Inflammation of the eye, with characteristic discharge, especially in scrofulous subjects. Intolerance of light (*Ferrum Phos.*).

EARS.—Aching pain, with swelling of the glands of face and neck. Earache, with characteristic albuminous, excoriating discharge. In scrofulous persons, where the glands are much swollen. Ears swollen, burning and itching.

NOSE.—Large, pedunculated nasal polypi. Nose swollen and greatly inflamed at the edges of nostrils (*Silicea*). Tip of nose cold. Coryza, cold in head, with albuminous discharge. Albuminous discharge, thick and tough, dropping from posterior nares, causing constant hawking and spitting: worse out-doors. Disposition to take cold in anemic persons (*Ferrum Phos.*). To prepare the way for other remedies in all cases of catarrh, *Calc. Phos.* has a decided tonic action on the membranes.

FACE.—Anemic, or chlorotic face. Dirty-looking face. Rheumatism of face, which is worse at night. Pimples on the face. Pains in face, with a creeping sensation; feeling of coldness and numbness. Face sallow, pale, earthy; skin cold and clammy. Lupus. Heat in face. Freckles, eruptions on the face of young persons, especially of young girls at puberty. Pains in face, of a grinding, tearing nature (*Magnes. Phos.*). Pale face in children, when teething is difficult.

MOUTH.—Bad, disgusting taste in mouth in the morning, caused by non-assimilation of food. Consider also *Natr. Phos.*

TEETH.—Retarded dentition (*Calc. Fluor.*). Phosphate of lime is a constituent of the teeth, and when this material is deficient, dentition will be slow and painful, often causing convulsions (*Magnes. Phos.*) and other ailments. Teeth decay as soon as they appear. Gums inflamed and painful (*Ferr. Phos.*). Toothache, which is worse at night (*Silicea*). *Chief remedy in all teething disorders.* "If the gums be pale this remedy is especially indicated" (Schuessler).

TONGUE.—Tongue swollen (*Kali Mur.*). Stiff and numb. Blisters and pimples on tip of tongue.

THROAT.—Enlargement of throat. Goitre (chief remedy) (*Natr. Mur.*). *Chronic enlargement of the tonsils.* "I have given it in the acute stage, when suffocation threatened, with excellent results" (Chapman). Glands painful, aching; deglutition painful. Thirst, with dry tongue and mouth. *Sticking pain in throat on swallowing.* Constant hoarseness. Hemming and scraping of throat when talking. Public speakers are greatly benefited by it (alternate with *Ferrum Phos.*). Burning and soreness in larynx and pharynx, in cases of chronic catarrh, when there is considerable dropping from the posterior nares.

GASTRIC SYMPTOMS.—Pain after eating. *Food seems to lie in a lump.* Heaviness and burning. Pains worse from eating even the smallest amount of food (*Ferrum Phos.*). Stomach sore to the touch. Abnormal appetite, but food causes distress. Cold drinks and food greatly aggravate the pains, while heat relieves (*Magnes. Phos.*). Faint, sinking feeling in region of stomach. Pain sometimes relieved by belching wind. Infants vomit sour, curdled milk (*Natr. Phos.*). Constant desire to nurse. Stomach feels bloated. A course of this remedy should be given after gastric or typhoid fever, and in all cases where digestion is poor, to aid assimilation of food. *Vomiting after cold drinks.* Headache, accompanied with indigestion. Belching of gas. Most of the gastric symptoms which come under this reemdy are due to non-assimilation of food.

Abdomen and Stool.—Diarrhea in teething children; stools slimy, green undigested, with colic (*Natr. Phos.*). Give injection of hot water. *Cholera infantum,* child craves food it should not eat. *Stool is hot, often noisy and offensive* (*Kali Phos.*). Summer complaint caused from inability to properly digest the food. Diarrhea after eating green fruit, abdomen sunken. Face pale and anxious, child fretful. Pain in the abdomen near the navel. Infant cries when it nurses. Marasmus, eats heartily but grows more emaciated all the time. *Frequent call to stool, but passes nothing* (*Kali Phos., Magnes. Phos.*). Diarrhea of school-girls, with the accompanying headache. Costiveness, with hard stool, in old people and infants. Itching piles, also protruding piles (*Calc. Fluor., Ferrum Phos.*). Hemorrhoids which ooze an albuminous substance resembling white of egg, especially noticeable in anemic persons. *Cracks and fissures of anus* (*Calc. Fluor.*). *Fistula without pain.* Offensive stools (*Kali Phos.*). Neuralgia of rectum and pain after stool. *Symptoms all worse at night or with change of weather* (*Silicea*). To prevent formation of gall-stones. Tabes mesenterica.

Urinary Organs.—Urine highly colored. Frequent urging to urinate, with sharp, shooting, cutting pains at the neck of the bladder and along the urethra (*Ferrum Phos.*). Increase in the quantity of urine. Albuminous urine calls for this salt (*Kali Phos.*).

Calc. Phos. has a chemical affinity for albumen. Bright's disease of the kidneys (*Kali Phos.*). Phosphatic deposit in the urine (as an intercurrent remedy). To prevent reformation of stone in the bladder. Gravel sediment in urine (*Natr. Sulph.*). Diabetes mellitus (as an intercurrent remedy).

MALE SEXUAL ORGANS.—Swelling of the testicles (*Orchitis*). Masturbation. Inguinal hernia (*Calc. Fluor.*). Scrotum itches and is greatly relaxed. Sweating and soreness of scrotum. Chronic gonorrhea and gleet, when the discharge is characteristic. Dropsy of the testicles. All albuminous discharges from the urethra are indicative of this salt.

FEMALE SEXUAL ORGANS.—*Weakness in uterine region from prolapsus uteri* and other *uterine displacements* (*Calc. Fluor., Kali Phos.*). "Calc. Phos. may not have the contracting power of Calc. Fluor., by acting directly upon the muscles and tissues involved, but it acts indirectly by building up the general health and aiding digestion, thereby restoring the tissues to a healthy condition and promoting the deposit of Calc. Fluor." (Chapman).

Aching in the uterus. Increased sexual desire, especially immediately before menstruation. Intercurrently in all cases of leucorrhea, to build up the general health. Leucorrhea, discharge albuminous, very tenacious (like white of egg). Acrid leucorrhea, worse after menstruating or with sexual excitement. Patient is dull and listless. Menses too early or too late in young girls with anemic conditions. Menstrual discharge bright red, and too frequent. Menses with pain in back. Labor-like pains at the time of menstruating (*Magnes. Phos.*); (to prevent, *Ferrum Phos.*). Menses, with flushed face and cold extremities (*Ferrum Phos.*).

PREGNANCY.—Aching in the limbs during pregnancy. Poor milk, watery, or with saltish taste (*Natr. Mur.*). Child refuses to nurse. Child vomits sour, curdled milk quite frequently. Sore nipples (*Ferrum Phos.*). *After pregnancy,* as a restorative; also *after long nursing,* when the patient is debilitated

(*Kali Phos.*). (Use locally a 10 per cent. unguentum of the second trituration and vaseline.)

Respiratory Organs.—Cough, with expectoration of albuminous mucus, not yellow. Chronic coughs. Incipient consumption. Intercurrently in all cases for the weakness and prostration. Chronic cases of whooping cough. *Rheumatic pains in lungs. Involuntary sighing.* Soreness and dryness in throat of consumptives. Aching in the chest. Night-sweats, especially about the head (*Silicea, Natr. Mur.*). Hawking to clear the throat. Cough in anemic persons or teething children.

Circulatory Organs.—Intercurrently in most cases of heart trouble. Poor circulation, with cold extremities. Palpitation of the heart, followed by weakness. Leukemia (excess of white corpuscles in the blood).

Back and Extremities.—Calc. Phos. being appropriately named "the bone remedy," plays an important part in the symptoms of disease located in the back and extremities, which are largely composed of this material. Curvature of the spine (with *mechanical supports*). *Numbness and coldness* of the limbs. Pains and aching in the joints. *Cold sensations in the limbs, as if cold water were being poured over them.* Pains in the bones, especially the shin-bones. Pain worse at night and in cold, damp weather. *Rheumatism of the joints, and in the back between the shoulders;* very severe and *worse at night* or *during rest.* Lumbago (*Ferrum Phos.*). Hydroma patella, cysts. Hydrops. Articular spinal irritation. Injuries of the coccyx. Infants are slow in learning to walk, and the bones are soft and friable. *Bow-legs* (with *mechanical supports.*) Neck thin in children. Broken bones; this salt is essential to facilitate deposit of extra material necessary for their union. Rickets: "this disease appears to consist essentially in the non-deposition of phosphate of lime in the osteoid tissues" (Thomas' Med. Dict.). Inflammation of the periosteum, of syphilitic origin. Ulcers and abscesses, when deep-seated on the bones or joints. Neuralgia, when deep-seated, as if on the bone, commencing at night (*Silicea*).

Pain in limbs, feel restless, asleep; better when moving them.

Nervous Symptoms.—Neuralgia (*nerve pains*) which are worse at night, colic, cramps, spasms, convulsions, etc. (after *Magnes. Phos.* fails to relieve). Convulsions in teething children, young girls, and in old people, when the lime-salts are deficient. Paralysis, when associated with rheumatism. Patient is tired and weary. *Pains very severe at night, with sensation of creeping numbness and coldness. Pains shoot all over the body like electrical shocks, and at other times like trickling of cold water.*

Skin.—Eruptions on the skin, when the discharge is albuminous. Pimples, acute or chronic, with itching. Itching of the skin, without eruptions. Eczema, with yellowish-white crusts. Face full of pimples. Scrofulous affections (*intercurrently*). Dry skin. Skin itching and burning, as from nettles. Perspiration on hands from spinal weakness. Lupus, with characteristic symptoms. Pruritus of vagina, with or without albuminous leucorrhea (*Natr. Mur.*). Freckles (apply a 10 per cent. solution in water to the face). Chafed skin (*Natr. Mur.*). Acne rosacea. Tubercles on the skin. Scaling herpes on the shins.

Tissues.—Bones weak and friable, easily broken; when broken will not unite, when new bone material is needed. Rickets. Tabes or atrophy of any organ or tissue. Poor nutrition through indigestion. Ulceration of bone substance. Stunted growth. Defective development, with pale, greenish-white complexion. All ailments dependent upon a deficiency or disturbance in the phosphate of lime molecules. Polypi. Disease of the pancreas. Emaciations, chlorosis, anemia. Intercurrently in all bone affections, constitutional weakness. As a tonic for delicate, anemic persons (*Ferrum Phos.*).

FEBRILE CONDITIONS.—Chilliness and shivering when beginning of fever (*Ferrum Phos.*). Perspiration excessive. *Night-sweats in phthisis. Cold, clammy sweat on the face and body.* After typhoid and other fevers, as the disease declines, to promote the deposit of new material in place of that destroyed.

SLEEP.—Restless sleep, due to worms (*Natr. Phos.*), drowsy, sleepy, hard to wake in the morning. Vivid dreams.

MODALITIES.—Symptoms are generally *worse at night in damp, cold weather,* and change of weather, getting wet, etc. *Better in warm weather* and in *warm room.*

CALCAREA SULPHURICA

SYNONYMS.—Calcii Sulphas, Sulphate of Calcium, Sulphate of Lime.

PRESENT NAME.—Calcium Sulphate.

COMMON NAMES.—Gypsum, Plaster of Paris.

FORMULA.—$CaSO_4 \cdot 2H_2O$.

MOLECULAR WEIGHT.—172.

ORIGIN AND PREPARATION.—The hydrated sulphate of calcium occurs native, forming gypsum, a transparent and regularly crystalline variety of which is called *selenite.*

It is prepared by precipitating a solution of calcium chloride with dilute sulphuric acid. The precipitate is to be washed with hot water and dried at about 30° C (86° F.).

PROPERTIES.—Precipitated calcium sulphate is a fine, white crystalline powder. It is soluble in about 400 parts of cold, and with more difficulty in boiling water; in alcohol it is insoluble. Heated to 200° C. (392° F.) it parts with its water of crystallization.

SULPHATE OF LIME is used to clean out an accumulation of heteroplasm in the interstices of tissue; to cause the infiltrated parts to discharge their contents readily, and to throw off decaying organic matter, so it may not lay dormant or slowly decay, and thus injure the surrounding tissue. A lack of this salt allows suppuration to continue too long. It controls suppuration. A decay of epithelial cells, after the infiltrated parts have discharged their contents, indicates a lack of this salt. The third stage of all catarrhs, lung troubles, boils, carbuncles, ulcers or abscesses need this cell-salt.

While Silicea hastens the process of suppuration in a normal manner, Calc. Sulph. closes up the process at the proper time if it is present in the blood in proper quantity.

The reason why Calc. Sulph. prevents the process or so promptly closes it up is because a lack of this vitalizer or inorganic worker in organic matter, allows the epithelial cells to break down—allows tissue to disintegrate; then the fluids from the blood (*serum*) take up the waste and carry it off through some natural or artificial orifice.

Other salts, of course, are of some importance in such conditions, but in true suppurations Calc. Sulph. is always the chief remedy, because there can be no true suppuration when this worker is present in proper quantity.

Exudations of albuminous, or fibrinous, or watery matter, may take place, because of a lack of other salts, even when there is no lack of Calcarea Sulph. (See Exudations.)

CHARACTERISTIC INDICATIONS

HEAD.—Suppurations of the head or scalp when the *discharge* is *yellow, purulent matter,* or when forming crusts of the same character. Discharges of a sanious nature. *Crusta lactea,* stage of resolution (after *Kali Mur.*).

EYES.—Inflammation of the eyes, when pus is discharging, third stage of the inflammation. Abscess of the cornea. Deep-seated ulcers of the eye (*Silicea*). Thick, yellow discharges from the eye. Hypopyum. Inflammation of the retina, third stage. Inflammation of the cornea or conjunctiva, with characteristic discharge.

EARS.—Discharges from the ear are thick, yellow, sometimes mixed with blood (*Silicea*). Deafness, when accompanied by these conditions.

NOSE.—Colds in the head in third stage or stage of resolution; when the discharge is thick, yellow, purulent and sometimes tinged with blood. Chronic catarrh of head, with purulent discharge from either the anterior or posterior nares (*Kali Sulph., Silicea*).

FACE.—Mattery pimples on face (alternate *Silicea*). *Pimples on the faces of young people at the age of puberty,* when the matter forms. Tender *pimples under* the *beard,* with *purulent bloody secretions.* Swellings and nodules on the face; to abort or control suppuration (*Kali Mur.*).

MOUTH.—Diseases of the mouth, if accompanied with purulent secretions.

TEETH.—Ulceration at the roots of the teeth, with swelled gums and cheeks; to abort or control the suppuration.

TONGUE.—Inflammation of the tongue, when suppurating (*Silicea*).

THROAT.—All ailments of the throat in the third stage of the inflammation, or when discharging mattery secretions. Sore throat, quinsy and tonsillitis, when suppurating, or before pus formed, to prevent its formation.

ABDOMEN AND STOOLS.—Discharge of pus, or blood and matter from the bowels. Pus-like, slimy discharges. Abscess of the liver, with purulent discharge. Soreness in region of liver. Diarrhea, dysentery, with characteristic evacuations.

Ulceration of the bowels. Bowels discharging mattery substance, or very constipated in latter stages of consumption.

URINARY ORGANS.—Chronic inflammation of the bladder, when passing sanious or bloody matter (*Ferrum Phos., Kali Mur.*).

MALE SEXUAL ORGANS.—Suppurating abscess of the prostate gland. Bubo, syphilis, or gonorrhea in the suppurative stage, with sanious, purulent discharge (*Silicea*). Ulceration of the glands, with characteristic discharges.

FEMALE SEXUAL ORGANS.—Leucorrhea, with thick, yellow, bloody discharge (*Silicea*). Gonorrhea, with the above conditions.

PREGNANCY.—Inflammation of the breast, when suppura tion has taken place and pus is discharging (*Silicea*).

RESPIRATORY ORGANS.—Last stages of consumption, when the expectoration is purulent, mattery and sometimes bloody. Pus falls to bottom of vessel and spreads out (*Silicea*). Cough, with hectic fever and sanious, mattery sputa. Last stage of croup, pneumonia or bronchitis. Generally indicated after *Kali Mur.* Pus forming in cavity of lung or pleura.

BACK AND EXTREMITIES.—Suppurations of the joints (*Silicea*). *All wounds, when in the suppurative stage* (if offensive, *Kali Phos.*). Hip-point disease (*Silicea*). *Ferrum Phos.* in the first stage, and institute rest. Ulceration of bones (*Silicea, Calc. Phos.*). *Burning of soles of feet* in consumption. Last stage of gathered finger, when the suppuration is superficial, to check the discharge (externally also on lint). Carbuncles on the back, to control the suppuration (*Kali Mur., Silicea*).

SKIN.—Skin affections, with yellow scabs (*Kali Mur.*) Pimples, when discharging pus. Pimples under the beard, with discharge of blood and pus. Mattery scabs forming on the heads of pimples. Crusta lactea (*scald-head*), with yellow crusts or secretions. Skin festers easily (*Silicea*). In small-pox, when the pustules are discharging. Boils, to abort them or to control suppuration. Neglected wounds, cuts, etc., when discharging pus, and when they do not heal readily. Burns and scalds (after *Kali Mur.*), when suppurating. Apply locally to the parts on lint.

TISSUES.—In all cases of suppuration, when the discharge continues too long and the sore is unhealthy. Follows *Silicea* well, and will cause the wound to heal. Thick, yellow or sanious discharge from any organ of the body. Suppurations and ulcerations of the glands (locally, also). Ulcers of lower limbs, etc., with characteristic discharges. Purulent discharges in gonorrhea, syphilis, bubo, leucorrhea, catarrh, consumption, etc.

FEBRILE CONDITIONS.—Typhoid, typhus, diarrhea, dysentery, etc., with sanious, bloody discharges from the bowels. Hectic fever in consumption and other diseases.

SLEEP.—Sleepiness and lethargy, when accompanied with hectic fever.

MODALITIES.—*Worse* from *getting wet*. A warm, dry atmosphere will greatly assist the action of the remedy.

FERRUM PHOSPHORICUM

SYNONYMS.—Ferroso-ferric Phosphate, Ferri Phosphas.

COMMON NAME.—Phosphate of Iron.

FORMULA.—$FeHPO_4+Fe_3(PO_4)_2$.

MOLECULAR WEIGHT.—725.

PREPARATION.—To ten parts of pure crystallized ferrous sulphate dissolved in sixty parts of cold, distilled water, is to be added a cold solution of thirteen parts of crystallized sodium phosphate in fifty of distilled water. The resulting precipitate is to be thrown on a filter and well washed with cold distilled water, then spread upon an unglazed tile or upon bibulous paper, and dried without the aid of artificial heat, when the dried mass is to be rubbed to a fine powder.

Properties and Tests.—The official phosphate of iron is a bluish gray powder without odor or taste. It is soluble in acids, but insoluble in water and alcohol. Its solution in hydrochloric acid has a yellow color, and when treated with barium chloride exhibits only a faint turbidity, and with hydrogen sulphide, shows no change. The powder becomes greenish-gray in color when warmed, and at a higher temperature grayish-brown. The influence of daylight upon the salt is to preserve its color.

IRON PHOSPHATE colors the blood corpuscles red, carries oxygen to all parts of the body, and thus furnishes the vital force that sustains life. Without a proper balance of iron in the blood, health cannot be maintained. When a deficiency in this cell-salt occurs, the circulation is increased, for the blood tries to carry enough oxygen to all the tissues of the body with the limited amount of iron at hand, and in order to do so must move rapidly; exactly as seven men must move faster in order to accomplish as much work as could ten, moving at a slower pace.

This increased motion being changed to heat by the law of the conservation of energy, is called fever. In no other medical writings will so simple and reasonable a definition of fever be found as the one offered by the biochemic pathology. It is not the fever or heat alone that causes the condition of unease in the patient, but the deficiencies in Ferr. Phos. and a subsequent lack of oxygen. The interference with metabolism thus caused soon prevents the functioning of other cell-salts, with the result that thev also lose their power of union with organic matter and are thrown out of the system. A deficiency in potassium chloride nearly always follows a deficiency in iron, unless the missing Ferrum Phos. be quickly supplied.

A lack of Ferrum Phos., or a proper balance in the blood, is the cause of "colds." When a deficiency of iron occurs, nature, or the natural law, draws the blood away from the outer parts, the skin, in order to carry on the process of life more perfectly about the heart, lungs, liver, stomach, brain, etc. This, on account of the closing of the pores of the skin, gives rise to accumulations of non-functional matters, which are thrown out by way of the mucous membranes, and forms the discharges of colds, catarrh, pneumonia, pleurisy, etc.

For all such conditions, whenever there is inflammation, under whatever name it may be known, Ferrum Phos. is the chief remedy.

Without subjecting his patient to the delay necessary to diagnose the type of fever from which his patient is suffering, the Biochemist gives Ferrum Phos., because he sees in the symptoms a call for that tissue-salt. Ferrum molecules toughen the cellular structure in the circular walls of the blood-vessels, hence a lack of iron frequently causes a breaking-down of the walls of minute blood-vessels, producing hemorrhage. Ferrum Phos. is indicated in hemorrhage from any orifice of the body. The alternating remedies are Natr. Mur., Kali Phos., etc., according to the symptoms.

CHARACTERISTIC INDICATIONS

MENTAL SYMPTOMS.—Rush of blood to the brain, causing delirium. Congestion of the brain from any cause. Maniacal moods; hyperemia. "Blood accumulated in any of the blood-vessels causes want of proper balance of the iron molecules in the *muscular* fibres, which are circularly arranged around these vessels; thus relaxed, they lose their tonicity, and do not support normal circulation" (Schuessler). Cerebritis, dizziness, wildness, madness, etc. (*Calc. Phos., Kali Phos.*). Delirium tremens (*Natr. Mur., chief remedy*).

HEAD.—Headache, with rush of blood to the head. Headache, when the pain is in the temples in front (*Natr. Phos.*); over the eye or on top of the head (*Natr. Sulph.*). Dull, heavy, bruising, throbbing, beating pains, generally accompanied by flushed face or fever. *Head sore to the touch;* pulling the hair causes pain; blind headache. Vertigo—cold applications relieve pains by momentarily contracting the excessively congested tissues. Nose-bleed relieves by lessening the quantity of blood. Sick headache, when the matter vomited is undigested food (*Natr. Phos.*). Headaches, with suffused eyes. Inflammatory conditions of the scalp. Tic-douloureux (*Calc. Phos., Magnes. Phos.*).

EYES.—Acute inflammation of the eye (*Kali Mur.*). *Inflammation of the eye in measles* and other eruptive diseases with great intolerance of light. Acute pain in the eyes, more when moving them, or attempting to use them. Dry inflammation, blood-shot, sometimes sore and watery (alternate *Natr. Mur.*). First stages of retinitis. Abscess of the cornea, for the pain. *Granulation on eyelids, with feeling as if grains of sand were there* (alternate *Kali Mur.*).

EARS.—Complaints of the ear, with inflammatory conditions. Earache, with beating, throbbing pain, due to catching cold. Sharp, stitching pains in the ear. Noises in the ear, roaring like running water, from an unequalization of the blood in the blood-vessels. *Inflammation of the ear, first stage,* fever and pain. Deafness from inflammatory action. Inflammation of the external ear, with *beefy redness* and burning. Tympanitis.

NOSE.—First or inflammatory stage of cold in head. Takes cold easily (alternate *Calc. Phos.*). Catarrhal fever. Bleeding from the nose, from injury or not, chief remedy. Predisposition to bleed, in anemic, poorly nourished or apoplectic subjects (*Calc. Phos., Kali Phos., Natr. Sulph.*).

FACE.—Face flushed and burning, with headache, or when precursor of recurring headaches. *Flushed face* with *cold sensation* in *nape* of *neck*. Pale, pallid face, from a lack of red blood corpuscles in the blood (*Calc. Phos.*). Inflammatory neuralgia of the face. *Florid complexion.* Pains and heat in the face, when cold applications are soothing. Erysipelas of the face, for inflammation and pain (*Natr. Sulph.*).

MOUTH.—Inflammation of mouth (*Stomatitis*). Gums hot, swollen and inflamed.

TEETH.—Toothache, when due to an inflammatory condition. Inflamed gums, or hot cheek. Toothache, when cold liquids are soothing. For feverishness in teething complaints, if *Calc. Phos.* does not suffice. Pains are generally aggravated by hot liquids and by motion.

TONGUE.—Clean and red tongue, showing an inflammatory condition. Tongue dark-red and inflamed, with swelling (alternate *Kali Mur.*).

THROAT.—Throat sore, with inflammation. *Throat dry, red and inflamed. Ulcerated throat,* with fever and pain. Inflammation of the tonsils (*Tonsillitis*). Quinsy (*Kali Mur., Calc. Sulph.*). First stage of throat diseases, when there is pain, heat or redness. This remedy reduces the inflammation; it should then be alternated with *Kali Mur.*, or if suppurating, *Calc. Sulph.*. Clergymen's sore throat, when it is due to irritation; sore throat of singers and speakers. *First stage of diphtheria,* and all other throat affections. Follow with *Kali Mur.* and other indicated remedies. Loss of voice after speaking or singing, from a strain.

GASTRIC SYMPTOMS.—Inflammatory conditions of the stomach, *pain after the smallest quantity of food.* Burning, sore pain in pit of stomach. Region of stomach tender to the touch. Heart-burn (*Calc. Phos., Natr. Phos.*). *Vomiting of undigested food,* or *bright red blood.* First stages of gastritis (*Kali Mur.*). Persistent vomiting of food. Belching of wind brings back taste of food. Cold drinks relieve pain. Hot, outward applications also relieve, by causing a counter-irritation, thereby relieving the inflamed and engorged blood-vessels of the stomach. Dyspepsia, with flushed face, and throbbing pain in the stomach. Vomiting of food, with sour fluids. "Stomachache from chill, with loose evacuation, caused by insufficient absorption, from relaxed condition of villi" (Schuessler). Headache, with vomiting of food. Gastric fever (*Kali Mur.*).

ABDOMEN AND STOOL.—First stage of all inflammatory conditions of the bowels. First stage of enteric fever, cholera, dysentery, peritonitis, etc., when patient complains of feeling chilly. Constipation, when there is heat in the colon or rectum, causing a dryness of the mucous membrane. Diarrhea, caused from lack of absorption. *Undigested* or *watery stools.* Dysentery (*Kali Mur., chief remedy*). *Bleeding piles, with* bright red blood, very sore and painful (*Calc. Fluor.*); also apply vaseline locally. Worms, with indigestion and passing of undigested food (*Natr. Phos., chief remedy*). Soreness and tenderness of the bowels, in acute diseases (*Kali Mur.*). Hepatitis. Hemorrhage of the bowels, when the blood is bright red, with tendency to coagulate quickly.

URINARY ORGANS.—*Incontinence of urine from weakness of the sphincter muscle.* First stage of inflammation of the bladder (*Cystitis*), causing retention of urine, with pain and smarting when urinating. Burning after urinating (*Natr. Mur.*). Cystitis is often caused by retaining the urine too long, which should be avoided. Burning, sore pain over the kidneys. Urine, high-colored, with feverish smell (*Natr. Phos.*). Bright's disease and diabetes, when there is feverishness, pain or congestion in any part of the system (*intercur-*

rently). Suppression of urine through heat frequently in children; also local applications. *Wetting the bed from weakness of the muscles of the neck of the bladder* (*Kali Phos.*). If from worms. (*Natr. Phos.*). *Constant urging to urinate,* if not chronic. Great quantity of urine (*Natr. Mur.*). Inflammation of the kidneys (*Nephritis*).

MALE SEXUAL ORGANS.—Irritation and inflammation of the prostate gland (follow with *Kali Mur.*). Varicocele, bubo, orchitis, etc., first stage, when there is feverishness, pain and throbbing. First stage of gonorrhea, for the inflammation; should be used in alternation with *Kali Mur.* as a preventive when exposure has occurred.

FEMALE SEXUAL ORGANS.—Inflammation of the womb and vagina, to remove the fever, pain and heat. Spasm of the vagina, with excessive dryness (*Natr. Mur.*). First stage of gonorrhea; also use local applications. Metritis. Dysmenorrhea (*painful menstruation, Magnes. Phos.*), when there is congestion and fever, also vomiting of undigested food. In dysmenorrhea it should be taken between the periods as a preventive (*Kali Phos.*). Menstrual discharge bright red.

PREGNANCY.—Morning sickness, with vomiting of food, sometimes with acid taste (*Natr. Phos.*). Inflammation of the breast, first stage; after-pains. If given immediately after the birth it will heal the lacerated parts, thereby generally preventing the dangers of puerperal fever.

RESPIRATORY ORGANS.—*All inflammatory conditions of the respiratory tract, in the first stage,* for the fever, heat and pain. Pneumonia, bronchitis, pleuritis, tracheitis, etc., in the inflammatory stage, and, indeed, as long as the pain lasts. It is followed well by *Kali Mur.* in the second stage or that of expectoration of white mucus. *Hemorrhages* from the lungs, *blood bright red.* Expectoration scanty, streaked with blood. Soreness of the chest. Breathing short and hurried at the beginning or during the course of the disease, when there is heat and fever present. Cold in the chest, with hard, dry cough and soreness in the lungs (*Kali Mur.*). Acute, painful, short, irritating cough. In the *beginning of all coughs and colds* this is the first remedy. Croup and whooping cough, for the febrile conditions. Asthma, for the soreness of the chest. Painful hoarseness and huskiness of speakers and singers, when due to the irritation of the bronchii (*Calc. Phos.*). Congestion of the lungs, acute or chronic, with oppression and pain; catch in breath, pleurisy, pain in the side, in first stage. Local applications of hot water or mustard should be used where the pain is deep-seated, to produce counter-irritation.

Circulatory Organs.—Inflammation of the blood-vessels. Full, rapid, quick pulse in fevers. Palpitation of the heart, when due to inflammatory conditions. Carditis, pericarditis, endocarditis, phlebitis, arteritis, in the congestive stage. Deficiency of red blood corpuscles (*Anemia*). Also *Calc. Phos.* Aneurism (*Calc. Fluor., chief remedy*). Dilatation of heart or of blood-vessels (alternate *Calc. Fluor.*). Naevi, varicose veins (*Calc. Fluor.*). Hyperemia, accumulation of blood in any of the blood-vessels.

Back and Extremities.—Inflammatory pains in the back over kidneys and through the loins. Lumbago (*Calc. Phos.*). Stiff back, movement increases the pain. Rheumatism, for the inflammation and fever. Rheumatic fever. Stiffness of the muscles or of the neck from cold. First remedy in gatherings and festers, to relieve heat, pain and congestion. Fingers painful or inflamed through rheumatism or other causes. Fractures of bones of the limbs, to meet the injuries sustained by the soft tissues, reduce inflammation, etc., In hip-joint diseases, for the fever, pain and inflammation (*Silicea*). *Rheumatic lameness of the joints,* when fever is present (*Kali Phos.*). Acute articular rheumatism, very painful. Rheumatism from catching cold. Pain is always aggravated by motion. Strains and sprains require this remedy in the first stage.

In all cases, where practical, local application of the remedy should be made.

NERVOUS SYMPTOMS.—Congestive neuralgia after catching cold, with inflammatory conditions. Epilepsy, with rush of blood to the head and febrile conditions. Convulsions, with fever, in teething.

SKIN.—*Inflammatory stage of all skin affections* needs this remedy. Abscesses, carbuncles, boils, felons, etc., require this remedy in the beginning, to relieve heart, pain and throbbing. Chicken-pox, small-pox, erysipelas, etc., in the initiatory stage, for the febrile conditions (either alternate or follow with *Kali Mur.*

TISSUES.—All injuries to the soft tissues, strains, sprains, cuts, blows, bruises, etc., require this salt internally and externally. It will reduce fever, pain and inflammation. In bone diseases or fractures, when the soft parts are inflamed and painful *Anemia* (*lack of red blood corpuscles*); it colors the blood-cells red. In *dropsy,* when the disease is caused *from loss of blood,* this remedy should be alternated with *Calc. Phos. Bleeding from the nose in children and anemic persons* (*Calc. Phos.*). *Hemorrhages* from any part of the body, *when* the *blood is bright red,* with *tendency to coagulate rapidly.* Hemorrhage from a small external vessel may be controlled by applying the remedy locally and binding on a compress tightly. In epistaxis, it should be blown up the nostrils, as well as taken internally. Plugging the nostril is sometimes necessary. In ulceration of the tissues, to control the fever and pain; should be used locally as well as internally, in all cases where practical.

FEBRILE CONDITIONS.—A feverish state at the commencement of any disease; should also be continued as long as fever and inflammation exist, to control and subdue the heat, inflammation and pain. It will, to a great extent, prevent the destruction of tissue. First stage of enteric, gastric, typhoid, typhus, rheumatic and scarlet fever, measles, chicken-pox, small-pox, etc., for the heat and congestion. Intermittent fever, with vomiting of food; catarrhal fever, with quickened pulse and chilly sensations.

SLEEP.—Sleeplessness, from an enfeebled or relaxed condition of the muscular fibres of the walls of the blood-vessels, allowing an accumulation of blood on the brain. If from worry or excitement, alternate *Kali Phos.*

MODALITIES.—Most of the ailments under this salt are of a congestive nature and are, therefore, *relieved by cold and aggravated by motion.* The cold should be applied directly to the congestion, or the relief will not be felt. If the inflammation is deep-seated, heat should be applied to relieve the engorgement of the deeper vessels.

KALI MURIATICUM

SYNONYMS.—Potassium Chloride, Kali Chloratum, Kali Chloridum, Potassii Chloridum.

COMMON NAMES.—Chloride of Potash, Chloride of Potassium

FORMULA.—KCl.

MOLECULAR WEIGHT.—74.5.

PREPARATION.—Potassium Chloride is a constituent of the mineral *carnallite*—a double chloride of potassium and magnesium found in large quantity at Stassfurth near Magdeburg, in Germany. The deposit is worked for the extraction of the chloride, by dissolving the double chloride in water and leaving the solution to cool; the greater part of the potassium chloride separates out, while magnesium chloride remains in solution.

Potassium chloride may be prepared by neutralizing pure aqueous hydrochloric acid, with pure potassium carbonate or hydrate. The solution is to be evaporated to crystallization.

PROPERTIES.—Potassium chloride crystallizes in cubes, often prismatically elongated, and occasionally in octohedrons. The crystals are colorless or white, are permanent in the air, decrepitate when heated, melt at a low red heat, and at a higher temperature volatilize without decomposition. The substance tastes like common or table salt. It is soluble in three parts of cold, and in two of boiling water, and is insoluble in strong alcohol.

TESTS.—According to German pharmaceutical authority, the presence of sodium chloride to an amount not exceeding two per cent., is permissible in potassium chloride for internal use. To determine the presence of a greater proportion of the sodium compound a handful of the crystals of potassium chloride is to be reduced to powder and quickly dried. Of this dry powder 0.2 grams, together with 0.49 gram of pure silver nitrate are placed in a test-tube with water, and dilute nitric acid added. The mixture is to be warmed, thoroughly shaken and after cooling, filtered. The filtrate, when treated with silver nitrate solution, should not exhibit the least turbidity, otherwise the proportion of the sodium compound is in excess of the limit prescribed.

POTASSIUM CHLORIDE should not be confounded with potassium chlorate or chlorate of potash, as it is an entirely different salt.

Fibrin is distinguished from albumen and casein by its separation, in a solid state, in delicate filaments in any fluid in which it is dissolved, shortly after the fluid is taken from the organism. It is clearly shown by Biochemistry that without the inorganic salt potassium chloride no fibrin can be made; and it is further shown that the normal amount of fibrin cannot be held in proper solution in the blood without the proper balance of that cell-salt.

Fibrin results from the union of certain fibrin-plastic substances (albuminoids), but this union does not take place in the absence of the chloride of potash molecules. In venous blood the fibrin amounts to three in 1,000 parts Arterial blood contains less, and lymph a still smaller amount. In inflammatory exudations we find fibrin in the serous cavities —such as pleura and peritoneum—and on the mucous membrane, as in croup, diphtheria, catarrh, etc. In all inflammatory conditions, Ferr. Phos., should be given in alternation with Kali Mur., for iron molecules carry oxygen, which becomes deficient when the proper balance is disturbed by the outflow of fibrin. It is quite clear that fibrin is created, or produced, by the action of the chloride of potash, with the assistance of oxygen, on certain albuminoids.

The *white* or *gray coating on the tongue, mucous lining or tonsils,* is the fibrin that has become non-functional because of a deficiency in potassium chloride and oxygen. We find the fibrinous exudations also in discharges or expectorations of a *thick, white slime or phlegm, from any of the mucous membranes,* or in *flour-like scaling of the skin.* The same material causes the enlargement in all soft swellings. (Hard swellings or lumps may be caused by the lime-salts and pure albumen, or silica.) The reason why Kali Mur. relieves the effect of burns is because the fibrin in the tissue first succumbs to the effects of heat, and the chloride of potash, by its union with albuminous substances, produces new fibrin and supplies the deficiency.

CHARACTERISTIC INDICATIONS

HEAD.—Headaches, with a thick, white coating on the tongue; vomiting of white phlegm, or hawking of thick, white mucus. Sick headache, arising from sluggish action of the liver—want of bile—frequently accompanied by constipation Secondary remedy in meningitis.

EYES.—All eye affections, when discharging a thick, white mucus (in alternation with *Kali Sulph.*), when the discharge is yellow-greenish matter). Sore eyes, with specks of matter on the lids, or yellow, mattery scabs (*Kali Sulph.*). Superficial, flat ulcer, arising from a vesicle. Secondary remedy in inflammations of the eye, with characteristic exudation. Granulated eyelids, with feeling as of sand in the eyes (alternate *Ferrum Phos.*). Retinitis, with exudations.

EARS.—Earache, with a swelling of the glands and gray or white-furred tongue. Earache, with swelling of the tonsils and eustachian tubes (*Ferrum Phos.*). *Catarrhal conditions of the middle ear* (*Ferrum Phos.*). Deafness from swelling of the internal ear; cracking noises in the ear on blowing the nose or swallowing. Deafness from swelling of the eustachian tubes or thickening of the drum of the ear. Dullness of hearing from throat affections or swelling of the middle ear. Granulations, moist, gray, or thick, white exudations from ear. Glands around the ear swollen; *noises in the ear; snapping and cracking* from unequalization of the air in the eustachian tubes (*Ferr. Phos.*).

NOSE.—Stuffy colds in the head, with thick, white discharges and gray or white-coated tongue. Catarrh, with characteristic white phlegm, not transparent. Dry catarrh, with stuffy sensation. Crusts in the vault of pharynx. Note also coating of the tongue.

FACE.—Cheek swollen and painful (alternate *Ferrum Phos.*). Faceache from swelling of cheek or gums.

MOUTH.—Canker of the lips or mouth, rawness of the mouth, swollen glands or gums. White ulcers (*thrush*) in the mouths of little children, observe color of tongue; with much saliva (*Natr. Mur.*).

TEETH.—Toothache, with swelling of the gums or cheek, this remedy to carry off the exuding, effete, albuminoid substance. Gum-boil, before matter begins to form (alternate with *Ferr. Phos.*) (*Silicea*).

TONGUE.—Coating of *tongue grayish-white, dry or slimy.* In inflammation of the tongue, for the swelling (*Ferrum Phos.*).

THROAT.—Ulcerated sore throat, with white or grayish patches, white or gray tongue. Inflammation of the tonsils, with swelling and grayish-white patches. Quinsy, acute or chronic; secondary remedy as soon as the swelling appears. In *diphtheria* this is *the sole remedy in most cases* (alternate with *Ferrum Phos.*). In diphtheria and all other throat diseases, a gargle of the same remedy should be used quite frequently (2x or 3x, ten to fifteen grains in glass of water). Loss of voice. Mumps (alternate with *Ferrum Phos.;* if there is much saliva or swelling of testicles, alternate with *Natr. Mur.*).

GASTRIC SYMPTOMS.—Poor appetite, with gray or white-coated tongue, indicating sluggish action of the liver. Dyspepsia, with white or gray-coated tongue, heavy pain under the right shoulder-blade, eyes look large and protruding. Fatty, greasy food disagrees; belching of gas, bringing back a greasy, sickening taste. Pastry or rich fatty food causes burning and pain in the stomach. Indigestion, with vomiting of greasy, white opaque mucus. Observe the white coating of the tongue. Gastritis, secondary stage, with white-coated tongue, or when caused by hot drinks, this remedy at once (*Ferrum Phos.*). Flatulence, with sluggishness of the liver. Stomachache, with constipation, vomiting or hawking thick, white phlegm. Vomiting of blood, dark and clotted.

ABDOMEN AND STOOL.—Evacuations are pale yellow, ochre or clay-colored, denoting a deficiency of bile. Sluggish action of the liver, with pale yellow evacuations; pains in region of liver or under right shoulder-blade. Sluggish action of the liver, with *constipation,* white-furred tongue and protruding eyeballs. Jaundice, when caused by a chill, resulting in catarrh of the duodenum, white-coated tongue, light-colored stools, etc. Typhoid or enteric fever, white-coated tongue and looseness of the bowels; stools light, pale color; swelling of the abdomen, with tenderness to the touch. Hemorrhage of dark, clotted blood. Constipation in typhus fever. *Diarrhea, with pale yellow, clay-colored stools;* swelling of the abdomen, slimy stools. Diarrhea after eating fatty, greasy food. Dysentery, purging, with slimy, sanious evacuations; pain in the abdomen, constant urging to stool; straining, with great pain in the anus, extorting cries. This remedy, alternated with *Ferrum Phos.,* generally cures (compare *Magnes. Phos.*). Constipation, light-colored stools, showing want of bile, sluggish action of the liver, etc. Second stage of inflammatory diseases of the abdomen and bowels, peritonitis, typhlitis, perityphlitis, enteritis, etc. (*Ferrum Phos. is the primary remedy*). *Hemorrhoids,* when the blood is dark and thick; alternate with other indicated remedies for the tumors, relaxed elastic fibres, etc.

URINARY ORGANS.—Cystitis, in the second stage, with swelling and discharge of thick, white, slimy mucus; also the principal remedy in the chronic form. Urine dark-colored; deposit of uric acid, when there is torpor and inactivity of the liver (*Natr. Sulph.*). Second stage of inflammation of the kidneys (*Ferrum Phos., primary remedy*).

MALE SEXUAL ORGANS.—The principal remedy in gonorrhea. Inflammatory swelling of the testicle (*Orchitis*) from suppressed gonorrhea (*Calc. Phos.*). Bubo, for the soft swelling. Chronic stage of syphilis, with characteristic white discharges, white or grayish tongue, soft chancres. Principal remedy, with local application of the same.

FEMALE SEXUAL ORGANS.—Leucorrhea, with characteristic discharge of milky-white, thick, non-irritating mucus. Ulceration of the os and cervix uteri, with thick, white, bland discharge; also injections or local applications of the same. Menstruation retarded or suppressed, too late or too early; when the discharge is dark-clotted, tough, black blood, excessive discharge. Neuritis, second stage. Congestion of the uterus, chronic, or second stage, menstrual periods too frequent (*Kali Phos.*); *note color of tongue.* Hypertrophy, second stage, to reduce the swelling; if very hard (*Calc. Fluor.*).

PREGNANCY.—Morning sickness in pregnancy, with vomiting of white phlegm and white-coated tongue. Inflammation of the breasts (*Mastitis*), secondary remedy, to control the swelling before pus has formed. Valuable remedy for puerperal fever in the early stage, with *Ferrum Phos.*; for mania, perverted brain functions, septic poison, etc. (*Kali Phos.*).

RESPIRATORY ORGANS.—Second stage of all inflammatory conditions of the respiratory tract; the characteristic indication is a thick, tenacious, white phlegm or milky sputa. Consumption, with the above symptoms and heavy cough. Loud, noisy, stomach cough, with white expectoration, white-coated tongue and protruded appearance of eyes. Short, spasmodic cough, like whooping cough (*Ferrum Phos.*). Cough, with croup-like hoarseness. Principal remedy in croup, for the exudation (*Ferrum Phos.*). Pneumonia, pleurisy, second stage, with thick, white, viscid expectoration (*note color of tongue*). Asthma, from gastric derangement, white tongue, mucus white and hard to cough up (for breathing *Kali Phos.*). Loss of voice. Hoarseness from cold (*Kali Sulph.*). Whooping cough, with characteristic expectoration, wheezing, rales or rattling sounds in the chest, caused by air passing through thick, tenacious mucus in the bronchi, difficult expectoration.

CIRCULATORY ORGANS.—Palpitation of the heart, in hypertrophic conditions, from excessive flow of blood to that organ; second stage of pericarditis, to complete the cure (*Ferrum Phos., chief remedy*). Embolism, for that condition of blood which favors the formation of clots which act as plugs (*Ferrum Phos.*).

Back and Extremities.—*Rheumatism* of any part of the body, *when there is swelling* of the parts or white-coated tongue. Rheumatic pains, which are felt only during motion or increased by motion (*Ferrum Phos.*). Chronic rheumatism, with swelling and pain from motion. Rheumatic fever, second stage, when exudation takes place, swelling around the joints; "this cell-salt will remove the swelling by restoring the non-functional cells of the excretory and absorbing structures to normal action." All swellings are controlled by this remedy; if exceedingly hard, alternate with *Calc. Fluor. Chronic swelling of the feet and legs.* Glands of neck swollen. Hip-joint disease, for swelling before pus formation has commenced. Ulcers on extremities, with characteristic fibrinous discharge (*Calc Fluor.*). Bunions; internally and externally (after *Ferrum Phos.*). Chilblains on hands or feet; also external use, for the itching (*Kali Phos.*). Creaking of the muscles at the back of the wrist or arm on movement (after *Ferrum Phos.,* if swelling remains).

Nervous Symptoms.—The specific or *chief remedy in epilepsy,* with white-coated tongue, protruding appearance of the eyes, etc. (*Magnes. Phos.*). Epilepsy, occurring with or after suppression of eczema or other eruptions. Wasting of the spinal cord (*Tabes Dorsalis*).

Skin.—All skin diseases, when the eruptions are filled with white, fibrinous matter, or when there exists white, flour-like scales on the skin. Skin diseases which arise from using bad vaccine lymph. Eczema resulting from deranged or suppressed uterine functions (*note coating of tongue*). Eczema, with dry, flour-like scales or albuminoid, whitish discharge, white-coated tongue; if very obstinate, alternate with *Calc. Phos.* Eruptions, acne, pustules, pimples, etc., with thick, white contents. Erythema (after *Ferrum Phos.*), for swelling and white-coated tongue. Scrufy eruption on the heads and faces of little children (*Crusta Lactea,* alternate *Calc. Phos.*). Vesicular, blistering *erysipelas, the chief remedy* (in alternation with

Ferrum Phos. for the fever). Abscess, boils, festers, carbuncles, etc., second stage, for the swelling before pus forms. Pimples on the face and neck, with thick contents. Herpes (*Shingles*), (*Natr. Mur.*). Irritation of the skin, similar to chilblains. Lupus, chief remedy. Measles, hoarse cough, glandular swelling, white-furred tongue. After-effects of measles, diarrhea, white-colored, loose stools, deafness from swelling of the throat, etc. Scarlet fever (alternate with *Ferrum Phos.*) Sycosis, principal remedy. Warts, low trituration, internally and externally.

TISSUES.—In anemia, this remedy should be used intercurrently, if skin affections be present. Cuts and bruises (after *Ferrum Phos.*, if there is swelling and exudation). Burns of all degrees—chief remedy—internally and externally; moisten lint with a strong solution and apply frequently without removing the lint. Fibrinous, thick, white, slimy exudations from any tissue; after inflammations, or when, not becoming absorbed, it causes swelling or enlargement of the parts. *Chief remedy in glandular swellings,* proud flesh, exuberant granulations. Enlargement of glands from scrofula. Sprains (after *Ferrum Phos.*). *Scurvy,* with hard infiltrations; *chief remedy.* Dropsy arising from heart, liver or kidney disease, or from obstruction of the bile ducts; generally a white coat on the tongue; whitish liquid (on aspiration). Dropsy of the extremities, when the limbs have a hard, shiny, glistening appearance, white mucous sediment in urine.

FEBRILE CONDITIONS.—Second stage of inflammations or congestions of any organ. In gastric, typhoid or enteric fever, second remedy, to restore the integrity of the affected tssue. In alternation with *Ferrum Phos.* in scarlet fever, also as a preventive. Typhus fever, for the constipation. Puerperal fever, an important remedy in the early stage, with *Ferrum Phos.* (*Kali Phos.*). In rheumatic fever, for the exudation. Intermittent fever, with characteristic symptoms. All febrile conditions, with grayish-white, dry or slimy coating of the tongue.

MODALITIES.—All stomach and bowel symptoms are *worse* after *eating fats, pastry or any rich food.* Pains are increased and *aggravated by motion.*

KALI PHOSPHORICUM

SYNONYMS.—Potassium Phosphate, Potassii Phosphas.

COMMON NAME.—Phosphate of Potash.

FORMULA.—$K_2 HPO_4$.

MOLECULAR WEIGHT.—174.

PREPARATION.—This salt is produced by mixing aqueous phosphoric acid with a sufficent quantity of potassium hydrate or carbonate until the reaction is slightly alkaline and evaporating.

PROPERTIES.—The salt crystallizes with difficulty in irregular forms. It is generally obtained as a white amorphous mass, is very deliquescent, is freely soluble in water, and is insoluble in alcohol. By ignition it is converted into pyrophosphate.

TESTS.—When prepared, as directed above, it is not likely to be contaminated. For identification, it may be dissolved in water and then treated with silver nitrate solution, when a yellow precipitate will be thrown down, showing the presence of orthophosphoric acid, and when treated with tartaric acid, a white crystalline precipitate is evidence of the presence of potassium.

THE GRAY MATTER of the brain is controlled entirely by the inorganic cell-salt, potassium phosphate. This salt unites with albumen, and by the addition of oxygen creates nerve-fluid, or the gray matter of the brain. Of course, there is a trace of other salts and other organic matter in nerve tissue, but potassium phosphate is the chief factor, and has the power within itself to attract, by its own law of affinity, all things needed to manufacture this vital tissue. Therefore, when nervous symptoms arise, due to the fact that the nerve-tissue has been exhausted from any cause, the phosphate of potassium is the only true remedy, because nothing else can possibly supply the deficiency. The ills arising from too rapidly consuming the gray matter of the brain cannot be overestimated, and if all who are inclined to nervous disorders would carry Kali Phos. with them, in tablet form, a large amount of sickness and suffering would be prevented.

Kali Phos. is one of the most wonderful curative agents ever discovered by man, and the blessings it has already conferred on the race are many.

Let the overworked business man take it and go home good-tempered. Let the weary wife, nerves unstrung from attending to sick children or entertaining company, take it and note how quickly the equilibrium will be restored and calm and reason assert themselves. We find this potassium salt largely predominates in nerve-fluid, and that a deficiency produces well-defined symptoms. The beginning and end of the matter is to supply the lacking principle, and in molecular form, exactly as nature furnishes it in vegetables, fruits and grain. To supply deficiencies—this is the only law of cure.

CHARACTERISTIC INDICATIONS

MENTAL SYMPTOMS.—Kali Phos., the great nerve and brain remedy, is indicated, and is the *chief remedy in all mental disorders,* when arising *from a want of nerve or brain power.* A deficiency of this salt is indicated by the following symptoms: *Brain-fag, from overwork. Depressed spirits, irritability, impatience* and *nervousness;* crossness of children, ill-tempered, fretfulness, crying and screaming; fear; poor memory (*Calc. Phos. intercurrently*). Screaming of children at night during sleep, sometimes from worms; note color of tongue. Anxiety, gloomy moods, fancies, nervous dread, forebodings, looks on the dark side of life. Dull, no energy. Fainting and tendency to fainting in nervous sensitive persons.

Insanity and other mental disorders. Delirium tremens (*Natr. Mur.*). Softening of the brain, mental illusions and aberrations, grasping at imaginary objects. Backwardness, shyness, sensitiveness; delirium during the course of any febrile disease (*Ferrum Phos., Natr. Mur.*). Puerperal mania, hysteria, fits of laughing and crying, melancholia, overstrain of the mind from continual mental employment, business worry, etc. Rest and *Kali Phos.* will keep thousands of such cases out of the insane asylum. Sighing, weariness and depression. Somnambulism in children requires a steady course of treatment with this remedy. Homesickness, haunted by visions of the past.

HEAD.—Headaches in nervous subjects, sensitive to noise, irritable. Headache, with confusion, nervousness, loss of strength, inability for thought, weariness, yawning and stretching, prostrated feeling and hysteria. Neuralgic headache, with humming in the ears; better under cheerful excitement, worse when alone; tearful moods. Pains and weight in back part of head, with weariness and exhaustion (after *Ferrum Phos.*). Headaches of students and those worn out with mental work and loss of sleep; gone sensation at stomach. Pains are generally relieved by gentle motion or cheerful excitement; concussion of the brain, asthenic conditions, dilated pupils, etc. Anemic conditions of the brain, causing nervousness, dizziness and swimming of the head, when from cerebral causes. Vertigo from exhaustion and weakness (*Ferrum Phos.*). Sleeplessness, noises in the head on falling asleep. Water on the brain (*intercurrently*).

EYES.—Excited, staring appearance of the eyes, dilated pupils, during the course of any disease. Drooping of the eyelids from weakness of the muscles. Squinting after diphtheria, when it is not spasmodic, but a weakness of the muscles. Partial or total blindness from decay of the optic nerve.

EARS.—Deafness from want of nervous perception, noises in the ears and head, with confusion. Deafness, with exhaustion of the nervous system. Ulcerations of the ear, when the discharge is foul, ichorous, offensive, sanious or mixed with blood. Dullness of hearing, with noise in the head.

NOSE.—Catarrh, with fetid discharge, foul odor, when the disease is located in the mucous membrane (*see also Silicea*). Ozena, with foul odor (*Silicea*). Bleeding from the nose in delicate constitutions, when the blood is thin, blackish, not coagulating; predisposition to bleed (*alternate with Ferrum Phos.*).

FACE.—Neuralgia of the face from exhaustion of the nervous system and poverty of the nerve fibres. Face livid and sunken, with hollow eyes. Pale, sickly and sallow face.

MOUTH.—Cancrum oris, water canker, gangrenous canker of the mouth (alternate with *Kali Mur.*). Ulcers of the mouth (*Stomatitis*), with very fetid, offensive breath and bad taste in the mouth; note also color of tongue.

TEETH.—Toothache in nervous, emotional subjects (*Magnes. Phos.*). Toothache after exhaustion, mental labor, or from loss of sleep, better with gentle motion. Gums bleed easily; predisposition of the gums to bleed, with a bright red seam or line. Chattering of the teeth of a purely nervous character—not from cold.

TONGUE.—*Tongue coated, like stale, brownish, liquid mustard.* Very offensive breath. *Tongue very dry* in the morning; feels as if it would cling to the roof of the mouth. Inflammation of the tongue, with excessive dryness or great exhaustion (*Natr. Mur.*).

THROAT.—After-effects of diphtheria, weakness of sight, partial paralysis, etc. Gangrenous condition of the throat, in the early stages. Croup, in the last stages, for syncope, nervous prostration, pale or livid countenance, etc., in alternation with the chief remedy, *Kali Mur.* Speech slow and indistinct, frequently indicating approaching paralysis. Paralysis of the vocal cords. In all throat diseases where there exists mental or nervous prostration.

Gastric Symptoms.—Inflammation of the stomach, when it comes too late under treatment, with weakness, debility and nervous prostration. Stomachache from exhaustion or depression, caused by grief, mental strains, worry, etc.; excessive hunger, unnatural appetite, frequently seen after febrile diseases. Hungry feeling after eating food; eats heartily, but appetite is not satisfied. Nervous depression, or "gone sensation" in stomach. Flatulence, with distress about the heart, or on the left side of the stomach.

Abdomen and Stool.—*Dysentery,* when the *stools* consist *of pure blood,* abdomen swollen, patient becomes delirious, stools have a foul, putrid odor, dryness of the tongue, etc. Diarrhea, with putrid, foul evacuations, depression and exhaustion of the nerves. In all diseases where bowel troubles are present, especially in foul or inflammatory conditions, the use of the indicated remedy in hot water injections should be resorted to. *Flatulence,* with weary pain in left side and distress about the heart; *cholera,* when the *stools* are *profuse* and have the appearance of *rice-water.* Typhoid fever, for the bowel troubles, malignant conditions, putrid blood, depression, etc. Prolapsus recti (alternate with *Ferrum Phos.* and *Calc. Fluor.*).

Urinary Organs.—Frequent urination, with passing of much water, frequently scalding. Inability to retain urine, from nervous debility. Incontinence from partial paralysis of the sphincter. *Enuresis* (wetting the bed) *of children,* alternate with (*Ferrum Phos.*), *chief remedy;* if from worms, (*Natr. Phos.*). Passing of blood from urethra; cystitis, for weakness and prostration. In diabetes (*intercurrently*), for nervous weakness, voracious hunger, sleeplessness, etc. Bright's disease, for the disturbance of the nerve centers (alternate *Calc. Phos.,* for the albumen).

Male Sexual Organs.—Phagedenic chancres; gonorrhea, when discharging blood. Spermatorrhea for the nervous symptoms arising from excessive sexual excitement.

FEMALE SEXUAL ORGANS.—Irregular menstruation, too late or too scanty, in pale, irritable, nervous, sensitive women. Too profuse discharge, deep red or blackish red; thin and not coagulating menses, with offensive odor. Colic at menstrual periods, in pale, lachrymose, nervous women (*Magnes. Phos.*). Suppression of the menstrual flow (*Amenorrhea*), with depression, nervousness and general debility. Hysteria at the menstrual period, nervousness and excitableness; also a feeling as of a ball rising in the throat. Hysterical fits of crying. Leucorrhea, when the discharge is scalding or acrid (alternate *Natr. Mur.*).

PREGNANCY.—Miscarriage, threatened in weak subjects (probably *Calc. Fluor.*). Mastitis, if the pus discharging is brownish, dirty-looking, with offensive odor; also external application of same. *Puerperal fever,* for the *mania* and *derangement of* the *mental faculties.* Labor pains, if feeble and ineffectual; also spurious labor pains. *Tedious labor, from constitutional weakness.* It will greatly facilitate labor, if given steadily for one month previous to the birth.

RESPIRATORY ORGANS.—Hoarseness from overexertion of the voice, exhausted feeling and nervous depression. Whooping cough, with the above symptoms. Asthma, large doses and often repeated, for the labored breathing and depressed system. Bronchial asthma, with characteristic expectoration and brownish coating of the tongue. Loss of voice from paralysis of vocal cords. Hay asthma, for depression and breathing (alternate with *Natr. Mur.,* for the watery conditions). Acute edema of the lungs, spasmodic cough, threatening suffocation (alternate with *Natr. Mur.,* for the watery, frothy expectoration). Last stage of croup, pale, livid countenance, extreme weakness; syncope (in alternation with *Kali Mur., chief remedy*). *Shortness of breath* from asthma, or with exhaustion or want of proper nerve power, *worse from motion or exertion.* Involuntary sighing, sighing or moaning during sleep.

Circulatory Organs.—Pulse sluggish and below normal standard from enfeebled nervous system. Intermittent, irregular pulse. *Palpitation,* with nervousness, anxiety, melancholia, sleeplessness and restlessness. Palpitation on ascending stairs, with shortness of breath, from a weakened condition or nervous excitement; poor circulation, fainting and dizziness, with uneasy feeling about the heart, from weak action. Fainting from fright, fatigue or weak heart action, pulse low and hardly perceptible. Intermittent action of the heart after violent emotion, grief or care.

Back and Extremities.—Idiopathic softening of the spinal cord, with gradual molecular deadening of the nervous centres. Paralysis or partial paralysis of the limbs. *Rheumatic pains,* lameness and stiffness, *worse from violent exertion,* but *relieved by gentle motion.* Pains during rest; a bruised and painful feeling in the part affected; gentle movement gradually relieves. Acute and chronic rheumatism, very painful; parts feel stiff, severe in the morning, after rest or when rising from a sitting position; worse from exertion or fatigue; relieved from gentle movement; neuralgic pains in the limbs, with feeling of numbness (*Calc. phos.*). Chilblains on the hands, feet or ears require this remedy, internally and externally, for the tingling or itching pains.

Nervous Symptoms.—*Paralysis of any part of the body,* and of all varieties, require *Kali Phos.,* the chief remedy. Partial paralysis, hemiplegia, facial, etc. Sudden or creeping paralysis of the vocal cords, causing loss of voice. Paralysis in which the vital powers are reduced, and stools have a putrid odor, fetid breath, bad taste, etc. Locomotor, facial or creeping paralysis. *"Neuralgic pains, occurring in any organ, with depression, failure of strength, sensitiveness to noise and light; improved during pleasant excitement and gentle motion, but most felt when quiet or alone."* Nervous affections; patient irritable, impatient, dwells upon grievances, despondent, cries easily, "makes mountains out of molehills," etc. Nervous sensitiveness, feels pain very keenly; better when the attention is occupied by pleasurable excitement. *Nervousness,* without any reasonable cause; patient *sheds tears while narrating her symptoms.* Hysteric attacks from sudden emotion, with feeling of a ball rising in the throat, nervous fidgety feeling. *Spinal anemia* from exhausting diseases. Infantile paralysis. Epilepsy, for the sunken countenance, coldness and palpitation after the fit (in alternation with *Kali Mur., the chief remedy*). Sciatica. Dragging pain down back of thigh to knee, accompanied by stiffness, great restlessness and pain. Exhaustion and weakness, from any cause, which has lowered the standard of the nervous system.

SKIN.—Eczema, with nervous irritation and oversensitiveness accompanying it (*intercurrently*). Felon, or any other skin disease, when the matter discharging becomes fetid. Pemphigus malignus. Blisters and blebs over the body, sanious, watery contents. Skin withered and wrinkled. Putrid conditions in smallpox, malignant pustules. *Itching of the skin, with crawling sensation;* gentle friction is agreeable, but excess causes soreness and chafing (*Calc. Phos.*). Greasy scales on the skin, with heavy odor. *Itching of the inside of the hands and soles of the feet* where the skin is thickest. Irritating secretions. Chilblains, for the itching and tingling pain (*Kali Mur., chief remedy*).

TISSUES.—*Wasting diseases,* when *putrid conditions* are present. Hemorrhages from any part of the body, when the blood is thin, dark, putrid and not coagulating. Anemic conditions, with characteristic symptoms of this salt. *General debility and exhaustion,* lack of energy. Exudations serous, ichorous, foul, offensive, sanious, mixed with blood. Exudations from the mucous linings, which are corroding or chafing (*Natr. Mur.*). *Gangrenous conditions,* early stages of mortification, to heal the conditions which give rise to it. Cancer, offensive discharges; greatly ameliorates the pain. Scurvy, gangrenous conditions. Suppurations, with characteristic discharge of offensive pus. Rickets, with putrid stools. Atrophic conditions in old people; tissues dry, scaly, lack of vitality. *Septic hemorrhages.* Persons suffering from suppressed sexual instinct, or from excessive sexual indulgence. General debility and exhaustion.

Febrile Conditions.—All febrile diseases, with low, putrid, malignant symptoms; typhus, camp, nervous or brain fevers, with low muttering. Sleeplessness, stupor, delirium, etc., high temperature, pulse below normal, or rapid and scarcely perceptible (*Natr. Mur.*). Intermittent fever, fetid, profuse, debilitating perspiration. Typhoid and scarlet fever, for the putrid, malignant conditions. Excessive and exhausting perspiration or sweating while eating, with weakness at stomach.

Sleep.—Walking in sleep (somnambulism). Hysterical yawning; yawning, stretching and weariness, arising from nervous causes, sometimes with feeling of emptiness of the stomach, although food is not needed. *Sleeplessness from nervous causes, often after worry or excitement.* Wakefulness from overpressure of blood to the head (*Kali Phos.*). Stimulates the gray nervous matter, thereby causing contraction of the arteries and diminished flow of blood to the brain.

Modalities.—Symptoms are generally *aggravated by noise, exertion, arising* from a *sitting position, etc.* Pains worse by continued exercise and after rest; symptoms are generally ameliorated by gentle motion, eating, excitement or pleasant company; worse when alone.

KALI SULPHURICUM

Synonyms.—Potassium Sulphate, Kali Sulphas, Potassæ Sulphas, Potassii Sulphas.

Common Name.—Sulphate of Potash.

Formula.—$K_2 SO_4$.

Molecular Weight.—174.

Preparation.—This salt occurs native in delicate needle-shaped crystals, or as a crust on many of the Vesuvian lavas, and is designated mineralogically as Glaserite, Arcanite, Aphthalose or Vesuvian salt. It is obtained as a by-product in several manufacturing processes, as in the preparation of nitric acid from nitrate of potassium, the acid sulphate usually obtained as a residue of this operation being converted into neutral sulphate by addition of potassium carbonate. It likewise crystallizes out from the mother liquors of sea water and salt springs.

Properties.—Potassium sulphate crystallizes in short, permanent, colorless, four and six-sided prisms, and by slow crystallization from a large quantity of its solution in double six-sided pyramids. It is soluble in 10 parts of cold and in 3 of boiling water, and is insoluble in alcohol. It has a sharp, bitter, saline taste; its specific gravity is 2.66. The crystals decrepitate strongly when heated.

Tests.—A solution of potassium sulphate should be manifested by treatment with hydrogen sulphide or ammonium sulphide (absence of heavy metals), by potassium carbonate (absence of earths), by antimonate of potassium (sodium), and by silver nitrate (chloride).

THE general field of action of this salt is the epidermis and the epithelium. In inorganic nature, sulphates and iron serve for the transfer of oxygen. When in the surface layer of the earth a sulphate and any oxide of iron come into contact with organic substances undergoing a decomposition, they surrender their oxygen and form sulphuret of iron. This may be again decomposed through the access of new oxygen, so that sulphuric acid and some oxide of iron will be formed, which under suitable conditions will again transfer oxygen. (Schuessler.) Thus is explained the *modus operandi* of Kali Sulph. as an oxygen carrier, in which function it co-operates with Kali Phos. The oxygen in the lungs is taken up by the iron in the blood and carried to every cell in the organism by the reciprocal action of Kali Sulph. and Ferr. Phos.

A deficiency of Kali Sulph. causing a lack of oxygen in the skin and epithelial cells, will give rise to symptoms of chilliness, heaviness and weariness, palpitation of the heart, anxiety, sadness, headache, and pains in the limbs.

Kali Sulph. is also applicable to ailments accompanied by profuse desquamation of the skin, including the stage of desquamation following scarlet fever, measles, erysipelas, etc. This is, of course, due to its action upon the skin cells.

CHARACTERISTIC INDICATIONS

HEAD.—Dandruff on the scalp (internally, and as a wash, *Natr. Mur.*). Falling out of hair. *Headaches,* which are *better in cool air, and worse in evening or heated room;* this is the characteristic modality for this remedy. Rheumatic headaches, with evening aggravations. Eruptions on the head, with secretions of decidedly yellow, thin matter; note color of tongue. Scaling of scalp, with sticky secretions.

EYES.—Discharge from the eyes or eyelids, of yellow-greenish, serous matter, or yellow, slimy secretions; sometimes water. Yellow crusts on the eyelids. Inflammation of the conjunctiva, with characteristic exudations. Cataract, with dimness of the crystalline lens (*Natr. Mur.*).

EARS.—*Earache, with yellow, watery discharge.* Sharp, cutting pains under the ears. Catarrh of the ear and throat involving the eustachian tubes, with yellow, slimy discharge, causing deafness. The ear should also be carefully syringed with the remedy once a day. *Deafness from swelling of the internal ear,* with characteristic discharge and evening aggravation; *note color of tongue.* After inflammation of the ear, when the secretion is thin, bright yellow or greenish.

NOSE.—Catarrhal conditions of the head and throat, acute or chronic, with discharges of slimy, yellow or watery greenish matter; worse in evening or in a heated room. In the commencement of colds (in alternation with *Ferrum Phos.*, to produce free perspiration); give frequently, and a majority of colds can be "broken." Colds, with dry, harsh skin, to induce perspiration. Stuffy colds, with large collections of greenish matter (*Silicea*).

FACE.—*Neuralgia* of the face, intermittent, shifting pain, evening aggravation; *better in cool air,* worse in heated room. Cancer of the face and nose (*Epithelioma*). *See "Tumors."*

MOUTH.—Epithelial cancer of the lip, with characteristic secretions. Dryness of the lower lip; skin peels off in large flakes.

TEETH.—Toothache; worse in the evening and in a warm room, better in cool air.

TONGUE.—*Coating of tongue yellow and slimy,* sometimes *with whitish edge.* Insipid taste.

GASTRIC SYMPTOMS.—Catarrh of the stomach, with yellow, slimy tongue. Dyspepsia, with characteristic coating on tongue. Indigestion, with sensation of pressure and fullness at pit of stomach. Indigestion, with pain (*Natr. Mur., Kali Mur.*). Colic pains in stomach, with slimy, yellow coating of tongue, or when *Magnes. Phos.* gives no relief. Dread of hot drinks. Thirstlessness. Gastric fever, with rise of temperature in the evening; *note tongue symptoms.* In gastric fever, when the skin is dry and hot (in alternation with *Ferrum Phos.,* to assist perspiration).

ABDOMEN AND STOOL.—In all abdominal troubles, with characteristic tongue symptoms and color of discharges from the bowels. Diarrhea, with yellow, slimy, purulent matter. Pains of a colicky nature, caused by sudden changes from heat to cold; *note color of tongue.* Abdomen cold to the touch. Sulphurous odor of gas from the bowels. *Piles* (in alteration with the *chief remedy, Calc. Fluor.*), *when the tongue has a slimy, yellow coating,* or the characteristic discharge from the tumors. "Pain in abdomen, just above the angle of the crest of the ileum, on a line toward the umbilicus, deep within, beside the right hip" (Dr. Walker). Bloating of the abdomen. Typhoid, enteric or typhus fevers, with evening aggravation and rise of temperature.

URINARY ORGANS.—Cystitis, with characteristic discharge of yellow, slimy matter from the urethra; third stage of the inflammation.

MALE SEXUAL ORGANS.—Gonorrhea, slimy, yellow or greenish discharge. Evening aggravation of syphilis, gleet, when yellow and slimy.

FEMALE SEXUAL ORGANS.—Gonorrhea, with characteristic discharges. Menstruation too late and scanty, with fullness and weight in abdomen; *note color of tongue.* Leucorrhea, discharge of yellow, slimy or greenish matter.

RESPIRATORY ORGANS.—Inflammatory conditions of the respiratory tract, when the expectoration is decidedly yellow-greenish and slimy. Bronchitis and consumption, with the characteristic expectoration or rise of temperature in the evening; *note the color of the tongue.* Bronchial asthma, with yellow expectoration, for the labored breathing, *Kali Phos. Cough,* with distinctly yellow sputa, which is *worse in the evening, or in a heated atmosphere; better in the cool, open air.* Cough when the expectoration is yellow, tenacious and ropy, causing it to slip back, and is generally swallowed. Croupy hoarseness (*chief remedy, Kali Mur.*). Sensation of weariness in the pharynx; speaking is fatiguing. In *whooping cough,* for the *yellow, slimy expectoration;* for the whoop, *Magnes. Phos.* Pneumonia, with yellow phlegm, great rattling and gurgling of mucus in the chest, suffocative, smothering feeling in the heated room, must go in the open air for relief.

Circulatory Organs.—Pulse quick, with throbbing, boring pain over crest of ileum; pallid face. Temperature rises toward evening. Pulse very slow and sluggish, sometimes met with in low fevers, which have a tendency toward blood-poisoning; *skin is hot, very dry and harsh.*

Back and Extremities.—Rheumatic pains in the joints, when they are disposed to wander. Rheumatism of any part of the body, when of a shifting or wandering nature, with other characteristic indications for this remedy. Neuralgic or rheumatic pains in the back, limbs or any part of the body, when worse in the evening or in a warm room; with amelioration in the cool, open air. Fungoid inflammation of joints.

Nervous Symptoms.—Pains of a neuralgic nature, with tendency to shift from one place to another.

Skin.—All sores on the skin, when exuding a thin, yellow, watery matter, sometimes with dryness and desquamation of the surrounding skin. Skin scales freely on a sticky base. Skin is dry, hot and burning, lack of perspiration. Scarlet fever, measles, smallpox, etc., when the rash has been suppressed, "struck in," skin is dry and hot. *This salt* also greatly *aids desquamation in eruptive diseases, and assists in the formation of new skin.* Diseased conditions of the nails, interrupted in growth (*chief remedy, Silicea*). Dandruff; epithelial cancer, with characteristic discharge of thin, yellow, purulent matter; also local applications of the remedy. Eczema, when the symptoms of this remedy are present, also when the eruption is suddenly suppressed. In fevers, when the skin is dry and hot (to promote perspiration, should be given in alternation with *Ferrum Phos.*).

Tissues.—*All inflammations,* when there is *watery, yellow, or greenish, purulent secretions.* Epithelial cancer, with characteristic discharges; serous, watery exudations from any membrane.

FEBRILE CONDITIONS.—Fevers, gastric, typhoid, scarlet, enteric fever, etc., when the *temperature rises in the evening.* In fevers, when blood poisoning threatens. It assists in promoting perspiration; it should, therefore, be given frequently in alternation with *Ferrum Phos.* In eruptive fevers, to aid desquamation.

MODALITIES.—Aggravation in a heated room or in the evening. Always better in the cool, open air. Rise of temperature in the evening until midnight.

MAGNESIA PHOSPHORICA

FORMULA.—Mg $HP.O_4$, $7H_2O$.

Two parts of sulphate of magnesia are dissolved in thirty-two parts of distilled water, mixed with a solution of three parts of phosphate of soda in thirty-two parts of distilled water and set aside to crystallize. The salt separates in the course of twenty-four hours in tufts of prisms or needles.

PROPERTIES.—Crystallized magnesium phosphate forms small six-sided needles, having a cooling, sweetish taste. It is sparingly soluble in water, 322 parts of water taking up one of the salt after long standing. By boiling the solution, the salt becomes decomposed through a partial separation of trimagnesium salt. Magnesium phosphate dissolves easily in dilute acids; its crystals effloresce in warm air, and when heated to 100° C. (212° F.) give off more than half of their water, and at 170° C. (248° F.) the remaining portion. At a red heat the basic hydrogen is driven off and magnesium pyrophosphate is left.

MOLECULES of magnesium phosphate are found chiefly in the white fibres of the nerves and muscles. Nerves and muscles are composed of many strands or fibres of different colors, each one acting as a special telegraph wire; each one having a conductile power or special affinity for certain organic and inorganic principles, and performing their varied functions through the operation of natural law. The white fibres are controlled by the molecular action of the magnesia cell-salt.

When a deficiency in this salt occurs, these white fibres contract, and produce a condition called spasms, or cramps. This symptom of cramps is merely the body's method of announcing a lack of magnesium phosphate, and showing the location where the deficiency has occurred. For convenience of description, different names are given to cramps and spasms in various parts of the body, but they are nevertheless all essentially the same, the result of a lack of magnesium phosphate.

When a deficiency of magnesium phosphate occurs in the muscular tissue of the walls of the stomach, the white fibres draw up, contract, and reduce the cavity of the stomach. Now, in order to meet this condition and prevent a collapse, gas is formed by a natural process from the material at hand, and by expansion produces a counter force. Magnesium phosphate relieves such conditions almost instantly.

The only exception to this rule in speedy cures by administering this remedy, is where the blood has furnished calcium phosphate as a substitute, in an effort to supply the deficiency. Calcium phosphate more nearly corresponds to magnesium phosphate than any other salt; therefore, when magnesium phosphate does not act very promptly, calcium phosphate should be given, in order to overcome the deficiency of that salt which has been caused in the blood.

Magnesium phosphate is the true antispasmodic remedy. It has cured cases of chorea, or Vitus' dance, in from two to four weeks. For all heart troubles, so called, caused by a distension of the cardiac portion of the stomach, and thus interfering with the action of the heart, it is the sovereign remedy.

But the question will arise: How can molecules of a certain mineral salt supply a certain white nerve or muscle fluid? There is certainly a difference between the particles of an inorganic salt and the fluid that controls white fibres. To answer these questions, and try to make the matter clear to the minds of everybody, is the object of these short articles. It is quite evident that the fluid in question is manufactured in the physiology of the body.

The particles of magnesium phosphate simply contain within themselves the power—the potency—to create this muscle and nerve fluid by uniting with albumen—using albumen as the basic organic material, then calling to its aid the spirit of life, oxygen. Each inorganic salt knows how to make some constituent of the human organism.

CHARACTERISTIC INDICATIONS

MENTAL SYMPTOMS.—*Illusions of the senses and mental disorders. Magnes. Phos.* is closely allied with *Kali Phos.*, as the latter acts upon the gray nerve fibres, while the former acts upon the white; these being so closely connected, it is evident that a molecular disturbance in one of them will be apt to cause a disturbance in the other, therefore, the characteristic indications of the two salts may, in some cases, be somewhat similar.

HEAD.—Headache of a nervous character, with illusions of sight. Headaches, with sharp, shooting, darting, intermittent and spasmodic pain. Headache, with chilly sensations, especially up and down the spine. *Neuralgia of head*, when the pain is sharp (*Ferrum Phos.*). All pain when heat relieves and cold aggravates. Excruciating pains in the head, rheumatic or neuralgic. Pain in nape of neck of a sharp character. *Trembling and involuntary shaking of the head* (*Kali Phos.*).

EYES —*Drooping of the eyelids* (*Kali Phos.*). Contracted pupils. Sparks, colors before the eyes. Illusions of the sense of sight. Sensitiveness to light, diplopia (*double sight*), *spectra, etc. Spasmodic twitching of the eyelids* (*Calc. Phos.*). Neuralgic pains in the eyes. Squinting. *Calc. phos.* should be used externally and internally in most diseases of the eye; will act better if applied hot. Great pain in the eyes, with flow of tears, requires *Natr. Mur.* Dullness of sight from weakness of the optic nerve (*Kali Phos.*).

EARS.—Dullness of hearing, from disease of the auditory nerve fibres. *Earache,* when *of a* purely *nervous or spasmodic character,* heat relieves, all pains worse from cold.

NOSE.—"Loss of sense of smell, or perversion of the sense of smell, under certain conditions, not connected with cold; a course of this remedy" (Schuessler).

FACE.—Neuralgic pains of the face, of a shifting, shooting, darting, spasmodic character. Pains, lightning-like, worse to the touch and by cold; relieved by warm applications. Faceache, of a rheumatic character. Faceache, with flow of tears, requires *Natr. Mur.* (if inflammatory, *Ferrum Phos.*). Pains worse in cold air, better in warm room.

MOUTH.—Twitchings of the mouth and lips, spasmodic. Tetanic spasms. *Spasmodic stammering;* speaks slowly and begins speaking with the teeth closed (*if nervous, Kali Phos.*). Lock-jaw, should also be rubbed into the gums very frequently; internally in hot water.

TEETH.—Convulsions, cramps, etc., during dentition (alternate *Calc. Phos.*). Toothache, sharp, shooting, rheumatic and spasmodic pain, when heat relieves. If cold relieves, *Ferrum Phos.* is the remedy, as it indicates an inflammatory condition of the nerve or some of the adjacent tissues. Teeth sensitive to cold air or to touch. *Toothache,* when *associated with neuralgia of the face,* heat relieves, pains darting, intermittent and change about. In toothache, if *Magnes. Phos.* fails, or the tooth is badly decayed, give *Calc. Phos.*

THROAT.—Spasms of the throat, spasmodic closing of the windpipe. *Choking on attempting to swallow.* Spasmodic cough. Constricted feeling of the throat. Closing of the larynx by spasm or cramp. Shrill voice coming on suddenly when speaking or singing, caused by spasm of the windpipe (*Kali Phos.*).

GASTRIC SYMPTOMS.—Neuralgia of stomach; tongue clean, pain relieved by heat or pressure. Spasms of the stomach, when the pain is constricted or griping. Indigestion, when food causes griping; tongue clean (*Calc. Phos., Ferrum Phos.*). Hiccough. Vomiting, when caused by excessive pain or constriction of muscles of stomach. *Pain is remittent and spasmodic.* Belching of gas with short, sharp, nipping pain; drinking hot water relieves; worse from drinking acid or cold drinks.

ABDOMEN AND STOOL.—Dysentery, when accompanied by sharp, griping pains in the abdomen, which are relieved by warmth, rubbing or pressure (*Kali Mur.*). Remittent and spasmodic pain. Colic of infants, with screaming and drawing up of legs. Gnawing pains in the bowels, with belching of wind. *Bloating of the abdomen* with passing of flatus. Griping pain in abdomen, with watery diarrhea, stools expelled with force. Hemorrhoids, with cutting, darting pains, very severe. Pain in the rectum and abdomen.

"In all cases of diarrhea, dysentery, neuralgia and inflammation of the bowels, copious injections of hot water should be given frequently; it will cleanse the unhealthy membrane, restore normal absorption, relax the abdominal muscles, wonderfully relieve pain and greatly aid in the restoration of the patient. Hot or cold applications should also be used" (Chapman).

Urinary Organs.—Spasmodic retention of the urine (alternate *Ferrum Phos.*). *Spasm of the bladder* and urethra, with *painful straining when urinating* (*Ferrum Phos., Kali Phos.*). Pain when passing gravel (*Natr. Sulph.*).

Male Sexual Organs.—Stricture, resulting from gonorrhea, sharp, spasmodic pains in the urethra.

Female Sexual Organs.—Dysmenorrhea (*menstrual colic*), at the time to relieve the pain (*Kali Phos.*). As a preventive (*Ferrum Phos.*). Very severe pain, of "labor-like character," heat generally relieves. *Neuralgia of the ovaries,* apply hot local applications also. Menstrual colic, when membranes are thrown off, or the discharge is stringy or fibrous. Vaginismus (*Ferrum Phos.*). Pain preceding the monthly flow.

Pregnancy.—Labor pains, when they are spasmodic, or with cramps in the legs and spasmodic twitchings. Excessive expulsive efforts. Convulsions (see *Kali Phos.*).

Respiratory Organs.—Asthma, with belching of gas, pain in the chest, and constrictive cough, must sit up (*give in hot water*). Spasmodic cough, coming in fits or paroxysms, without expectoration. Sudden, shrill voice. Sharp pains in the chest, shortness of breath (*Ferrum Phos.*). Whooping cough (*Kali Mur.*). Must be given persistently in chronic cases. Spasm of the glottis. *Convulsive fits of coughing,* with *constriction of* the *chest* and little or no expectoration. Spasmodic coughing at night, worse on lying down.

Circulatory Organs.—Neuralgic spasms of the breast (*Angina Pectoris*). When pain is severe in any organ, the remedy should be given in hot water, and very frequent doses.

Back and Extremities.—Pains in the back and extremities, of a neuralgic character, very sharp, darting, or remittent. Pain in small of back and neck, heat relieves. Convulsions, with stiffness of the limbs, clenched fingers (*Calc. Phos.*). Painful joints. *Neuralgia of the limbs.* Violent pains in rheumatism of the joints. Local applications. Sciatic rheumatism, with violent pains. *Shooting sensation in the limbs resembling electric shocks.* Power of motion deficient.

Nervous Symptoms.—Trembling and involuntary motion of the hands. Paralysis agitans (*Kali Phos.*). Involuntary shaking of the head. *Epilepsy, from any cause,* for the spasm (*Kali Mur., chief remedy* for the disease). Chorea (*St. Vitus' dance*). Lock-jaw, frequent doses in hot water; also rub it into the gums. Compare with *Kali Phos.* in all nervous diseases. Writer's cramp. Cramps in the limbs at night. *Patient* is *tired and exhausted,* caused by insufficient nutrition of the nerve tissues (*Kali Phos.*). Want of sensibility.

Tissues.—Spasms and neuralgic pains in any tissue, due to a deficiency of unequalization of the *Magnes. Phos.* molecules.

Febrile Conditions.—Nervous chills, with chattering of the teeth (*Kali Phos.*). Fever, when chills and cramps are present (*Ferrum Phos.*). Intermittent fever, with cramps of the calves of limbs. Chills run up and down the spine.

Sleep.—Yawning, with spasmodic straining of the lower jaw, sometimes throwing the jaw out of its socket. Drowsiness.

Modalities.—All the symptoms of this remedy are relieved by heat, pressure and rubbing, and are aggravated by cold, cold air, draughts, etc. If practical, hot applications should always be used when this remedy is exhibited.

NATRUM MURIATICUM

Synonyms.—Sodium Chloride, Chloruretum Sodium, Natrium Chloratum Purum, Sodii Chloridum Chloride of Sodium.

Common Names.—Common salt, table salt.

Formula.—NaCl.

Molecular Weight.—58.5.

Origin and Preparation.—Sodium chloride occurs very abundantly in nature, both in the solid state as rock salt, forming extensive beds in rocks of various ages, and in solution in sea-water, salt-lake and salt springs. The salt is mined from the solid deposits or taken from the open cuts, while from saline waters it is obtained by evaporation or by first freezing; the latter mode is followed in Northern countries of Europe, since salt water separates on freezing, into ice containing no salt and a strong saline lye. After the crystallizing out of sodium chloride the mother liquors containing potassium, sodium, calcium and magnesium sulphates, chlorides and bromides are utilized for the extraction of these compounds and their derivatives.

Properties.—Pure sodium chloride chrystallizes from aqueous solutions at ordinary temperatures or higher, in colorless, transparent, anhydrous cubes, but an aqueous solution exposed to a temperature of 10° C. yields hexagonal plates containing two molecules of water; when the temperature rises the water of crystallization is expelled and the crystals are changed into a heap of minute cubes. Ordinarily, sodium chloride is found as a white powder, made up of small, glistening, hard cubes, without reaction to test-paper, without odor and possessing a pure saline taste. The crystals are anhydrous, have a specific gravity of 2.16, decrepitate when thrown on red hot coal or when heated upon platinum foil; in a very damp atmosphere they become moist. Salt is soluble in less than three parts of water in the cold, and is scarcely more soluble in boiling water, but the admixture of other salts increases its solubility. It is not taken up by absolute alcohol, and 100 parts of 90 per cent. dissolve only two parts of it. At a red heat it melts, and on cooling solidifies to a crystalline mass; at a white heat it volatilizes. Its watery solutions have the property of dissolving several bodies insoluble in water, *e. g.*, calcium phosphate, calcium sulphate and silver chloride.

TESTS.—The aqueous solution of sodium chloride should be perfectly neutral (absence of carbonate and of free hydrochloric acid); it should not be precipitated by hydrogen sulphide nor by ammonium sulphide (absence of metals), nor by ammonium oxalate (absence of calcium), nor by barium chloride (absence of sulphate), nor by sodium carbonate (absence of the earths, especially magnesia).

WITH the exception of the phosphate of lime, the human system contains more sodium chloride than any other inorganic salt. The reason for this may be readily understood when we realize that our bodies are about 70 per cent. water, which, in the absence of sodium chloride, would be inert and useless. It is the power that this salt has to use water that renders it of any value to man. The same principle holds good in plants and vegetable life.

Sodium chloride uses water to build up and carry on the functions of life, and also as a vehicle to eliminate waste substances. Any deficiency in this cell-salt at once causes a disturbance of the water in the human organism, because it has lost that element which renders it fit to perform its allotted task. In sun-stroke, a deficiency in sodium chloride allows the moisture to be drawn from other parts, especially the nape of the neck, and cause a pressure against the base of the brain, producing dangerous and sometimes fatal results. The above named salt relieves the unpleasant condition called sun-stroke, surely and quickly.

In delirium tremens, the continuity of water is broken up, due to a deficiency of sodium chloride molecules, and the symptoms incident to this disease follow. Very severe cases of delirium tremens have been relieved in one hour by administering frequent doses of this remedy. The coming physician will wish to know more than the mere fact that a certain agent has curative properties; he will demand to know "how and why." And if the remedy is the true one, the "how and why" can always be explained. It is necessary to make clear the *modus operandi* of the twelve inorganic salts; to show that each one has a special building or creative power. This salt may be compared to a brick-mason or carpenter. The brick-mason has the power to build up a brick wall when he is supplied with brick and mortar. So the carpenter can create a wooden structure, when lumber and other material necessary for the work is furnished. The carpenter is the workman, or vitalizer, of the inert organic material and possesses the creative power to produce a building. So the inorganic salts possess the creative power to make something out of organic matter; and thus the chemistry of life goes on.

CHARACTERISTIC INDICATIONS

MENTAL SYMPTOMS.—*Delirium at any time, with muttering and wandering,* when the tongue has a frothy appearance, or is dry and parched. Stupor and sleepiness. Low delirium in typhoid or typhus fevers. Delirium tremens; this salt is the chief remedy to overcome the dryness which exists in the brain (*Kali Phos.*). Melancholy, hopeless, with dejected spirits. Despondent moods, with constipation or excess of watery symptoms, weeps easily.

HEAD.—*Chief remedy in sun-stroke;* this disease, like delirium tremens, is due to an excessive dryness of the tissue of the brain, owing to a disturbance of the sodium chloride molecules. Headaches, with dryness of some of the mucous membranes and excessive secretion from others. Headaches, with constipation. *Headaches, with profusion of tears* or frothy coating on the tongue; hopeless, dejected spirits.

Headaches, with vomiting of frothy, watery phlegm. Headaches of girls about the time of puberty; patient is dull and listless. Dull, heavy, hammering headaches, with drowsiness and unrefreshing sleep. Eruptions of the scalp, with watery contents. Dandruff. White scales on the scalp (*Kali Sulph., Kali Mur.*).

EYES.—Neuralgic pains in the eyes, with flow of tears (*Magnes. Phos.*). Flow of tears from the eyes, when associated with fresh colds in the head. Weak eyes, with tears when going into cold air or when the wind strikes the eyes. All eye affections with flow of tears. Granulated eyelids, with or without secretion of tears (*Ferrum Phos., Kali Mur.*). Blisters on the cornea (*Kali Mur.*); should also be syringed daily with a solution of the salt, to produce absorption of the spot. Stoppage of the tear-duct from colds. Pain in the eyes, with tears; recurring daily at certain times. Scrofulous conditions of the eyes, thick lids, acrid, smarting secretions, with tears. Muscular asthenopia (*Magnes. Phos.*). Conjunctivitis, with mucous secretions and lachrymation.

EARS.—Deafness from swelling of the eustachian tubes (*Kali Mur., Kali Sulph.*). Ear affections, with excessive secretion of saliva or characteristic discharge from the ears.

NOSE.—Fresh colds, with discharge of clear, watery, transparent mucus and sneezing. Dropping of watery, salty secretion from the posterior nares (*Calc. Phos.*). Chronic catarrh of anemic persons, with salty mucus. Hay fever, influenza, with sneezing and watery discharges from eyes and nose. Coryza (*running cold*), with watery, slimy discharge. Loss of smell, with dryness and rawness of the pharynx. Bleeding of the nose in anemic persons; the blood is thin and watery (*Ferrum Phos.*). Excessive dryness of the nose, with tendency to form scales or crusts in the nose.

FACE.—Faceache, with constipation; tongue covered with a clear mucus, slime and frothy bubbles at its edge. Faceache, with vomiting of clear phlegm or water. Neuralgia of the face. with excessive discharge of clear mucus from the eyes (local application of the same). Sycosis; whiskers fall out; if the watery symptoms correspond. *Perspiration on the face while eating.* Chlorosis, sallow, dirty-looking face.

Mouth.—Excess of saliva, alone or during the course of any disease. Salivation. *Catarrhs* of the mouth and pharynx, *with watery, transparent, frothy discharges* (albuminous *Calc. Phos.*). Aphthe (*thrush*), with flow of saliva (alternate *Kali Mur.*). Swelling of glands under the tongue. Ranula. Inflammation of salivary glands when secreting excessive amount of saliva. *Constant spitting* of *frothy mucus.*

Teeth.—Toothache, with excessive flow of tears or saliva. *Neuralgia of teeth* and facial nerves, with characteristic secretions. Teething in infants and drooling.

Tongue.—*Tongue has clear, slimy, watery coating,* with small, frothy bubbles of saliva on the sides. Small blisters on the tip of the tongue. Dryness of the tongue in low fevers, with watery discharge from the bowels.

Throat.—Inflammation of mucous lining of the throat, with characteristic watery secretions. Uvula relaxed when there is much saliva (*Calc. Fluor., chief remedy*). Goitre, with watery symptoms (*Calc. Phos., chief remedy*). Sore throat, with excessive dryness or too much secretion of saliva. In *diphtheria,* when there is drowsiness, *watery stools,* flow of saliva or vomiting of water; face is puffy and pale. Mumps, when watery symptoms are present (*Kali Mur., chief remedy for the swelling*). Thin neck, with chlorotic conditions.

Gastric Symptoms.—All conditions and diseases of the stomach, where excess of saliva or watery vomit is present; tongue has a clear, frothy, transparent coating. *Indigestion, with watery vomiting* and salty taste in the mouth. Patient sometimes has a great *craving for salt or salt food.* Indigestion, with pain in stomach and watery gathering in the mouth, sour or salt taste in mouth. Great thirst. Dyspepsia, with pain after eating, if watery symptoms are present. Vomiting of transparent, watery, stringy mucus, or watery fluids and froth (*not acid*). Jaundice, with drowsiness and watery symptoms. Water-brash, not acid, frequently accompanied with constipation, from dryness of the intestines.

ABDOMEN AND STOOL.—Looseness of the bowels, with watery stools. Diarrhea, alternating with constipation. Constipation from dryness of the mucous membranes of the bowels, with watery secretion in other parts. *Constipation, with dull, heavy headache, profusion of tears,* or vomiting of frothy water. Stools are dry and often produce fissure in rectum, burning pain in rectum, or torn, bleeding, smarting feeling after stool. Constipation, with drowsiness and watery symptoms from eyes or mouth. *Diarrhea,* stool frothy, glairy slime, *causing soreness and smarting.* Hemorrhoids, with constipation, caused from dryness of the bowels. Stinging piles. Weakness of bowels and muscles of the abdomen. An occasional injection of hot water, with *Natr. Mur.,* will be found very beneficial. *Natr. Mur.* not only controls the watery secretions of the bowels, but it has a stimulating effect, and will strengthen the muscles of the viscera and abdomen

URINARY ORGANS.—Catarrh of the bladder, when secreting watery, transparent fluid. Polyuria. Cutting and burning after urinating. Diabetes insipidus; great thirst and excessive flow of watery urine.

MALE SEXUAL ORGANS.—*Chronic gonorrhea, with transparent, watery, scalding slime.* Chronic syphilis, with serous discharge. Hydrocele. Preputial edema (*Natr. Sulph.*). Discharge of prostatic fluid.

FEMALE SEXUAL ORGANS.—Gonorrhea and syphilis, with characteristic discharges, indicating this remedy. *Menstrual flow thin, watery blood.* Menstruation too late, accompanied with sadness, headache and weeping. Delayed menstruation in young girls, when there is headache, dullness and sadness, or when the person is emaciated or chlorotic. Soreness and smarting in vagina after urinating. Itching of the vulva. Menses mixed with leucorrhea; discharges are smarting, scalding and watery. Watery, slimy, excoriating leucorrhea. Dryness of vagina; sexual connection causes great pain. Vaginal douches of about one-half ounce of salt to quart of warm water, of much benefit. Smarting, burning, sticking pain in vagina; inflammation caused by dryness of the mucous membrane.

PREGNANCY.—Vomiting of watery, frothy phlegm, not acid.

RESPIRATORY ORGANS.—Asthma, with watery, frothy mucus (alternate *Kali Phos. for the breathing*). Bronchitis; mucus frothy and watery. Sometimes coughed up with difficulty. Acute inflammation of the windpipe, with characteristic expectoration, constant spitting of frothy water. *Edema of the lungs,* with *watery expectoration,* sometimes tasting salty. Catarrh of the bronchi, "winter cough," with characteristic symptoms (*note appearance of tongue*). Chronic coughs of consumptives, with frothy discharges, salty taste. Cough, with headache and excessive lachrymation. Cough, with flow of tears and spurting of urine (*Ferrum Phos.*). In whooping cough, note the expectoration. *Pneumonia, with* characteristic expectoration and much *loose, rattling phlegm in the chest;* note also tongue symptoms. Pleurisy, when serous effusion has taken place. Hoarseness. Pain in chest from coughing (*Ferrum Phos.*).

CIRCULATORY ORGANS.—Palpitation of the heart, in anemic persons, with watery blood, or dropsical swellings. Enlargement of the heart, with characteristic indications. Poor circulation, cold hands and feet (*Calc. Phos.*). Pulse rapid and intermittent; *pulsations of heart felt all over the body.* Blood thin and watery; will not coagulate.

BACK AND EXTREMITIES.—Weak and languid feelings, with drowsiness. Blisters on the hands of fingers, containing watery, serous fluid. *Involuntary movement of the legs;* fidgets; cannot sit still. Starting and jerking of limbs during sleep (*Magnes Phos.*). Rheumatic, gouty pains, if tongue and watery secretions correspond. Rheumatism of the joints; joints crack; note appearance of tongue and watery symptoms. Pains in the back and extremities; *backache relieved by lying on something hard.* Hang-nails, when there is dryness of the skin. Rheumatic gout, coming on periodically. Feeling of coldness in the back.

NERVOUS SYMPTOMS.—Neuralgic nerve pains, with flow of saliva or tears, or when recurring periodically (*Magnes. Phos.*). Sensation of numbness in parts affected; spine, cannot bear to have it touched, oversensitive to pressure; paralytic pain in small of back. Neuralgia; pains shoot along the nerve fibres, but accompanied by flow of saliva or tears. Hysterical; feels worse in the morning or in cold weather. Hysterical spasms and debility. Restlessness and twitching of the muscles.

SKIN.—All skin diseases, where there is a watery exudation, or an excessive dryness of the skin. Eczema, with white scales; external applications also. *Eruptions of the skin, with watery contents;* poor in albumen; note tongue and watery symptoms. Colorless, watery vesicles. Herpes in bend of knee. Herpetic eruptions on any part of the body, or occurring during course of a disease. Chafing of skin in small children, with watery symptoms (alternate *Natr. Phos.*). White scales on the scalp (*Kali Sulph., chief remedy*). Warts in palm of hands. Hang-nails. Stings of insects; apply locally as soon as possible. Small-pox, with drowsiness and flow of saliva. Shingles, with characteristic symptoms calling for this remedy. Rupia, blisters with watery contents. Intertrigo between thighs and scrotum, with acrid and excoriating discharge. Scarlet fever, with watery vomiting, drowsiness, twitchings. *Exudations* on the skin or mucous lining, after inflammations, when *watery and serous.* Blisters and blebs on the skin, with watery contents. *Nettle-rash, with violent itching;* appears after becoming overheated, causing an unequalization of this salt. Nettle-rash in intermittent fever. Eczema from eating too much salt. Chronic skin diseases, especially urticarious and miliary eruptions.

TISSUES.—Dropsy in any part of the body (*Natr. Sulph.*). Accumulations of serum or water in the areolar tissues. Dryness of some of the mucous membranes, with excess of secretions in others. Anemic conditions, with thin, watery blood. Chlorotic conditions; chlorosis, with dirty, torpid skin. Face pale and sallow, when watery symptoms are present. Effusions serous, poor in albumen, slimy, like boiled starch. Note also tongue and watery secretions. Chronic inflammation of lymphatic glands, with watery secretions from some of the membranes. Mumps. Emaciations, especially of the neck; acts upon cartilage, mucous follicles, glands, etc. Emaciation while living well. Cachexia following ague from excessive use of quinine. The *slimy, frothy appearance of the tongue, with watery secretions,* is the "keynote" for this remedy. It regulates the proper degree of moisture of solids and proper amount of water of the fluids in the organism.

Febrile Conditions.—In all kinds of fevers, when there are malignant symptoms, such as stupor, drowsiness, watery vomiting, twitchings, etc. Typhoid, typhus, scarlet fevers, with the above symptoms. *Intermittent fever, after the abuse of quinine;* living in damp regions or on newly-turned ground (in alternation with *Natr. Sulph., chief remedy*). Chill coming on in the morning about 10 o'clock and continuing till noon, preceded by intense heat, increased headache and thirst, sweat weakening and sour, backache and headache, great languor, emaciation, sallow complexion, and fever blisters on the lips. Profuse night-sweats; bathe once a day in salt water. Feeling of chilliness, especially in the back; watery saliva; full, heavy headache, increased thirst, etc.

Sleep.—Excessive sleep, if traced to an excess of moisture in the brain. *Constant desire to sleep,* drowsy, dull and stupid, when accompanied by the characteristic symptoms of this salt. Natural amount of sleep does not refresh, patient feels tired and stupid in the morning.

Modalities.—Symptoms are generally worse in the morning, in cold weather, or in a salty atmosphere; feels better in the evening. Complaints after the free use of poisonous drugs. Complaints coming at regular periods.

NATRUM PHOSPHORICUM

SYNONYMS.—Sodium Phosphate, Natri Phosphas, Phosphas Natricus, Sodæ Phosphas, Sodii Phosphas.

COMMON NAME.—Phosphate of Soda.

FORMULA.—Na_2 HPO_4, $12H_2O$.

MOLECULAR WEIGHT.—358.

PREPARATION.—To 10 parts of bone, calcined to whiteness and in fine powder, add 6 parts of sulphuric acid in an earthen vessel and thoroughly mix the ingredients; 22 fluid ounces of water are to be added to the mixture, and the whole thoroughly stirred. The mixture is to be set aside to digest for three days and during that time is to be frequently stirred and enough water added from time to time to replace that lost by evaporation. At the end of the time, 22 fluid ounces of boiling water are to be added, and the whole thrown upon a muslin strainer, and repeatedly washed by boiling water in small amounts till the liquid comes through tasteless. The strained liquid is then to be set aside to permit the newly formed precipitates to settle. When the precipitation is complete, the clear liquid is decanted off and boiled down to 22 ounces. This concentrated liquid is to be decanted from any fresh precipitate and heated in a vessel of iron, and there is gradually added to it a hot solution of sodium carbonate as long as effervescence ensues, and until the liberated phosphoric acid is entirely neutralized; the liquid is now to be filtered and set aside in a cool place to crystallize. The first crop of crystals is the purest, but a subsequent crop may be obtained by adding sodium carbonate to the liquid as long as crystals are formed; the crystals of the secondary crop must be repurified by solution and recrystallization.

The salt should be kept in a well-stoppered bottle.

PROPERTIES.—Official sodium phosphate crystallizes in oblique rhombic prisms and tabites, which are transparent and colorless, and have a mild, cooling, saline taste. They are soluble in two parts of hot water, and in four or five of water at medium temperatures; they are insoluble in alcohol.

The solutions are slightly alkaline in reaction. Heated to 35° C. (95° F.) they melt in thin water or crystallization, and solidify to a crystalline mass on cooling at 100° C. (212° F.) they give up their water of crystallization, and above 300° C. (572° F.) the salt is converted into pyrophosphate. The aqueous solution of the salt, when treated with silver nitrate solution, precipitates yellow orthophosphate of silver, and the filtered fluid has an acid reaction; the aqueous solution, upon the addition of barium chloride, gives a white precipitate of barium phosphate; both these precipitates are soluble in nitric acid. The solution of the salt after acidulation with HCl should not be changed in any way by hydrogen sulphide (absence of metals, and especially arsenic). The neutral solution should not effervesce upon the addition of an acid (absence of carbonate) and should give no precipitate or turbidity when treated with ammonia (absence of magnesium), or with ammonium oxalate (calcium).

THE fluids of the body contain both alkali and acid; but a deficiency in acid never occurs, because it is organic, and, like albumen, is always present in sufficient quantities, when proper food is taken. As it is necessary, absolutely necessary, that a proper balance of lime phosphate molecules be present to work with albumen and properly distribute it and incorporate it into bone and other tissue, so it is absolutely necessary that a proper amount of the phosphate of soda be present as a worker with acid, to combine with it and thus form *new compounds*. Thus it will be seen that "an excess of acid" is a misnomer, and that the true way to put it is: "A deficiency exists in the phosphate of sodium." And here again comes in the *creative* power inherent in the inorganic salts.

Organic matter has no creative power, no more than has brick. The brick-mason, given a supply of brick, possesses the power to create the brick wall.

The inorganic mineral salts have the power to create, when furnished with the proper material. But the material is always present; it is the laborers that are scarce in disease. The only trouble that ever arises is a deficiency in workmen. A lack of proper balance of the alkaline cell-salt in gastric juice will allow ferments to arise and so retard digestion that the lining quickly becomes involved. An inspissation of bile occurs, and bilious diarrhea or other bilious disorders follow. For such conditions Natr. Sulph. must be given also, although Natr. Phos. would have prevented such results.

CHARACTERISTIC INDICATIONS

HEAD.—Headache on the crown of head or in the forehead, with feeling as if the skull were too full. Sick headache, with vomiting of sour fluids (alternate *Ferrum Phos.*). Headache on awakening in the morning. *Note color of the tongue*; if there is a creamy deposit on the back part, this salt is indicated. Very severe headaches on top of the head, with intense pressure and heat (*Ferrum Phos.*). Some gastric troubles usually exist and should be relieved. Headaches, with pain in the stomach and ejection of frothy, sour fluid. Giddiness, when gastric derangements are present (alternate *Ferrum Phos.*).

EYES.—*Inflammation of eyes,* when *secreting a golden-yellow, creamy matter.* Eyes glued together in the morning with a creamy discharge. Any disease of the eyes, when accompanied with the characteristic creamy discharge (*note also color of root of tongue and palate*). *Squinting,* when caused by irritation *from worms,* to remove the cause (*Magnes. Phos.*).

EARS.—"One ear red, hot and frequently itchy, accompanied by gastric derangement and acidity" (Dr. Walker). Outer ears sore and scabby, with creamy discharge, or the scabs have a creamy, yellow appearance (*note color of tongue*). Heat and burning of the ears, with gastric symptoms (*Ferrum Phos.*).

NOSE.—Picking at the nose, generally a symptom of worms or of an acid condition of the stomach. Cold in the head, with yellow, creamy discharge from the nose; *itching of the nose,* with acidity. *Note color of tongue, palate and roof of mouth.*

FACE.—Face red and blotched, without fever; blotches come and go suddenly; white about the mouth and nose, indicating worms or acid condition of the stomach, associated with *cream-colored tongue* and sour, acid risings.

MOUTH.—Creamy, yellow coating at the back part of the roof of mouth. Creamy, golden-yellow exudation from tonsils and pharynx. *Sour, acid taste in the mouth,* sometimes accompanied with canker sores (*Kali Mur., Kali Phos.*).

TEETH.—Children grind their teeth during sleeping, associated with gastric derangements or worms. *Gastric derangements during teething.*

TONGUE.—"The great keynote for this remedy is the moist, creamy or golden-yellow coating at the back part of the tongue" (Drs. Boericke and Dewey).

THROAT.—Sore, raw feeling in the throat; tonsils and throat inflamed, with creamy, yellow, moist coating. Catarrh of the throat; tonsils covered with the characteristic exudation of this salt, usually associated with acid condition of the stomach. *False diphtheria,* with *creamy coating of the palate* and back part of the tongue.

GASTRIC SYMPTOMS.—All conditions of the stomach where there are sour, acid risings or the tongue has a moist, creamy, yellow coating. Dyspepsia, with acid risings (alternate with *Ferrum Phos.,* to strengthen digestion). Gastric abrasions, superficial ulcerations, pain after eating, calls for this remedy if the accompanying acid conditions are present (*Calc. Phos., Ferrum Phos.*). Gastric derangements, causing flatulence, headache and giddiness. *Morning sickness,* with *vomiting of sour fluids.* Nausea, with sour risings. Stomachache from the presence of worms or acidity of the stomach. Ulceration of the stomach, when the *least amount of food causes pain* and the tongue and palate have the characteristic creamy, yellow coating. Ulceration of the stomach, with vomiting of sour, acid fluids or substance like coffee-grounds; follow with *Ferrum Phos.* and *Calc. Phos.* Vomiting sour, acid fluids (*not food*). Infants vomit curdled milk.

ABDOMEN AND STOOL.—Diarrhea, especially of children, with green, sour-smelling stools, caused by an acid condition. Flatulent colic, with green, sour-smelling stools or vomiting of curdled masses. *Diarrhea,* when there is *much straining at stool or constant urging to stool,* with passing of jelly-like masses of mucus, indicating acidity (*Kali Mur.*). Worms of all kinds, with accompanying symptoms of picking the nose, itching at the anus, pain in the abdomen, acidity of the stomach, restless sleep, etc. (injections of same remedy). Ulceration of the bowels, when characteristic symptoms are present (*Ferrum Phos.*).

URINARY ORGANS.—Frequent urination, with *inability to retain urine,* with corresponding symptoms of acidity; more frequently seen in children (*Ferrum Phos.*). Dark-red urine, with rheumatism (*Ferrum Phos.*).

MALE SEXUAL ORGANS.—Seminal emissions, without dreams, or when followed by weakness and trembling. Irregularity of sexual desires, either gone or increased, when there are other indications of acid condition of the system.

FEMALE SEXUAL ORGANS.—All secretions from uterus or vagina which are acid, creamy, yellow and watery. *Sterility caused by acid secretions* from the vagina, proving fatal to the spermatozoa. Leucorrhea, with watery, creamy, yellow, acid discharge, causing itching, rawness and soreness of the parts. Discharges smell sour and sickening. Irregularity of the monthly periods, when accompanied with acid leucorrhea and frontal headache; also vomiting of acid fluids (*not food*).

PREGNANCY.—Morning sickness of pregnancy, with sour, acid vomit (*not food*), or other acid conditions. Nausea, with sour risings.

RESPIRATORY ORGANS.—In consumption, when the expectoration causes soreness of the lips or rawness of the tongue and mouth.

CIRCULATORY ORGANS.—Palpitation and irregularity of heart's action, caused from imperfect digestion. *Trembling about the heart;* always *worse after eating.* The diet and bowels should be looked to carefully.

BACK AND EXTREMITIES.—In all cases of acute or chronic articular rheumatism this remedy is indicated and should be prescribed alternately or intercurrently with other remedies. *Natr. Phos.* is a remedy for the acid diathesis, which many believe is (if not the sole cause) at least a formidable attendant upon this distressing disease. *Rheumatic pains in the joints,* weak feeling in the legs. Acid, sour-smelling perspiration. Cracking and creaking of joints, with pain and soreness. Gout (*Natr. Sulph.*).

NERVOUS SYMPTOMS.—Squinting and grinding of teeth, with intestinal irritation from worms. Nervousness, with trembling and palpitation of the heart, from acid condition of the stomach.

SKIN.—*Eczema* of the skin, when accompanied *with acid, creamy, yellow secretions.* Chafing of the skin, with soreness and rawness in little children; *note characteristic symptoms* of this salt (*Natr. Mur.*). Erythema, "rose-rash" (alternate with *Ferrum Phos.*). Crusta lactea. Pimples all over the body, like flea-bites, with itching and acid symptoms. Hives.

TISSUES.—Exudations from any mucous membrane or sore in the flesh, of a creamy, yellow or honey color, which can be traced to a disturbance of the molecules of sodium phosphate, is said to favor the deposit of calcium phosphate in bone diseases. Rheumatism, with acid symptoms.

FEBRILE CONDITIONS.—Acid, *sour-smelling perspiration* during any disease. Fever, with vomiting of sour fluids. Acid symptoms during the course of any febrile disease. Flashes of heat from indigestion, often causing frontal headache.

SLEEP.—Restless sleep from worm troubles, gritting the teeth and screaming in sleep, with itching of anus and picking of nose.

MODALITIES.—No characteristic modality has as yet been discovered for this salt.

NATRUM SULPHURICUM

SYNONYMS.—Sodium Sulphate; Sodæ Sulphas, Sodii Sulphas.

COMMON NAMES.—Glauber's Salt, Sulphate of Soda.

FORMULA.—Na_2 SO_4+, $10H_2O$.

MOLECULAR WEIGHT.—322.

ORIGIN AND PREPARATION.—This salt occurs rather abundantly in nature, either anhydrous as *Thenardite*, crystallized in right rhombic prisms, or with ten molecules of water as Glauber's salt, in monoclinic prisms. It occurs more abundantly in combination with calcium sulphate as *Glauberite;* it is also found in sea-water, in the waters of most saline springs, and it exists in large quantity in many salt lakes in Russia. Sodium sulphate is prepared in enormous amount by the action of sulphuric acid on common salt, as a preliminary step in the manufacture of sodium carbonate and as a secondary product in many other chemical processes. It is purified by recrystallization.

Properties.—Pure sodium sulphate forms large, colorless, transparent, glistening, oblique rhombic or irregularly six-sided prisms, whose specific gravity is 1.35. They possess a cooling, bitter, saline taste, and in the air, especially in a warm place, they effloresce, becoming a white powder. At 30° C. (86° F.) they melt in their own water of crystallization, and at a higher temperature are rendered anhydrous by the loss of that water. Their behavior to solvents is remarkable with increase of temperature, their solubility increases in water to a certain limit, and decreases again if heated beyond that. The point of greatest solubility is 33° C. (91.4° F.), so that a saturated solution at this temperature will, if either further warmed or cooled, deposit some of the salt as crystals; at this maximum solubility one part of water will take up more than three of the salt.

Tests.—Pure sodium sulphate should be free from other salts, and its solution should undergo no change when treated with hydrogen or ammonium sulphide. In German pharmacy a trace of chloride is permissible, but the precipitate in watery solutions with silver nitrate should not be more than a mere opalescence. The solutions of the salt must be neutral to test-paper, and 100 grains of it dissolved in distilled water and acidulated with hydrochloric acid should give, by the addition of chloride of barium, a white precipitate which, when washed and dried, weighs 72.2 grains.

THIS inorganic salt is found in the intercellular fluids, and its principal office is to regulate the water in the tissue, blood and fluids of the body. A deficiency of this salt prevents the elimination of such water from the tissue as is produced by oxidation of organic matter, while sodium chloride properly distributes the water in tissue, as has been shown. Sodium sulphate regulates the amount by having the power to eliminate any excess that may, from any cause, be present. *First,* Decomposition of lactic acid with sodium phosphate leaves a residue of water to be gotten rid of, and sodium sulphate must be present in proper quantity, or a hydrogenoid condition will arise. *Second,* In hot weather, where water is present, it is held in solution, by the heat of the sun, in the atmospheric air, and thus enters the blood through the lungs. Those who are weakly, whose digestion is any way impaired, are then liable to malarial troubles, because the circulation is not able to eliminate the excess of water from the blood because of a lack of proper quantity of sodium sulphate molecules to do the work. To speak from a chemical view, one molecule of sodium sulphate has the power to take up and carry out of the organism two molecules of water.

Biochemistry has established the fact that chills and fever (or ague), cholera, yellow fever and all ailments incident to hot weather, are basically caused by an excess of water in the blood, and probably in intercellular fluids: and that all such conditions arise from the inability of the digestion and assimilation to furnish sufficient quantity of sodium sulphate to carry off the excess of water breathed into the blood through the lungs. Let us take a case of malaria. Hot weather causes a rapid evaporation of water, especially in low, marshy districts, and regions where there are many ponds and other small bodies of water. This water is held in solution in the atmosphere, and is, of course, taken into the blood through the lungs by the act of breathing; thus the blood becomes overcharged with water.

The cell-salt Natrum Sulph. has an affinity for oxygen, and oxygen has an affinity for water, and thus, in health, Natrum Sulph. is able to eliminate this excess of water from the system. If, however, from any cause, a deficiency of Natrum Sulph. exists in the system, this surplus water cannot be carried off.

Thus a suitable breeding place in the blood is supplied for the plasmodium malariae or haematozoa of Laveran, a vegetable micro-organism to which the active manifestations of malarial fever are due. The plasmodium is introduced into the human system by a species of mosquito, the anopheles, which carries the organism in its blood, and transmits it through its bite.

When once established in the blood, the plasmodium causes a series of paroxysms, nearly always occurring with remarkable regularity, either at the end of 24, 48 or 72 hours. If occurring at the expiration of 24 hours from the beginning of the preceding paroxysms, the fever is said to be of the quotidian type. If the interval between paroxysms is 48 hours, the paroxysms occurring every third day, the fever is of the tertian type. If the interval is 72 hours, the paroxysm recurring on the fourth day, it is a quartan fever. The quotidian and tertian types of intermittent fever are the most common, the quartan being comparatively rare.

There is also a form of malarial fever known as remittent fever, in which the temperature varies, but never gets as low as normal. This fever ranges from mild to severe, and lasts from one to two weeks.

Quinine seems to possess a specific action against the plasmodium malariae, but as its maximum effect is not obtained from four to six hours after its administration, it should be given in the quotidian type eight hours, in the tertian twelve hours, and in the quartan type fifteen to eighteen hours before the expected chill, and repeated. Ten to 15-grain doses are usually sufficient in the milder types, while in the more severe types 30 to 60 grains are often required. The quinine should be given in powder in soft capsules easily dissolved.

Quinine is not, however, the only nor the most important remedy in malarial fever. The basic cause of the trouble is an excess of water in the blood, which has provided a suitable breeding place for the plasmodium malariae, and this excess of water must be removed, so that a recurrence of the disease may be prevented, and a permanent restoration to health assured.

This excess of water is due to a deficiency of the cell-salt Natrum Sulph., and it is only by supplying this lacking salt that the condition can be overcome. Natrum Sulph. is thus the chief remedy in malarial fevers. When the trouble has continued for some time, the nervous system is frequently affected by a lack of Kali Phos., and this salt is also needed. The fever, too, always calls for Ferrum Phos.

So we find that among the inorganic salts in the human economy, sodium sulphate works with water, keeps bile and pancreatic juice at normal consistency, regulates the supply of water in intercellular fluid, and eliminates the excess of water from the blood.

CHARACTERISTIC INDICATIONS

MENTAL SYMPTOMS.—Irritation due to biliousness; tendency to suicide, with wildness and irritability, from an excessive secretion of bile. *Feels discouraged* and *despondent;* worse in the morning and in damp weather.

HEAD.—Headache on top of head; very severe, burning and throbbing (*note color of tongue*). Sick headache, with bitter taste in the mouth, vomiting of bile or bilious diarrhea. *Headache, with dizziness* or drowsiness; often the precursor of jaundice. Vertigo, giddiness from excessive secretion of bile; *tongue* has a *dirty, greenish-gray or greenish-brown coating* at the back part; bitter taste in the mouth. Violent pains at base of brain. Spinal meningitis, with determination of blood to head; spasmodic symptoms and delirium (*Ferrum Phos., Magnes. Phos.*).

EYES.—Yellowness of the conjunctiva. *Burning of the edges of the lids,* with lachrymation. Chronic conjunctivitis, with large blister-like granulations on the lids.

EARS.—Earache, lightning-like pain through the ears; worse in damp weather.

NOSE.—Ozena syphilitica, worse in damp, wet weather. Nasal catarrh. Dryness and burning in the nose. Pus changes to green when exposed to light.

FACE.—Yellow, sallow or jaundiced face, due to biliousness. (*Note appearance of tongue.*) *Erysipelas* of the fact, *smooth, red, shiny swelling* (for the fever, *Ferrum Phos.*).

MOUTH.—Bad taste in the mouth, always full of slime, thick and tenacious, greenish-white. Bitter taste in mouth. Constant hawking of foul, slimy mucus from the trachea, esophagus and stomach.

TONGUE.—*Dirty, greenish-gray or greenish-brown coating on the root of the tongue,* with slime. Bitter taste in the mouth.

THROAT.—When *vomiting* of *green water occurs in diphtheria,* this remedy should be given intercurrently with the chief remedy (*Kali Mur.*). *Throat sore,* with *feeling of a lump when swallowing.* Catarrh of the pharynx and throat, with thick, tenacious, grayish mucus, if tongue symptoms correspond.

GASTRIC SYMPTOMS.—Biliousness, caused from the liver secreting an excess of bile. The tongue should be noted carefully; a greenish-gray or greenish-brown coating indicates an excess of bile, while a white or gray coating denotes a deficiency of bile, and requires *Kali Mur. Bitter taste in mouth. Mouth full of slime.* Bilious colic, with bitter taste in mouth (*see tongue symptoms*). Lead colic (very frequent doses and low triturations). Vomiting of bile, with bitter taste, dizziness and headache. Vomiting of greenish water, tasting bitter. Jaundice from vexation, oversecretion of bile, with coated tongue, bilious, green evacuations, yellow eyeballs or sallow skin. Sick headache from gastric derangement (*note tongue*). Cutting pains in region of liver. *Enlargement of the liver;* worse lying on the left side. Irritable liver (*Kali Phos.*). Pain in left hypochondriac region, frequently accompanied by a cough.

Abdomen and Stool.—*Diarrhea,* with *dark, greenish, bilious stools,* or vomiting of bile (*note coating of tongue*). Loose morning stool; worse in cold, wet weather. Heat in the lower bowels and rectum, accompanied by bilious evacuations. Flatulent colic, irritable liver, frequently after a mental strain (*Kali Phos.*). Liver sensitive, sore to touch, with sharp, shooting pains. Congestion of liver (*Ferrum Phos.*). Cutting pains in abdomen (*Magnes. Phos., Ferrum Phos.*). Typhlitis, to aid in reducing the inflammation (in alternation with *Ferrum Phos., the chief remedy*). Looseness of bowels in old people. *All symptoms worse during,* or after a spell of, *wet weather.*

Urinary Organs.—*Diabetes, chief remedy,* for the sugar and general waste from the kidneys. Lithic *deposit* in the urine; *looks like brick-dust and clings to the sides of the vessel.* Gravel, with gouty symptoms, in bilious persons. *Excessive secretion of urine,* when diabetic. Sandy deposit in the urine. (*Note color of back part of the tongue.*)

Male Sexual Organs.—Hydrocele (*Calc. Phos.*). Preputial edema (*Natr. Mur.,* in alternation). Chronic syphilis, when corresponding symptoms are present. Condyloma, of syphilitic origin, internally and externally. Chronic gonorrhea, with characteristic discharge.

Female Sexual Organs.—*Profuse menses, with morning diarrhea,* or colic and constipation. Note color of tongue and other characteristic symptoms.

Pregnancy.—Morning sickness, with vomiting of bilious fluids, bitter taste in the mouth.

Respiratory Organs.—Asthma, violent attacks, with greenish, purulent expectoration; very copious. *Asthma, worse in damp, wet weather,* with loose evacuations in the morning. Bronchial catarrh, harsh breathing. All symptoms worse in damp, rainy weather. Observe coating on root of tongue and color of expectoration.

CIRCULATORY ORGANS.—Vertigo, with giddiness; *feeling of pressure and uneasiness in region of heart.*

BACK AND EXTREMITIES.—Rheumatism, for the bilious symptoms, when present; intercurrently or in alternation with the chief remedy. Gout, acute or chronic cases (*Ferrum Phos.*). *Spinal meningitis,* for the drawing back of the neck, spasm in the back, and violent determination of blood to the head; violent pains in neck and back of head. Arthritis, acute; patient should abstain from intoxicating liquors.

NERVOUS SYMPTOMS.—Lassitude; tired and weary feelings, when accompanied by bilious symptoms, jaundiced skin, yellow eyeballs, etc. *Hands and feet twitch during sleep.*

SKIN.—All diseases of the skin, with exudation of yellowish water; generally accompanied by other bilious symptoms. Inflammations of the skin, with yellow, watery exudation. Skin affections, with vesicular eruptions containing yellowish water; *moist, yellowish scales on the skin,* with bilious symptoms. Chafed skin of infants (*Natr. Mur., Natr. Phos.*). Pemphigus, watery vesicles all over the body containing yellowish, watery secretions. Eczema, with watery exudations and bilious symptoms. Erysipelas ("rose"), smooth, red, shiny, tingling, or painful swelling of the skin (alternate with *Ferrum Phos.; note condition of tongue*). Fistulous abscess of long standing; discharging watery pus, surrounded by a broad, bluish border.

TISSUES.—Dropsy invading the areolar tissues of the body. Infiltration. Yellowish, watery secretions from any tissue. Smooth, edematous swellings. *Consumption,* when the *expectoration* is *yellow, watery and green;* also when corresponding bilious symptoms exist.

FEBRILE CONDITIONS.—*Intermittent fever* (*ague*); this is the *chief remedy* in all its stages. Vomiting of bile, also brown or black fluids, with bitter taste. Bilious fever. Yellow fever, if it assumes the severe, bilious, remittent fever form, with greenish-yellow, brown or black vomit (alternate *Ferrum Phos.*, for the fever). *Observe* carefully the *characteristic* dirty, greenish-gray or greenish-brown *coating of the tongue* in all febrile conditions.

Sleep.—Drowsiness and weariness, with bilious symptoms, frequently preceding attacks of jaundice. (*Note coating of tongue.*) Dull, sleepy and stupid in the morning; better in the evening. Much dreaming, with *heavy, anxious dreams.* Attacks of "nightmare," with bilious symptoms (*Natr. Mur., Kali Phos.*).

Modalities.—All symptoms are worse in the morning and in damp, rainy weather; feels better in dry, warm atmosphere. Complaints from living in damp buildings, basements, etc., or from eating water-plants, fish, etc. *Symptoms aggravated by* the use of *water* in any form. Conditions which tend to increase the water in the system, such as living in low, marshy places, "ague districts" will cause a molecular disturbance of *Natr. Sulph.*

SILICEA

Proper Name.—Silicic Oxide.

Synonyms.—Silica, Silicea Terra. Silex. Acidum Silicium.

Formula.—SiO_2.

Common Names.—Pure Flint, Silicious Earth.

Preparation.—The classic method of preparation is as follows: "Take half an ounce of mountain crystal and expose it several times to a red heat, or take pure white sand and wash it with distilled vinegar; when washed mix it with two ounces of powdered natrum, melt the whole in an iron crucible until effervescence has ceased, and the liquefied mass looks clear and smooth, which is then to be poured upon a marble plate. The limpid glass which is thus obtained is to be pulverized while warm, and to be filled in a vial, adding four times its own weight of distilled water (the vial being exactly filled to a level and a stopper being put in immediately). This mixture forms a solution which remains always clear; but upon pouring it into an open vial, which is loosely covered with paper, it becomes decomposed, and the snow-white silica separates from the natrum and falls to the bottom of the vial."

The following process, which does not differ in any essential particular from the above is generally adopted: Take of silica, in powder, one part; dried carbonate of sodium, four parts. Fuse the four parts of dry sodium carbonate in a clay crucible, and gradually add to the fused mass the powdered silica; at each addition an escape of carbonic oxide takes place, so that a roomy crucible should be used. When the carbonic oxide ceases to come off, pour the fused mass upon a clean marble slab, and while slightly warm break it in a mortar into small pieces and transfer to a wide-mouthed bottle, adding sufficient distilled water to dissolve it; the stopper is to be capped with wet bladder. The following day the solution may be diluted and rapidly filtered through cotton wool to remove particles of dirt, etc.; then add to the filtered liquid hydrochloric acid gradually in small quantities. The hydrated silica is precipitated in the form of a bulky gelatinous white precipitate, which is collected and washed with distilled water upon a square frame filter. The washing must be continued until the filtrate is without taste and no longer precipitates solutions of nitrate of silver. The precipitate, when thoroughly washed, may be advantageously dried upon a porcelain water bath, when it shrinks, to an impalpable powder, which has neither taste nor smell.

THE chemical action or function of silica as a worker in the human organism has never been clearly explained. Writers on Biochemistry have heretofore been content to state its general action, and give it its place in the repertories, according to certain symptoms. It is a constituent of common quartz, and found in the hair, nails, skin, periosteum, neurilemma (nerve sheath), and a trace in the bone tissue. This salt is indicated in all suppurative processes until the infiltrated parts have fully discharged the heteroplasm or accumulation of decaying organic matter that may have arrived at a given point during nature's effort to eliminate it from the system. In the first stage of any swelling, Ferrum Phos. and Kali Mur. should be given (for reasons explained in biochemic pathology), but should these salts fail to abort the process, Silicea should at once be employed. When silica is present in proper quantities, the process of suppuration is carried on in a normal manner. When a deficiency of silica occurs, suppuration is retarded; the greater the deficiency, the greater and more stubborn and painful the swelling where the matter is attempting to escape, or, more correctly speaking, the point at which nature attempts to cast it off.

CHARACTERISTIC INDICATIONS

MENTAL SYMPTOMS.—*Patient* rather *despondent* and *disgusted with life.* Mental abstraction; difficulty of thought.

HEAD.—Headache, when small lumps or nodules, about the size of a pea, appear on the scalp. *Scalp sensitive and sore to touch.* Painful pustules, suppurating wounds, with characteristic thick, yellow discharge of pus. Eruptions and nodules on the scalp; falling out of hair (*Kali Sulph.*). *Sweat on head of children,* also *Calc. Phos.*

EYES.—Stye on the eyelid; internally and externally, to promote painless discharge of pus (if there is much inflammation, alternate *Ferrum Phos.*). Disease of the lachrymal apparatus. Lachrymal fistula. Inflammations of the eye, with discharge of thick, yellow matter. Injuries of the eye, neglected cases, with subsequent suppuration of thick, yellow matter. Boils and indurations around eyelid. *Cataract after suppressed foot-sweats or eruptions.*

EARS.—Inflammatory swelling of external meatus. Dullness of hearing, with swelling and *catarrh of the eustachian tubes* and tympanic cavity. Boils and cystic tumors around the ear. Suppurative otitis, when the discharge is thick, yellow matter. Otorrhea, with caries of the mastoid process. Daily injections of the remedy—in water.

NOSE.—Catarrh of head, with characteristic discharge of fetid, thick, yellow matter. *Ozena,* when the affection is seated in the periosteum or in the submucous connective tissues; *fetid, offensive discharge.* Nose sore, with little boils around edges of nostrils; very itchy. Caries of the nasal bones, with very offensive discharge (*Kali Phos.*). Dryness of the nostrils, with formation of scales and sores. Tip of nose red; itching of the tip of the nose.

FACE.—Faceache, with small lumps or nodules on the face and scalp. Lupus, with discharge of thick matter. *Eruptions on the face,* from any cause, with discharge indicative of this remedy. Caries and necrosis of the bones of the jaw. Induration of cellular tissues, after boils, etc.

MOUTH.—Suppurations of the glands of the mouth, with characteristic discharges.

TEETH.—Toothache, very violent, at night, when heat nor cold gives relief, caused by chilling of the feet. *Toothache caused by sudden chilling of the feet when damp with perspiration.* Gum-boils on the jaw. Toothache, with ulceration of the tooth; pain deep-seated in the periosteum.

TONGUE.—Hardening of the tongue. Ulcers on the tongue.

THROAT.—Ulcerations of the throat, with thick, yellow, mattery discharges. *Tonsilitis,* after pus has begun to form, to produce suppuration; if it will not heal and infiltration has ceased, *Calc. Sulph.* is the remedy. Goitre.

Gastric Symptoms.—Induration of the pylorus. *Chronic dyspepsia,* with *acid eructations,* with heartburn and chilliness (*Natr. Phos., Calc. Phos.*). Child vomits as soon as it nurses; not sour (*Ferr. Phos., Calc. Phos.*).

Abdomen and Stool.—Abscess of the liver, with induration. *Sweating of the head in children,* with swollen abdomen and fetid, very offensive stools. Very painful piles, with discharges of thick, yellow matter. Fistula in ano, etc., with above symptoms.

Urinary Organs.—Suppurations of the kidneys, with urine loaded with pus and mucus. After febrile diseases, with the above discharges in the urine.

Male Sexual Organs.—Chronic syphilis, with suppurations and hardening of the tissues. Prostatitis, when suppuration has commenced. Hydrocele. Chronic gonorrhea, with thick, yellow, mattery discharges. *Itching of the scrotum, with much sweat.*

Female Sexual Organs.—*Menses,* when *associated with fetid sweating of the feet;* constipation; icy coldness all over the body. *Leucorrhea,* with characteristic discharge. *Metrorrhagia from standing in cold water.* Abscess of the labia, with tendency to fistulous openings. Burning and itching of pudenda.

Pregnancy.—Mastitis (*gathered breast*), when suppurating, to control the formation of pus (*Kali Mur. in first stage*). Hard lumps in the breast, threatening suppuration (*Kali Mur.*). *Fistulous ulcers of the breast,* with thick, yellow discharge.

Respiratory Organs.—Inflammations of the respiratory tract, when tissue destruction has gone to that stage in which there is a copious expectoration of thick, yellow or greenish-yellow pus, accompanied with hectic fever, *profuse night-*

sweats and great debility (*Calc. Phos., Natr. Mur.*). Consumption, with the above symptoms. Abscess of the lungs, to promote suppuration and heal the ulcers, after suppuration has begun; sputa abundant, thick and pus-like. Pneumonia, bronchitis, etc., suppurative stage (*Calc. Sulph.*).

BACK AND EXTREMITIES.—Neglected injuries, when festering or threatening to suppurate. Deepseated wounds of the extremities, when discharging thick, yellow matter. *Hip-joint disease, to abort* or control *suppuration* and heal the parts. Whitlow (*felon*), to assist formation of pus and control suppuration, also to stimulate the growth of new nails (local application of the same). Carbuncles (after *Kali Mur.*), to mature the tumor and discharge matter. *Fetid perspiration of the feet,* very offensive smell. Caries of the bone, with fistulous openings; discharging pus; if bony fragments, alternate *Calc. Fluor.* Psoas abscess, Pott's disease.

NERVOUS SYMPTOMS.—Obstinate neuralgia, occurring at night, when neither heat nor cold gives relief. Epilepsy and *spasms occurring at night,* or from slight provocation; very obstinate cases (*Magnes. Phos., Calc. Phos., Kali Mur.*).

SKIN.—Inflammation of, or injuries to, the skin, at that stage when thick, yellow pus is being discharged. *Tendency to boils* in any part of the body, especially *in the spring-time.* Carbuncles, boils, ulcers, felons, etc., if deepseated and discharging thick, heavy, yellow pus. Skin heals slowly and suppurates easily after injuries. Ulcers around nails, with unhealthy-looking skin. Scrofulous eruptions. Pustules on face and neck; extremely painful. Leprosy, for the nasal ulceration, nodes and coppery spots.

TISSUES.—Abscess, easily bleeding after matter has begun to form, chief remedy, to promote the discharge of pus (*Kali Mur.,* before matter forms). Swellings of the glands (if *Kali Mur.* does not abort them and matter has formed). *Suppurating glands, with thick, yellow, offensive discharge* of matter. Scrofulous, enlarged glands. Neglected cases of injury, with suppuration. Ulceration and caries of bone. Malignant, gangrenous inflammations (*Kali Phos.*).

FEBRILE CONDITIONS.—*Copious night-sweats, with prostration* in phthisis, or when no other disease is apparent. *Sweat about the head in children.* Hectic fever, with burning in soles of feet. *Offensive sweat of feet and armpits.* Fever during suppurative processes.

SLEEP.—Sleeplessness from orgasm of blood; *wakefulness in old people,* with phthisis. *Jerking of limbs during sleep.*

MODALITIES.—Symptoms are always worse at night. Better by heat and in warm room. *Worse from chilling of the feet.* Worse in open air.

PART III.

THERAPEUTICAL APPLICATION

OF THE

Twelve Biochemic Remedies

PART III.

THERAPEUTICAL APPLICATION

OF THE

Twelve Biochemic Remedies

ABSCESS

ETIOLOGY

A DEFICIENCY in any one of the inorganic salts in the blood, is immediately and necessarily followed by an excess of organic matter in the tissues, the nature of this excess varying in accordance with the particular salt which is lacking, and with which it has a natural tendency to unite.

As an example, let us consider Kali Mur. (potassium chloride): the molecules of this inorganic salt have an affinity for and unite with certain organic fibrin-plastic substances (albuminoids) to form fibrin, which is then deposited in the various parts of the body where it performs its functions.

A scarcity of the organic constituents of fibrin practically never exists, as its components, together with other organic matter, oil, sugar and albumen, are always being absorbed by the system from the food.

This is not true, however, of the inorganic salts, which are frequently omitted in the modern methods of preparing foods, and thus not supplied to the system in a sufficient quantity. Indigestion and poor assimilation also play their part here.

Should, therefore, a deficiency arise in the inorganic salt, potassium chloride, there would naturally be a certain quantity of organic fibrin-plastic substance in excess in the blood, depending in amount upon the lacking potassium chloride.

This non-functional organic substance is practically a foreign matter in the system, and an attempt is made to expel it through the glands and skin. If a considerable quantity accumulates at any one spot, an abscess results. In case the abscess delays opening readily, a few doses of Silicea should be administered, which will frequently assist the abscess in forcing its way to the surface, and thus avoid the necessity of operative interference.

Furthermore, of course, Kali Mur. must also be prescribed, so that by uniting with the free organic fibrin-plastic substances in the blood it may cut short the continuation of the abscess present, and prevent the formation of new ones.

BIOCHEMIC TREATMENT

Ferrum Phos.—*In* the *first* or *inflammatory stage of abscess, boils, carbuncles or felons,* for the heat, pain, congestion and fever; given early, in alternation with *Kali Mur.,* this remedy will often abort suppuration.

Kali Mur.—*In* the *second stage of abscess, boils,* etc., when there is swelling, but no pus formation, *Kali Mur.* is indicated. If given steadily, in alternation with *Ferrum Phos.,* very often the swelling will disappear and no pus will form. The remedy should also be used locally on lint. Abscess of the breast, very much swollen, but no pus formation; rub it with vaseline or, preferably, a lotion of *Kali Mur.* on lint.

Silicea.—After the use of *Kali Mur.,* and when the pus formation has commenced, *Silicea* is the indicated remedy; it greatly assists suppuration, causes the abscess to ripen and often break without surgical interference. *After the tumor has broken, Silicea* should be used internally and externally, as long as infiltration remains. In felons it is indispensable to control the formation of pus and promote the growth of new nails, which are largely composed of this salt, if they have been affected.

Calc. Sulph.—After the use of *Silicea,* and when infiltration has disappeared, should the *discharges* still *continue* until the condition of indolent ulcer is produced, *Calc. Sulph.* is indicated and should be used until the wounds heal. While the lack of *Calc. Sulph.* gives symptoms somewhat resembling those caused by a lack of *Silicea* in suppurative processes, there remains the following distinguishing feature: *Silicea,* by promoting the formation of pus, ripens the abscess; while *Calc. Sulph.,* by restraining suppuration, causes the wound to heal. It is useful in boils, felons, gathered breasts, etc., under the above conditions. Owing to its power of restraining the discharge of pus, it will often abort suppuration, if given in the early stage, before pus has formed; but when this is not possible, *Silicea* must be used to bring it to the surface.

Calc. Fluor.—*When the suppurative process affects the bone,* causing it to throw off splinters. *Suppurating wounds, with hard, callous edges.* Pelvic abscess, proceeding from caries of the bone.

Natr. Sulph.—*Fistulous abscess of long standing,* especially of the lower limbs, when the *discharge* is *watery pus,* and the wound is *surrounded by a dark, bluish border.*

Kali Phos.—When the suppurative process becomes unhealthy. Pus is bloody, ichorous, offensive and dirty-looking. *In gathered breasts, with discharge of foul, dirty matter.*

CLINICAL CASES

Calc. Sulph. to abort Suppurations:

Carrie A., æt. 16, came to me with a severe pain in the middle left ear, with all the symptoms of a gathering. Reasoning from the fact that *Calc. Sulph. cures* suppurations, I concluded to test its power to abort suppurative processes before suppuration had set in, so gave her *Calc. Sulph.,* two small powders each day. On the second day she reported her ear well, and has had no symptoms since.

Silicea in Boils:

In August, a young man, who had suffered from sciatica years ago, and had been in the habit of having subcutaneous injections of morphia, developed a boil on the gluteal muscle. This discharged freely and would not heal. When, at last, it seemed to be healed and was comparatively well, the patient took cold. Suppuration began again, and at this time the discharge was excessive. His mother became alarmed, as he was very weak and had no appetite. His sleep was disturbed and he felt a constant thirst. I prescribed *Silicea*—a dose every morning on an empty stomach. After one week the mother was able to furnish favorable report: "The discharge of matter has been reduced so much that at one time it seemed gone altogether. The great thirst has left him, and his appetite has returned; his sleep is sound, and the shivery, chilly feeling he had has completely gone." *Silicea* has here furnished a brilliant demonstration of its power over suppuration, and with its characteristic accompanying symptoms.
(Dr. Goullon, Jr.)

Calc. Sulph. in Chronic Abscess:

Helen C., age 30, had an abscess of two years' standing at lower border of axilla, right side. The discharge of pus was so great that a large roll of cotton had to be kept in place to take care of the discharge. She had consulted several doctors, and had taken much treatment resulting in no improvement. *Calc. Sulph.* made a permanent cure in six months.
(Dr. Wm. B. Deffendall, Washington, Indiana.)

Silicea in Suppurations:

Silicea has proved an excellent remedy. Within the last month I was able to cure a young lady, æt. 16; I did not see her myself. The mother came to me and told me her daughter had been suffering for the past few months from her right foot. The medical men treating her declared that the foot

must be amputated. It was fearfully swollen; the discharge of matter was excessive. Her leg was almost bent to a right angle at the knee-joint, and could absolutely not be stretched out. I advised her to give up all internal as well as external remedies, and prescribed *Silicea,* to be taken once daily. Three months later the patient came herself, walking without any assistance. The foot was almost completely healed, with only a slight discharge of matter. Then, I succeeded in a case of discharge of matter from the ear, which had been treated for a long time ineffectually, and caused the patient severe pain day and night. This case was also cured with *Silicea.*
(From Schuessler.)

ACCIDENTS

(See Mechanical Injuries.)

ADDISON'S DISEASE

Natr. Mur.—Tension and heat in the region of the kidneys; yellowish, pale color of the face; brown spots on back of hands; *excessive lassitude, relaxation of mind and body,* with *trembling of lower limbs; dimness of sight, nausea,* vomiting; pressing pains in the stomach; loss of appetite, with aversion to animal food; constipation, pain in the abdomen and hypochondria; aversion to motion or labor; *frequent yawning and stretching, with sleeplessness,* still he cannot sleep; cold extremities; vertigo, when rising up or trying to walk, with faint feeling; cross and irritable.
(Lillienthal.)

AGUE

(See Intermittent Fever.)

ALBUMINURIA

ETIOLOGY

This term is applied to urine in which is found serum albumin, serum globulin and other urinary proteids.

In most cases albuminuria indicates inflammation or congestion of the kidneys, as albumin being a colloid substance and so not diffusing readily through animal membranes, it does not pass through the blood vessels of the kidneys and renal tubules unless these structures have undergone some degenerative change, or are subjected to a pressure which they cannot withstand. It may also be due to changes in the blood itself, whereby its albuminous ingredients are altered, or the renal texture is secondarily affected.

It occasionally occurs also from contamination in the lower urinary tract by blood or pus from disease of the pelvis, ureter or bladder. The disorders most often causing albuminuria in the urine when disease of the conducting apparatus can be excluded, are chronic parenchymatous nephritis or chronic interstitial nephritis, or possibly a subacute nephritis complicating one of the acute infectious diseases.

As a general rule, the quantity of albumin is in direct ratio to the severity of the renal lesion.

Congestion of the kidneys due to cardiac failure frequently causes albuminuria. It may also develop after severe exercise. as in soldiers after long marches, or athletes after severe exercise. The ingestion of excessive quantities of albumin in food will also cause temporary albuminuria in some persons.

In detecting albuminuria several different tests may be employed. The simplest is the heat test, in which a test-tube is two-thirds filled with urine, which if cloudy should be filtered and if alkaline acidified, and the upper part of it is held over a lighted alcohol lamp so that the fluid in this part of the tube soon boils. If albumin is present the upper part of the urine becomes clouded from coagulated albumin, but the portion below remains clear until the coagulated albumin is precipitated. Some cloudiness of the fluid may develop if earthy phosphates are present, but the addition of a few drops of nitric acid disperses the cloud if due to phosphates, but not if it is due to albumin.

Another somewhat less accurate method consists in placing one-half to one drachm of nitric acid in a test-tube, and allowing an equal quantity of urine to trickle down the side of the tube so that it overlies the acid. If albumin is present a layer of albumin will appear at the point of junction of the two fluids.

A delicate test may be made by the potassium ferrocyanide method. To a test-tube half full of urine there should be added 5 or 6 c.c. of a freshly prepared solution of potassium ferrocyanide of the strength of one in twenty, adding 10 to 15 drops of acetic acid. The tube should then be shaken when, if albumin is present, tiny flocculi may be seen floating in the liquid, which settle to the bottom of the test-tube when it is placed at rest.

If the specimen of urine is very alkaline, an extra quantity of acid solution should be added. If cloudiness be produced, the urine must be heated. If the reaction is due to albumin the precipitate remains undissolved.

In an emergency the urine may be acidified with vinegar, boiled in a spoon or cup, and poured into a glass for inspection.

Physiological albuminuria may occasionally occur, but it is not common.

The fact that albumin is found in the urine is evidence of the lack of the cell salt Calc. Phos. in the system, as this salt has the property of uniting with albumin. Occasionally, also, there will be a lack of Natr. Phos., which has been called on by the system to make up for the missing Calc. Phos., while if the lining of the kidneys or bladder has been affected, Kali Mur. may be called for. If the trouble has extended to the nervous system, Kali Phos. should be given.

BIOCHEMIC TREATMENT

Calc. Phos.—Urine highly colored. Albumin in the urine. Increase in the quantity of urine.

Natr. Phos.—Frequent urination, with inability to retain urine. Symptoms of overacidity of system.

Kali Mur.—Mucus in the urine. Urine dark colored.

Kali Phos.—Frequent urination with excessive secretion of urine from nervous weakness. Paralysis of the muscles, with inability to retain the urine.

CLINICAL CASES

Complete Cure in Case of Albuminuria:

Mrs. L. G., aged 23. The first test showed 12 per cent. albumen. She had been under the care of another physician for three weeks, and showed no improvement. I put her on *Calc. Phos., Kali Mur.*, of each three doses a day, and an occasional dose of *Kali Phos.* for the nerves. At the second test, ten days later, she gave only 3 per cent. albumen. In two weeks she was entirely cured.

(Dr. W. Whisler, Tingley, Iowa.)

AMENORRHEA

Calc. Phos.—This remedy is indicated especially in anemic conditions.

Kali Phos.—Retention or delay of the monthly flow, with *depression of spirits, lassitude* and *general nervous debility.*

Kali Sulph.—Menses too late or scanty, with fullness and weight in abdomen; *note color of tongue.*

Kali Mur.—Lymphatic constitutions; *white coated tongue;* inactivity of the glandular system.

CLINICAL CASES

Kali Phos., Calc. Phos., in Menstrual Irregularities:

Miss Anna W., æt. 20, consulted me, in company with her mother, regarding menstrual irregularities, with either an en-

tire absence of the menstruation, or else it was very scant and delayed almost every month. She was of a nervous temperament, blonde, pale, waxy skin, irritable, easily exhausted, headache, sleepy during day; slight edema of lower limbs and feet; dyspnea. Nervous, fidgety, at times must be held; depressed in spirits; desires to avoid company, especially the opposite sex. DIAGNOSIS: Amenorrhea, with history of chorea. *Calc. Phos., Kali Phos.,* every night and morning a powder. Her history revealed the non-appearance of the menstrual flow till her eighteenth year, but very scant since then. Has had mild attacks of hysteria in past two years. Has taken the medicine now for about six weeks, with marked improvement, the last period being at the proper time, and more normal than before, while there has been a cessation in the severity of the other symptoms.
(C. R. Vogel, M. D.)

Kali Sulph. in Amenorrhea:

Mrs. V., æt. 23; widow, with fifteen-months-old child, nursing. Since its tenth month menses regular, but weaned child at fourteen months; missed menses and fourteen days passed. *Kali Sulph.,* tablets, one every two hours, taken over a period of hardly two days, re-established menses, and with little or no pain, where formerly quite a dysmenorrhea.
(O. D. Whittier, M. D.)

Kali Sulph. in Amenorrhea (non-occurrence):

Miss S., æt. 19; plethoric habits; a foreigner. *Kali Sulph.,* tablets, one every two hours, established menses inside of three days. Had tried other remedies without success.
(O. D. Whittier, M. D.)

ANEMIA

ETIOLOGY

Anemia may be either a reduction in the quantity or the quality of the blood, or even both. It is an underlying factor in many acute and chronic diseases, and its elimination is absolutely necessary before a complete restoration of health can be expected. An anemic condition denotes an initial lack of calcium phosphate and iron phosphate in the system, possibly followed by a resultant lack of other cell salts.

The lack of calcium phosphate is directly responsible for the deficiency in red blood cells, as it enters largely into the formation of bone, in the marrow of which the red blood cells are created.

A lack of iron phosphate shows immediately in a deficiency of hemoglobin. By giving the needed cell salts the blood can be quickly brought up again to its normal amount and quality.

BIOCHEMIC TREATMENT

Calc. Phos.—This remedy supplies new blood-cells. Face pale or chlorotic, greenish-white. *Anemia, where nutrition is defective.* Excess of white corpuscles in the blood (*Leucemia*), *after wasting or exhausting diseases,* chief remedy

Ferrum Phos.—After the new blood cells have been supplied by *Calc. Phos.,* if there still appears to be a deficiency of hemoglobin, *Ferrum Phos.* should be prescribed, as it is a vital constituent of this component of the blood, and without it the exchange of oxygen and carbonic acid between the lungs and tissues could not be carried on.

Iron has long been the accepted remedy in anemia, but one of the great objections to most iron preparations is that they are not properly assimilated, but simply pass through the digestive system, and are excreted from the body unused. Another drawback is that they attack the teeth, causing a black, ugly discoloration. Furthermore, they are practically all nauseous and disagreeable in taste, and it is very difficult to induce patients to continue their use for the requisite amount of time.

Ferr. Phos. possesses none of these drawbacks. It is quickly and easily assimilated by the blood, does not discolor the teeth, is practically tasteless, and an increase in the proportion of hemoglobin is shown almost invariably soon after its prescription in anemia.

Natr. Mur.—In chlorotic conditions, where the *blood is thin and watery, not coagulating. Chlorosis in young girls at puberty,* when the menses do not appear or are irregular. Skin has a dead, dirty look; characteristic tongue, indicating this salt; constipation combined with mental depression.

Kali Phos.—Anemia from long-continued mental strains, causing depression of the mind. *Spinal anemia, after exhausting diseases.* Cerebral anemia.

Kali Mur.—When eczema, eruptions of the skin, etc., exist in connection with anemia, this remedy should be given in alternation or intercurrently with the chief remedy.

Natr. Sulph.—Hydremia, sycosis, hydrogenoid constitution of the body, depending upon dampness of weather or dwelling in damp houses; sycosis and hydremia.

Natr. Phos.—*Anemia,* accompanied *with indigestion acid risings,* etc., to aid in the proper assimilation of the food; intercurrently with *Calc. Phos.*

Silicea.—*Anemia in infants,* when improperly nourished; thin, delicate and puny; intercurrently with other remedies indicated.

CLINICAL CASES

Calc. Phos. in Anemia of school-girls:

Young lady, æt. 17, became anemic and chlorotic, after long continuance at school, becoming so debilitated that she could attend no longer; had no appetite and desired only to lie about the house, having no ambition to go anywhere or do anything. Her study made her head ache and she had to give it up entirely; her menses were irregular; absent for months, then a flow varying in quantity. I gave her *Calc. Phos.*, as principal remedy, giving also, at times, *Ferrum Phos.* as well. After a few months she became well enough to resume her studies,

and could walk anywhere she desired to go, and her color improved.
(C. T. M.)

Calc. Phos. and Ferrum Phos. in Anemia from menstrual irregularities:

Miss Nellie C., æt. 15; anemia; face very pale and waxlike; dull and listless; poor appetite; menstruation irregular and scanty. *Calc. Phos., Ferrum Phos.* for the menstrual troubles, made a permanent cure in six weeks.
(J. B. Chapman.)

ANEURISM

ETIOLOGY

Aneurism is the term used for the localized dilatation of an artery. It may be due to a stretching of the arterial wall or to a rupture of one or more coats of the blood vessel. In either case the basic cause is a relaxation of elastic fibres, due to a deficiency in Calcarea Fluor., and a consequent weakening of the wall of the artery.

BIOCHEMIC TREATMENT

Ferrum Phos.—To establish normal circulation and *to remove* those *complications arising from excessive action of the heart.* It should be resorted to early, and may be given in alternation with *Calc. Fluor.*

Calc. Fluor.—*Chief remedy for aneurism;* will keep it in check, if taken at an early stage, providing iodide of potassium has not been used. Give in alternation with *Ferrum Phos.*

ANGINA PECTORIS

BIOCHEMIC TREATMENT

Magnes. Phos.—For the *neuralgic spasms* and *sharp pains.* It will act best in hot water, and in very frequent doses.

Kali Phos.—In asthenic conditions, weak or *intermittent action of the heart;* tendency to fainting, etc.; alternate with *Magnes. Phos.,* the chief remedy.

Ferrum Phos.—With rush of blood to the head, flushed face, burning heat, etc., in alternation with *Magnes. Phos.*

CLINICAL CASES

Magnes. Phos.:

Mrs. W., æt. 25; severe pains in left breast; cutting, stabbing pains. Pulse almost imperceptible, and her friends thought her dying. *Magnes. Phos.,* in hot water, for the pain and spasmodic symptoms, alternated with *Kali Phos.*, for the feeble action of the heart. The pulse returned to normal condition, and the pains quickly ceased. Nothing could have acted more satisfactorily.
(J. B. Chapman.)

APHONIA

(See Hoarseness and Throat.)

ETIOLOGY

Aphonia, or loss of voice, usually follows overexertion in speaking, or exposure to cold. A deficiency of *Kali Mur.* allows an oversecretion of mucus in the throat, which irritates and causes inflammation of the vocal cords. A deficiency of *Ferrum Phos.* will allow this inflammation to continue, and it will generally prove necessary to prescribe *Ferrum Phos.* and *Kali Mur.* in alternation in order to overcome the condition completely.

BIOCHEMIC TREATMENT

Ferrum Phos.—Painful aphonia of singers or speakers, caused by overexertion of voice, from draughts, cold and wet. Aphonia coming on in the evening. Frequent scraping of the throat.

Kali Mur.—Loss of voice, hoarseness, and huskiness from cold. If obstinate and not yielding to this remedy, alternate with *Kali Sulph.*

CLINICAL CASES

Ferrum Phos. in Aphonia resulting from dampness:

Mr. C., æt. 52, a minister, contracted laryngeal troubles through sleeping in a damp room. Was cured in a short time by the use of *Ferrum Phos.*, ten grains once a day. Speakers and singers with accumulation of phlegm in the larynx, with scraping of the throat, have been generally benefited by the use of the above.

APHTHAE, THRUSH

(See Mouth, Diseases of.)

BIOCHEMIC TREATMENT

Kali Mur.—Aphthae, thrush, which occurs in the mouth of little children or nursing mothers.

Natr. Mur.—Aphthae, with profuse flow of saliva; salivation.

APOPLEXY

(See Hemorrhage.)

ETIOLOGY

Apoplexy, when caused by hemorrhage, cannot be materially benefited by medicinal treatment. If nature does not form a clot to plug the bleeding vessel, the hemorrhage must continue until it has done so much damage that death is inevitable unless the vessel is on the surface or in the meninges, when surgical relief should be given. Again, the pressure with which the blood escapes into the soft textures of the brain is so great that if the leak is of any size the mechanical injury to the cerebral tissues must be very great, and for this reason the organ is permanently disabled.

If the cause is an embolus or thrombus, treatment is equally unavailing, as acute softening of the brain will develop. If a tumor or abscess is the causative factor, there is hope for a partial return to normal conditions; never with a perfect use of the affected parts, however, and often with contractures.

APPETITE

(See Gastric Derangements.)

ARTHRITIS

(See Rheumatism.)

BIOCHEMIC TREATMENT

Ferrum Phos.—For an *acute attack Ferrum Phos.* is the *first remedy,* for the fever, heat, congestion and pain. Very painful joints, worse on movement. Give frequent doses at first, but as the febrile symptoms disappear, intercurrently with the remedy indicated; also local applications.

Natr. Sulph.—Should be given in alternation with *Ferrum Phos.* in acute cases, but in *chronic cases* it alone will suffice. Gout in the feet, acute and chronic. *Arthritis, gout, brought on from high, rich living—chief remedy for the chronic stage,* especially if there be bilious symptoms present. Note also the color of the tongue.

Natr. Phos.—According to Dr. M. D. Walker, of Scotland, *Natr. Phos.* is indicated in all cases of *rheumatism of the joints,* especially in those cases where there is an acid diathesis, shown by acid taste and *golden-yellow coating at the root of the tongue.*

ASCITES

(See Dropsy.)

ASTHMA

ETIOLOGY

A deficiency in certain salts causes certain organic matter, such as albumin and fibrin, to become waste material, which may be thrown off through the lungs, and sometimes causes reflex neuroses and spasms of the muscular tissue of the bronchial tubes. The elastic fibre in muscular tissue being deficient, allows the tubes to close, hence, the difficulty in breathing. The molecules of certain inorganic salts, by uniting with albumen, make, *i. e.*, create, elastic fibre, and thus supply the want.

BIOCHEMIC TREATMENT

Calc. Phos.—*Bronchial asthma,* intercurrently; secretion *clear and tough.* Child gets a suffocative attack on being lifted up from cradle (*Natr. Phos.*). Asthma, with thick, yellow expectoration.

Kali Phos.—*Chief remedy for the breathing,* in large and frequent doses. Nervous system depressed; nervous asthma. from the least food.

Kali Mur.—*Asthma, when gastric derangements are present,* white-coated tongue, confined bowels and sluggish action of the liver. Expectoration is thick, white, tough, mucus, hard to cough up. Alternate with *Kali Phos.,* for the breathing.

Kali Sulph.—*Bronchial asthma,* with light, yellow sputa, rather loose and easily coughed up. *Worse in warm room* or during the summer time; better in the cool air.

Natr. Mur.—*Asthma* with *characteristic expectoration of clear, frothy mucus,* watery discharges from the eyes and nose, etc. Alternate with *Kali Phos.,* for the breathing.

Magnes. Phos.—Asthma, with troublesome flatulence or constrictive sensation in the chest.

Calc. Fluor.—When the mucus coughed up consists of tiny, yellow lumps. Matter raised with much difficulty. Alternate with *Kali Phos.,* for the breathing.

Natr. Sulph.—According to the reports of Schreter, and the experience of others, *Natr. Sulph.* is an *important remedy in asthma of young people,* worse from damp weather or wet surroundings, with characteristic expectoration, coating of tongue, loose morning stools, etc.

Silicea.—*Breathing very difficult; must be in fresh air.* Possibly as a constitutional remedy, with *Natr. Sulph.*, in order to eradicate the disease. Alternate with *Kali Phos.*, for the breathing.

CLINICAL CASES

Natr. Sulph. in chronic Asthma:

Female, married, æt. 42; subject to attacks for years; expectoration greenish and remarkably copious; *Natr. Sulph.* every three hours. Improvement began after a few doses, expectoration becoming paler and less abundant; has felt better since than for years, and one noteworthy fact is that the expectoration stopped in a few doses, whereas in previous attacks it had continued for weeks, thus indicating that the *Natr. Sulph.* had gotten at the root of the evil.

(Wm. J. Guernsey, M. D.)

Natr. Sulph. in Asthma from exertion:

Mr. C. has for years had an attack of asthmatic breathing, so marked as to herald his approach at some distance, and coming on after any unusual exertion. He is a tall, strong man. with no family history of lung trouble, albeit rather narrow-chested. Examination of the lungs during a period of remission disclosed no lesion or abnormal sounds, except coarse rales along the larger bronchi. An especially severe attack, brought on by severe physical exertion, "the worst spell" he has ever had, was promptly relieved by *Natr. Sulph.*, and occasional doses since have caused the attacks to disappear almost entirely for the first time in many summers.

(Wm. E. Leonard, M. D.)

Kali Phos., Kali Mur. in Asthma:

A young gentleman, J. G., the son of a landed proprietor, had been subject to severe attacks of asthma for several years, and all the various usual remedies had failed. Shortly after commencing with the Biochemic remedies, his sister writes: "My mother wishes me to say that she provided herself with a small store of the Biochemic remedies, and my youngest brother having an attack of asthma on Saturday and yesterday, tried the *Kali Phos.* and *Mur.* with, we think, *very* great success, relief having been experienced more quickly than by any other remedy he has tried. He goes abroad with my father and mother this week, and it is comforting to think he will have such a portable and effectual remedy in case of suffering."

(From Schuessler.)

ATROPHY

(See Marasmus.)

BACKACHE

(See Pain.)

BIOCHEMIC TREATMENT

Silicea.—Spasmodic pain in the back, compelling patient to lie still. *Constant aching in center of spine.*

Ferrum Phos.—Pains in the back and loins and over kidney. Rheumatic pains, felt only on moving. Lumbago.

Calc. Fluor.—Backache simulating spinal irritation. Tired feeling and pains in the lower part of the back, with a sensation of fullness and burning pain and confined bowels. *Lumbago aggravated on beginning to move,* but improved after continuous motion.

Natr. Mur.—Pains in small of back, *relieved by lying on something hard,* with characteristic tongue, bubbles of frothy saliva. Pain after prolonged stooping, as if bruised. Weak back, worse in the morning. Spine very sensitive. Neck stiff and emaciated. Great weakness and weariness.

Magnes. Phos.—Pains in the back, of a neuralgic character. Pain in small of back and neck—heat relieves, convulsive drawing in the back.

Natr. Sulph.—Pain in the back, as if ulcerating, all night; can lie only on the right side. *Soreness up and down spine and neck.*

Natr. Phos.—Pains across loins on awakening in morning.

CLINICAL CASES

Calc. Fluor. and Natr. Mur. in Backache:

James H., æt 29, plasterer, complained of having a severe backache, lasting sometimes only in the forenoon; at other times all night; could not bear to reach above his head for any length of time while at work, as it made him feel as if his back were bruised, as if it would break. Much better on working in front of him, and by constant motion; also by lying for a short time against the edge of his scaffolding. Neck stiff from looking above head. *Calc. Fluor.* and *Natr. Mur.* were prescribed in alternation; a powder every four hours for two weeks. Began to get better after taking two or three doses, and in a few weeks was completely relieved.

(C. R. Vogel, M. D.)

BLADDER

(See Urinary Disorders.)

BOILS

(See Abscess.)

BIOCHEMIC TREATMENT

Ferrum Phos.—In first or inflammatory stage of boils, for heat, pain, congestion and fever; this remedy will often prevent suppuration.

Silicea.—When pus-formation has commenced, *Silicea* greatly assists suppuration, causes the boil to ripen and often break without surgical interference.

CLINICAL CASES

Silicea in Boils:

Here is a case of boils on the neck, treated with Silicea. Mr. E., a lawyer of this city, had been suffering for some time, and had not been relieved by lancing. He came to me. On examination I found two abscesses, molars. A new boil was forming, and his neck was too sore to do any extracting. I put him on treatment of *Silicea* for five days with great relief. The following week I extracted both molars. I gave him another course of *Silicea* and the boils have not returned. (Dr. L. O. Hope, Hutchinson, Kansas.)

BONES, DISEASES OF

ETIOLOGY

By referring to *Calc. Phos.*, it will be seen that a lack of this salt is the primary cause of all bone diseases not brought about by injury.

Caries of the bone shows quite clearly, according to Biochemistry, that while enough albumen (used as cement to build bone tissue) is present, the lime molecules are not; therefore, the true and only scientific mode of procedure is to supply the lime—just the form in which nature uses it.

Any heteroplasm or decaying organic matter that may have accumulated will be thrown off or absorbed without the necessity of bone-scraping.

BIOCHEMIC TREATMENT

Calc. Phos.—*Calc. Phos.*, owing to its predominance in the bones, becomes one of the chief remedies in affections involving this part of the system. When the *bones are weak and soft, Calc. Phos.* will give them solidity. Fractures, to aid in uniting the broken parts (also surgical aid). Bow-legs in children (also mechanical supports). Rickets, spinal curvature, etc., owing to lack of power to extract the *Calc. Phos.* from the food. Intercurrently in ulceration of bones.

Silicea.—*Silicea* is indicated in nearly all bone diseases; the *chief symptom* calling for its use is the *thick, yellow, offensive, mattery discharge* from ulcerations of the bone. Hip-joint disease. All excretions very offensive.

Calc. Fluor.—Exudations from the bone, forming hard, rough, corrugated elevations on the bone surface, require this remedy. Bruises on the bone surface, with hard, uneven lumps. *Catarrhal affections,* when the *nasal bones* are *affected,* with bad odor. Ulcerations of bone surface; spina ventosa (*Magnes. Phos.*). "This remedy is even better than *Silicea* in cases of cephalohematoma (so-called blood tumors) on the parietal bones of new-born children." (Schuessler.)

Calc. Sulph.—Ulceration of bone, with characteristic indications for this remedy.

Ferrum Phos.—In bone diseases, when the soft parts are inflamed, hot and painful. *Hip-joint disease, first remedy.* Ostitis, periostitis, with painful soft parts.

Kali Mur.—Second stage of ostitis and periostitis.

Kali Phos.—Atrophy of bones, with foul diarrhea.

Natr. Sulph.—Pain in bones, cracking of joints, knee stiff.

CLINICAL CASES

Kali Phos. and Calc. Phos. in deficient Osseous Development:

Ida P., æt. 5 years, could not walk or lift up her head; fontanel open; spasms nearly every day; did not appear any more advanced in bone material than a babe five months old. TREATMENT: *Calc. Phos., Magnes. Phos.* and *Kali Phos.* In a few months the child was so much benefited, the parents

lavished their thanks upon me; but having removed, have lost sight of the case.
(Wm. Chapman, M. D.)

Kali Phos. and Calc. Phos. in delayed Dentition:

Daisy C., æt. 18 months; was taken from the Orphans' Home; she was exceedingly small and deficient in bone material, having cut but four teeth, and could not walk a step; fontanel open; very pale and nervous. TREATMENT: *Calc. Phos.* and *Kali Phos.*, every day, was given in water. Report was given in two months after commencement of the above treatment; cut eleven teeth; fontanel closed, and could walk, having passed through her teething without the sickness usually accompanying such cases, and was so far cured that she became the remark of all who knew her.
(Wm. Chapman, M. D.)

Silicea saved her foot from Amputation:

In the case of a poor orphan girl, æt. 14, *Silicea* saved her from having her foot amputated. She had been under treatment for a long time for bone abscess. Her physician saw no alternative, as the evil only grew worse, but to make arrangements with the infirmary surgeon to have the foot taken off. This was agreed upon six days before removing her. Her friends were greatly distressed, and applied for the new remedies. *Silicea,* a dose every hour, was steadily taken, and lotion on lint externally applied. On the fifth day the ankle-bone and surrounding tissues presented such a healthy appearance that all cause for amputation was removed. She continued the treatment a short time longer, and her case was pronounced perfectly cured.
(M. D. W., from Schuessler.)

Calc. Phos. in slow union of Fracture:

Man, æt. 60, had a fracture of the shaft of the femur. It remained movable, in spite of great care; after two months. *Calc. Phos.* was given; at first every night; later, every second night. At once the fracture grew firm and was soon well.

This is certainly better than instrumental interference. Eighteen months later the same femur sustained another fracture in the lower portion. The same salt was given in like manner, as before, but from the beginning. It was well in two months. (J. C. Morgan, M. D.)

Calc. Fluor. in Osteosarcoma:

Injury of the tibia of some years' standing; a painful growth appeared on the seat of the injury. This was diagnosed as an osteosarcoma by a prominent physician, who advised an operation. *Calc. Fluor.* relieved the pain and reduced the growth.
(L. A. Bell.)

Calc. Fluor. in Osseous Growths:

Dr. C. F. Nichols reports a number of cases of osseous growths cured and benefited by *Calc. Fluor.*
(Organon.)

BOWELS

(See Diarrhoea, Dysentery, etc.)

BRAIN

(See Meningitis and Delirium.)

BIOCHEMIC TREATMENT

Kali Phos.—To restore lost nerve-power. *Brain-fag, from overwork,* with loss of appetite, depressed spirits, irritability, impatience, *loss of memory or sleeplessness.* Softening of the brain from inflammations, alternate with *Kali Mur.;* if connected with water on the brain, alternate with *Calc. Phos.* Nervous prostration.

Ferrum Phos.—*First stage of all inflammatory diseases of the brain,* meningitis, brain fever, etc., to reduce fever, heat and congestion.

Calc. Phos.—Brain-fag, with pale, emaciated countenance, coldness of the limbs, numb sensations, night-sweats, loss of virile power, etc.

Natr. Mur.—*Depressed spirits,* gloomy thoughts, looks on the dark side of everything, tearful moods, easily exhausted, etc.

Natr. Sulph.—*After injuries to the head,* mental troubles following. Intense pain in occipital region. Determination of blood to the head.

Magnes. Phos.—Diseases of the brain, when convulsive symptoms are present.

CLINICAL CASES

Kali Phos. wrought a complete cure:

E. A. S., bookkeeper for large manufacturing company, working much after night, was compelled to give up position on account of his mental faculties becoming impaired; could not sleep at night; worried over accounts till he became a physical and mental wreck. Did not want any one about him; could not eat; everything seemed to annoy; impatient with every one about him. Condition bordering on brain fever. Change of scenery, rest and *Kali Phos.,* worked a complete cure

(C. R. Vogel, M. D.)

Kali Phos. in inflammation of Brain:

The following is from an elderly gentleman, Mr. J. M., who had suffered from a prolonged attack of acute and subacute inflammation of the brain. He recovered slowly, but symptoms of softening of the brain set in. He was anxious to give the new remedies a trial. His speech was affected; he seemed to lose momentary consciousness; could not hurry, though he saw himself in great danger of being run over or stop walking when dangerously close to the quay, and could not be trusted alone. I prescribed *Kali Phos.,* and in a letter of recent date he says: "I think it is time I were again informing you that I still continue to improve; indeed, I have little to complain of, except occasionally a feeling of mental stupor, the best remedy for which I have found to be *Kali Phos.,* which you recommend to me."

(M. D. W., from Schuessler.)

BRAIN-FAG

(See Brain.)

ETIOLOGY

The condition known as brain-fag, or mental exhaustion, may be due either to a deficiency of Kali Phos., causing a breaking down of nerve cells in the brain, with a consequent impairment of its efficiency, or it may follow some systemic condition such as that brought about by a deficiency of *Calc. Phos.* with a resulting loss of albumen. In any event, the symptoms present should indicate the cell salt or salts that are lacking.

BIOCHEMIC TREATMENT

Calc. Phos.—*Nervous prostration,* with depression of spirits; profuse night-sweats; pale, wan and emaciated countenance; *loss of virile power;* habitual coldness and venous congestion of the extremities from debility, *sleeplessness* and loss of appetite; numb sensations.

Silicea.—Confusion, difficulty of fixing attention. Fatigue from mental exertion. Patient has sense of great debility and is subject to anxious moods.

Kali Phos.—To restore lost nervous energy. Covers the whole field of neurasthenia. Sleeplessness.

Natr. Mur.—With sleeplessness, gloomy forebodings, *exhaustion after talking.*

CLINICAL CASES

Kali Phos. in Brain-fag from mental strain:

Case of a man under great mental strain; engaged in literary work; nervous; worn-out; exhausted; inability to think. Prescribed *Kali Phos.;* reported almost immediate relief, with amelioration of all the adverse symptoms.
(J. B. Chapman.)

Silicea, in Brain-fag of school-girls:

Marie S., æt. 16, attending school, became very easily fatigued from study; must stop frequently during exercises, on account of tiring; compelled to rest; cannot think clearly; cannot bear to think; becomes confused during recitations, because she cannot concentrate her thoughts; wants to think, but cannot. Emaciation, accompanied by great debility. Advised taking out of school and change of scenery, and gave *Silicea,* a powder every four hours for one week. Discontinued a week, then continued for one week longer. Her mother reports her much improved in every way, and anxious to again resume her studies.
(C. R. Vogel, M. D.)

BRIGHT'S DISEASE

(See Kidneys, Affections of.)

ETIOLOGY

The Biochemic pathology of albumen in the urine is as follows:

Of the twelve inorganic salts in human blood, the phosphate of lime has an affinity for albumen. Albumen adheres to the molecules of lime phosphate, and is thus carried to the bone structure, and is used as a cement in building up the organic structure of bone, which is 53 per cent. lime.

Biochemists have clearly demonstrated the fact that when a deficiency in one or more of the cell-salts of the blood occurs, the organic matter with which those salts have been associated is thrown out of the vital circulation. If this organic matter in making its way to the outer world reaches a membrane or orifice, or clogs in connective tissue, an irritation is caused.

When the phosphate of lime molecules fall below the standard in quantity, the albumen with which they are associated is, of course, thrown out of circulation, and if this albumen reaches the outer world by the kidney route, a case of albuminuria is developed.

Of course, the remedy is Calc. Phos.

Bright's disease is simply a chronic form of albuminuria. Nature, not having a sufficient supply of calcium phosphate, draws upon the potassium phosphate and leaves the patient with nervous prostration. Then, again, there is frequently a breaking up of the proper balance of water in the tissue, caused by the drain in carrying off the lime and albumen, which is always indicated by a frothy urine, or by bubbles rising on the urine.

BIOCHEMIC TREATMENT

Calc. Phos.—Is the principal remedy to control the albumen in the system; weakness, emaciation, loss of appetite, etc.

Kali Phos.—To control the nervous symptoms, as they arise. Sleeplessness, prostration, irritation, etc.

Natr. Mur. and **Natr. Phos.**—When characteristic symptoms are present; acid conditions.

Ferrum Phos.—For all the inflammatory or febrile symptoms.

CLINICAL CASES

Calc. Phos. in Bright's Disease following Scarlatina:

I have had two cases of Bright's disease following scarlatina. Tube-casts were present. Albumen; general anasarca; heart weakness; retinitis; albuminuria. There seemed to be extensive destruction of tissue, and as the cases also presented

a profuse desquamation, I gave them *Calc. Phos.*, which speedily brought about a cure.
(C. E. Fisher, M. D.)

BRONCHITIS

ETIOLOGY

This disease is an inflammation of the bronchial tubes. It may be acute or chronic, but the former is much more serious, in its immediate results, than the latter. Bronchitis may appear as a separate disease, but it may exist with some other, such as measles, scarlatina, whooping cough, small-pox, etc. The cause is the same as that of common catarrh, which is "catching cold," thereby causing a deficiency of some of the cell-salts.

The disease is usually ushered in with chilliness, followed by fever. Tightness, constriction or oppression of the chest; hoarseness, difficulty of breathing; severe, hacking and distressing cough, dry at first but afterward becomes copious and at times streaked with blood; loss of appetite; weakness; foul tongue; anxious countenance; loud wheezing; sometimes a loud crackling or whistling sound, harsh and broken, is heard when the ear is applied to the chest. Bronchitis frequently attacks young children, but the disease, although the symptoms differ in some respects from those in the adult, can easily be recognized by the peculiar crackling sound in the chest, immediately over the bronchial tubes.

This disease, in the acute form, should be treated similarly to inflammation of the lungs. Ferrum Phos. should be given frequently in the first stage, till the fever and acute inflammation has subsided, and then not so frequently, but in alternation with the remedy indicated by the expectoration, etc.

BIOCHEMIC TREATMENT

Ferrum Phos.—In the *first stage of bronchitis, Ferrum Phos.* is the remedy for the febrile conditions, heat, fever, pain and congestion. It should be alternated with the remedy indicated by the expectoration, until all inflammatory symptoms disappear. Inflammatory irritation of the bronchial tubes; short, painful cough, without expectoration. Breathing short and oppressive.

Kali Mur.—Should be given in the *second stage* in alternation with *Ferrum Phos.*, when the *expectoration is thick, white tenacious* phlegm, and tongue has a white or grayish white coating.

Kali Sulph.—In the *third stage,* or stage of resolution, when the *expectoration* is *light-yellow, watery* and *profuse,* or greenish, slimy yellow; in alternation with *Ferrum Phos.,* if febrile symptoms are still present. Evening aggravation.

Silicea.—When the expectoration is thick, yellow and heavy, pus falls to bottom of vessel. *Cough worse from cold drinks* and better from warm. Night sweats.

Natr. Mur.—Acute bronchitis, with characteristic *expectoration of clear, watery, frothy phlegm.* Chronic bronchitis, "winter cough," with watery symptoms. Phlegm is loose and rattling, and sometimes coughed up with difficulty; at other times it swells up into the mouth, causing constant spitting. Patient is generally worse near sea-shore, from breathing the salt air.

Calc. Phos.—Expectoration of albuminous mucus (not watery). Bronchitis in anemic patients, with the above symptoms. As a restorative after the disease.

Calc. Sulph.—Mattery expectoration, or mattery mixed with blood. Last stage. Expectoration heavy, purulent matter.

Natr. Sulph.—Where exudation causes soreness and chafing. *Patient must hold his chest in coughing.* Asthmatic spells, worse towards morning. Worse in cold, damp, rainy weather.

CLINICAL CASES

Ferrum Phos. and Kali Mur. in Acute Bronchitis:

F. S. C. Acute bronchitis. Age 3 years, temp. 103, resp. 20, pulse 118. Hard cough with rales all over the chest. *Ferrum Phos.* alternated with *Kali Mur.* Next temp. 99, cough much better. Finished case with *Kali Sulph.*
(Dr. G. A. Budd.)

Ferrum Phos. in recurring Bronchitis:

Lady Louise has been subject to attacks of bronchitis for several winters; the first attack, of pneumonia, proving very serious. Her husband wrote to ask which of the biochemic remedies should be given. *Ferrum Phos.*, a dose every hour, and a few doses of *Kali Phos.*, for exhausted condition, were steadily taken for a few days, and then *Ferrum Phos.* and *Kali Mur.*, alternately. Shortly after this I received a letter dated London, October 6th, in which she says: "I must write to thank you more than I can say, for your remedies have done me untold good. The doctor who has called yesterday states all the bronchial symptoms are gone."
(Dr. Walker.)

Kali Mur. and Ferrum Phos. in chronic Bronchitis:

Archibald Herbert, suffering from chronic bronchitis had an attack of pneumonia. An iron moulder by trade, he was exposed to great heat; he had laid down on a form in a state of perspiration, took a severe chill, and inflammation in the right lung set in. His case was a bad one, complicated by bronchial affection; fever high; cough distressing; a pain, deep-seated, in the right side; expectoration tenacious, rusty-colored. *Ferrum Phos.*, in alternation with *Kali Mur.*, a dose every half hour was taken for twenty-four hours, then every hour. For his prostration and sleeplessness, a few doses of *Kali Phos.* were taken now and then. The improvement every way was very marked in two days. As the color of the sputa changed to yellow, he took *Kali Sulph.* instead of *Kali Mur.*; and as this condition was remedied, *Natr. Mur.* and *Calc.*

Phos. completed the cure in little more than ten days. (From Schuessler.)

BURNS AND SCALDS

BIOCHEMIC TREATMENT

Ferrum Phos.—May be applied at first till the pain ceases, but as soon as the pain stops, *Kali Mur.* should be used to restore the destroyed tissues.

Kali Mur.—Burns and scalds of any degree must be treated with this remedy, internally and externally. Moisten lint with a strong solution of the remedy. Apply the remedy frequently without removing the lint.

Calc. Sulph.—Second remedy, after *Kali Mur.*, when suppurating.

Natr. Phos.—Burns, with suppuration; also apply locally.

CANCER

(See Tumors and Cancer.)

CANKER

(See Mouth, Diseases of.)

CARBUNCLES

(See Abscess.)

BIOCHEMIC TREATMENT

Ferrum Phos.—In first or *inflammatory stage of carbuncles,* for heat, pain, congestion and fever; will often abort suppuration.

Kali Mur.—In the *second stage of carbuncles.* If given in alternation with *Ferrum Phos.*, the swelling will very often disappear and no suppuration ensue.

Silicea.—When the pus formation has commenced. *Silicea* promotes suppuration. Externally and internally after the tumor has broken and while infiltration remains.

CATARACT

(See Eye, Diseases of.)

BIOCHEMIC TREATMENT

Calc. Fluor.—Cataract of the eye. Blurred vision.

Calc. Phos.—In checking the progress of cataract, it has appeared to be of decided service, and will be of value when the following symptoms are present: Headaches, especially of the right side, pain around the eye, aching pain in the eye, tired feeling of the eye. These have all been relieved by *Calc. Phos.* Other symptoms noted were: *Eyes feel stiff and weak,* dizziness, rheumatic pains, etc. (Norton.)

CATARRH

ETIOLOGY

It may affect any mucous membrane of the body, and wherever found the treatment will be the same. The cause is that of any other disease, *i. e.*, a deficiency of one or more tissue-salts; however, there are certain primary causes which are responsible for the deficiency. Catarrh is of two varieties, viz.: acute and chronic. The acute form is generally known as a common cold. This disease consists of a mild inflammation of the mucous membrane, which is induced by exposure to sudden changes of temperature, or to a damp, chilly atmosphere. Sometimes—quite often—when a deficiency in certain salts occurs, the organic matter controlled by them is thrown out through the nasal passages.

Natr. Mur. controls water; hence, a deficiency in that salt causes a watery discharge. Kali Mur. controls fibrin, and a deficiency in that salt causes a fibrinous discharge, known by the exudation, being whitish, sticky, viscid, etc.

An albuminous exudation indicates a lack of the lime phosphate, because the particles of that salt attract albumen.

Potassium Sulphate, or Kali Sulph., works with oil. A yellow exudation indicates an oily substance, caused by a lack of the potassium molecules. (See article on Exudations.)

BIOCHEMIC TREATMENT

Ferrum Phos.—First or *inflammatory stage,* or cold in head; *takes cold easily* (with *Calc. Phos.*). Catarrhal fever. Congestion of nasal membranes.

Kali Mur.—*Second stage* of catarrhal troubles, *with white, thick, tenacious phlegm* (not transparent). Catarrhs of the head, with stuffy sensations, with whitish or gray-coated tongue. Dry coryza.

Natr. Mur.—*Catarrhs of the head, with watery, transparent discharges,* poor in albumen. Catarrhs of anemic patients, with frothy discharges, sometimes having a salty taste. *Chronic catarrh,* with the above symptoms. Bronchial catarrh, with frothy mucus. Influenza, with sneezing and watery symptoms. Dry catarrh.

Calc. Phos.—*Calc. Phos.* is one of the most important remedies in the treatment of catarrhal affections, especially of anemic persons and chronic cases. *Catarrh,* when the *discharges* are rich in albumen, transparent, *like white of egg,* before it is cooked. *Calc. Phos.* has also a tonic action and is very beneficial as a preparatory remedy, or intercurrently with the chief remedy.

Kali Sulph.—Catarrhs in the *third stage,* or stage of resolution; generally follows after *Kali Mur.,* if the *expectoration* or secretions are *yellow, slimy* or *watery matter;* thin, yellow discharge from the nose. In catarrhal conditions, when the skin is dry and hot, in alternation with *Ferrum Phos.,* to promote perspiration. Symptoms worse in a warm room or in the evening.

Calc. Fluor.—Catarrh of head, stuffy cold or dry coryza *Bronchial catarrh,* when tiny, yellow lumps of mucus are coughed up with difficulty. Ozena. Diseases of the nasal bones, with very offensive odor; *Calc. Fluor.* will take away the odor.

Kali Sulph.—Thick, yellow, mattery discharges, sometimes mixed with blood.

Kali Phos.—*Ozena,* with *foul, offensive discharge;* other characteristic symptoms correspond.

Natr. Phos.—Catarrh, with acid condition of the system (intercurrently). Note also coating of the tongue, and the creamy, golden yellow discharge.

Natr. Sulph.—Nose-bleed during menses. Ozena syphilitica; worse every change from dry to wet weather. *Catarrhs* of mucous membranes *in general,* characterized by a tendency to profuse secretion of greenish mucus.

Magnes. Phos.—Loss or *perversion of the sense of smell.* Alternate dry and loose coryza. Gushing flow from nostrils.

Silicea.—"Ozena, with fetid, offensive discharge from the nose, when the affection is seated in the sub-mucous connective tissue or periosteum; also syringe with a solution of the remedy." (Dr. Walker.) *Excessive, chronic dryness* or ulceration of the edges of the nostrils. *Itching of the tip of nose.*

CLINICAL CASES

Kali Sulph. restored the Senses of Taste and Smell:

Case of thick, yellow, offensive ozena, with watery discharge; has been affected with it for eighteen months; has lost taste and smell; left nostril worse. Catamenia occurs every three weeks. Takes cold very easily; still-born child three years ago. Gave three doses of *Kali Sulph.*, in water, to be taken once a day. In one month reported catarrh entirely well; has regained much of lost senses of taste and smell (W. P. Wesselhoeft, M. D.)

Kali Sulph. in Catarrh involving Antrum of Highmore:

Case of gentleman; light complexion. About once a week a thick, dark-brown, semi-fluid accumulation of pus formed in the left nostril; on being blown out it emitted a terrible stench. About a month previous a piece of carious bone was taken from the antrum of Highmore, through an upper left alveolus, from which a tooth had been drawn. Three weeks after, having taken *Kali Sulph.*, in water, morning and evening a table-spoonful for four days, nothing more remained of the discharge, and the alveolus closed so that no probe entered. (W. P. Wesselhoeft, M. D.)

Natr. Phos. in Post-Nasal Catarrh:

Dr. H. Goullon (*Pop. Zeitschrift*) praises *Natr. Phos.* in chronic post-nasal catarrh, giving as indications the golden-yellow exudation and yellow tongue, etc., and relates a case cured by *Natr. Phos.* after *Kali Bich.* had failed, as well as everything else, and the patient had become hypochondriacal.

CEREBRAL CONGESTION

(See Brain, Meningitis.)

CLINICAL CASES

Ferrum Phos. in Cerebral Congestion from overeating:

Drug: *Ferrum Phos.* History of case: Cerebral congestion, caused by excessive eating and drinking, followed by cold. Clinical symptoms: Headache. Pain running from left ear to nape of neck. Movement of right hand and arm difficult. Pulse full and hard. Remarks: *Ferrum Phos.* given with prompt disappearance of symptoms in one night.

Ferrum Phos. and Natr. Sulph. in Cerebral Congestion of children:

Having a case that interested me very much, I thought I would report it. On Friday morning, August 5th, my little boy, 11 years old, was taken with a violent fever, and rush of blood to the head, accompanied with severe pain in the back of the head and neck. I immediately commenced giving him *Ferrum Phos.* and *Natr. Sulph.*, alternately every half hour, a small powder dry on the tongue, and to temporarily ease the pain I sponged the back of his head and neck with cold water quite often. I gave *Ferrum Phos.* for the fever, *Natr. Sulph.* for the tendency of blood to the head. I followed this treatment steadily until Sunday morning, when the fever had completely left him, and until the congestion of blood had stopped. He was as well as ever, excepting a trifle weak. It was the first severe case of the kind I have had; and I felt more elated over the triumph of the Biochemic remedies when I knew that a leading physician of the city had lost last year one patient having the same disease, and had another in bed with it for over two months, who only finally recovered on account of his strong constitution.

CHICKEN-POX

ETIOLOGY

The basic cause of chicken pox is a deficiency in the inorganic cell salt Kali Mur., which sets free a corresponding quantity of organic matter. The system tries to eliminate this waste matter through the skin, and thus provides a breeding place for the micro-organism which causes the characteristic symptoms of chicken pox.

The micro-organism exhausts itself in a few days, and it is only necessary to supply the lacking cell salt to insure a speedy return to health.

BIOCHEMIC TREATMENT

Ferrum Phos.—For the febrile conditions connected with this disease, alternated with the remedy indicated by the tongue or eruption.

Kali Mur.—Second stage, with white or grayish-white coated tongue.

Kali Sulph.—For suppression of the rash; in alternation with *Ferrum Phos.*

Natr. Mur.—With corresponding watery symptoms, drowsiness, stupor, etc.

Calc. Sulph.—When the nature of the eruption indicates this remedy.

CHLOROSIS

(See Anemia.)

CHILD-BED FEVER

(See Puerperal Fever.)

CHOLERA

ETIOLOGY

Cholera is a Greek term, and is derived from *Chole,* or bile. It is now used in medicine as indicating one of two or three forms of disease, characterized by purging and vomiting, followed by great prostration.

Cholera is a condition characterized by violent emesis, diarrhea, abdominal pains and cramps. In Asiatic cholera there is also a germ present, but this is not true of cholera morbus, the form of cholera found in this country. But this is not a diagnosis clear enough to base the remedy on, according to Biochemistry. The character of the alvine discharges must be known. The discharge from the bowels resembling rice-water, with flocculent sediment, indicates a great disturbance in the gray matter of the nervous system, and, of course, breaking up the continuity of the molecules of water throughout the entire organism, or, more properly speaking, a deficiency in sodium chloride, without which water would be inert and could not be held in the blood. The chief cause of the acute attack is the breaking away of the water from the blood and blood-serum. But the primary cause is an over-supply of water in the blood, caused by an atmosphere heavily charged with water. Cholera does not continue in a temperature below seventy degrees, although cases of cholera sometimes appear after the weather becomes much cooler. The cause is produced by the moisture in the atmosphere during hot weather; for it is only those who have been exposed to a high temperature that ever yield to such conditions in a low temperature. Those who have not been exposed to a high temperature do not yield, although they come in contact with a cholera patient. The supply of sodium sulphate in the blood regulates the amount of water in the blood and the blood-serum; but should the blood receive more water from any source than there is sodium sulphate present to eliminate, an abnormal condition prevails, because the blood must furnish the nerves, muscles and all tissue of the body that water which it has in hand.

Now, if the amount of water in the blood be still greater, and from a certain combination of causes be discharged through the bowels, a watery diarrhea or cholera is the result. The liver seems first to empty its contents, the bile having become thinned by the excess of water in the system. The first discharges in cholera are colored with bile, but later on the discharge becomes clear or colorless. All the outlets of the body seem to be closed against the outflow of water, except the bowels. The urinary secretions become dried at their source, and the pores closed.

As long ago as 1852 Peyton wrote that "very remarkable effects have been found to follow the injection into the veins of a dilute solution of saline matter, resembling, as nearly as possible, the *inorganic salts of the blood, which have been drained away.*"

Natr. Sulph. is a preventive of cholera, because it regulates the water in the blood, and should be taken in hot weather, especially in low districts. because the moist air is found there.

Cholera, malaria, etc., do not prevail in a high altitude. It is the damp air, or water in the air, that causes these conditions, and not swamps, poor drainage, miasma, etc. For, the same people, living in the same locality, cease to suffer from these complaints as soon as the temperature falls below seventy degrees; or, in other words, as soon as the atmosphere becomes dry, these symptoms disappear.

Treatment of cholera, with biochemic remedies, is as follows:

Preventive: *Natr. Sulph.;* at commencement of disease, *Ferrum Phos.* and *Kali Sulph.;* for cramps, *Magnes. Phos.*

After a case has progressed two hours or more, *Ferrum Phos., Kali Phos.* or *Magnes. Phos.,* in combination, and *Natr. Mur.* in alternation.

Dose should be given every five minutes, and the patient be urged to drink as much hot water (just plain, common, hot water) as possible. A copious injection of hot water should be given every hour until relief is obtained, which will be in from two to four hours. A half teaspoonful of salt should be added to each quart of water. The moment there is a favorable change, give light nourishment, but *no stimulants.*

BIOCHEMIC TREATMENT

Ferrum Phos.—For the febrile symptoms and vascular disturbance. *Cholera infantum,* with *watery stools,* from relaxed state of the villi not taking up the proper amount of moisture; child has high fever and stupor.

Natr. Sulph.—As a preventive, to eliminate the excess of water in the blood. During the disease for the same purpose, in alternation with other remedies indicated. Note color of tongue; taste, and other characteristic indications of this remedy.

Kali Phos.—*Stools have the appearance of rice-water;* very offensive. Collapse, with livid, bluish countenance and low pulse.

Magnes. Phos.—Cramps of the bowels and limbs in cholera. Vomiting and watery diarrhea. "In cholera or any other bowel complaint, an injection of hot water, with the appropriate remedy, should be given at once. It will relieve spasms, clean the mucous membranes, cause normal absorption and greatly ameliorate all unfavorable symptoms." (Chapman.)

Natr. Mur.—To regulate the distribution of water in the system, watery coated tongue and other characteristic symptoms.

CLINICAL CASES

Kali Phos. cured Cramps and Diarrhea:

Old man, attacked with severe vomiting and diarrhea, cramps in calves, and rice-water discharges. *Kali Phos.* cured. (Schuessler.)

Kali Phos. in rice-water Stools:

An old man was attacked by a severe case of vomiting and diarrhea, accompanied by exceedingly painful cramp in the calves. Evacuations had the appearance of rice-water. One dose of *Kali Phos.* effected a cure after six hours. The speedy cure of this case of choleric diarrhea would justify the belief that *Kali Phos.* is a specific against cholera. (Schuessler.)

CHOLERA INFANTUM

(See Diarrhoea.)

ETIOLOGY

This is a disease which most frequently appears among teething children in the after part of the summer, when the system is weakened and debilitated by the preceding hot weather. Improper diet, chilling of the abdomen, and similar causes have much to do with this trouble, but the basic reason for its occurrence is a deficiency in Calc. Phos., which brings about a general systemic weakness, with consequent indigestion and malassimilation, and a lack of Magnes. Phos., which affects the stomach and abdominal muscles, and gives rise to cramps and pains. An acid condition from the lack of Natr. Phos. may also be present.

SYMPTOMS

Violent and copious vomiting, accompanied with diarrhea, are the most prominent symptoms. At first the vomiting may be of food, but later it changes to a sour liquid. The child is restless, tosses from one side of the bed to the other. The head is hot; pulse rapid, but feeble; extremities cool; eyes sunken, and half open; eyelids heavy; drinks greedily; great weakness, and sometimes emaciation. The discharge from the bowels usually consists of a colorless, or sometimes greenish, and watery fluid, occasionally with shreds of mucus. The stools are generally discharged without effort, sometimes unconsciously—or are squirted out, as if thrown from a syringe. Sometimes there is pain, straining, and the infant cries plaintively, and draws up its limbs. As the disease advances, the discharges from the bowels become more frequent, resembling dirty water or the "washings of meat," and are offensive. The eyes become languid and dull, or hollow and glassy, and take no notice of the surroundings. The lips are dry and shriveled. It frequently happens that the brain becomes involved, and the child rolls its head and moans piteously. In fatal cases, the patient falls into a complete state of stupor, and convulsions may appear.

BIOCHEMIC TREATMENT

Ferrum Phos.—Is the remedy for the fever; watery, frequent, undigested stools, feverish thirst; vomit of undigested food. Brain symptoms, delirium, rolling of the head, moaning, etc. Alternate with remedy indicated by the color of the stools.

Natr. Phos.—When the stools are sour-smelling and green. Cholera infantum, when associated with worms, acid conditions, lack of digestive power, or from eating unripe fruit. Note the color of the tongue, the acid, sour vomit, and other acid symptoms.

Calc. Phos.—One of the most valuable remedies for bowel complaints in teething children, due to non-assimilation of food, or in emaciated children, where the lime salts are at fault. Stools are hot, watery, offensive, profuse and sputtering; sometimes green and undigested.

Kali Phos.—Stools are like rice-water; great depression and exhaustion; stools very offensive and putrid.

Magnes. Phos.—Cholera infantum accompanied with cramp-like pains in the bowels, flatulent colic, drawing up of the legs, convulsions, spurting stools, etc. Alternate with remedies indicated by color of the stools.

SUGGESTIONS

The child must be kept as quiet as possible. If the extremities or abdomen should become cold, efforts should be made to create artificial warmth by the application of warm, woolen cloths, gentle friction, etc. At the beginning, and during the course of the disease, an injection of quite warm water into the bowels is very beneficial; it washes the tissues and promotes healthy secretion. A quantity of the indicated remedy should be used in the water. The child will not have much appetite, but care must be taken in selecting such food as will not irritate the bowels.

During attacks the child should receive very little food, and especially *no milk*. The diet of nursing mothers should be very simple and non-irritating. Feeding should be resumed very gradually and in very small quantities at a time. The mistake in giving a child too much food as soon as it recovers is often made. This may cause a dangerous relapse. Barley water with a little cream or the white of an egg in warm water is recommended. Give about one or two teaspoonfuls every one-half to one hour. Severe attacks of colic are sometimes relieved by hot applications over the abdomen.

Water may be given in small quantities, but not too cold; and if it excites vomiting or purging, it should be discontinued entirely. Hot water drinks can do no harm. and will be beneficial if the infant will take them.

CLINICAL CASES

Ferrum Phos. in Cholera Infantum:

Mary B., 18 months old; green, watery stools, mixed with mucus, every few minutes, producing great weakness and emaciation. She rolled her head about as if it was too heavy; eyes half open; constant moaning or starting up in sleep; pulse rapid; respiration accelerated; complexion of a dirty, white appearance; watery vomit. *Ferrum Phos.,* in hot water every hour for six or eight, then *Calc. Phos.* in alternation, every hour, cured the case completely in less than two weeks.
(C. R. Vogel, M. D.)

A mother brought her child to my office, with the following symptoms: temperature, 104; pulse, 130; flushed and staring; great thirst; frequent green, slimy discharges from the bowels, with occasional vomiting; pain in the abdomen and stomach. I prescribed one grain each of *Ferrum Phos.* and *Magnes. Phos.* every half-hour in alternation. I heard no more of the case for two weeks, when the mother reported "that from the first dose the child began to obtain relief, and was sleeping nicely in two hours, and continued to improve rapidly until entirely well.
(Dr. W. E. Keimett.)

CHOREA (St. Vitus' Dance)

ETIOLOGY

St. Vitus' Dance is a nervous disorder manifesting itself in convulsive and involuntary twitchings of the muscles, fits, spasms, etc. This disease, usually found in children, especially girls, is due to a deficiency of the cell-salt Magnes. Phos., which controls the white fibres of nerves and muscles. The deficiency may arise from a number of causes: vicious habits, great fear, overtaxing the nervous or muscular system, worms, acid conditions, eating indigestible foods, etc.

The cure consists in supplying Magnes. Phos. alone or in alternation with other indicated Biochemic Remedies.

The symptoms are regular and uncontrollable movements of portions of the body; sometimes one side, at others the face, lower jaw, one arm, etc. These motions are strange and fantastic, making the sufferer appear crazy to those unfamiliar with the cause.

BIOCHEMIC TREATMENT

Magnes. Phos.—For the spasms, *involuntary movements* and *contortions of the limbs, Magnes. Phos.* is the remedy. Mute, appealing looks for sympathy. This is the *chief remedy.*

Calc. Phos.—To follow *Magnes. Phos.,* if relief is not obtained; also intercurrently *in scrofulous or anemic subjects.*

Silicea.—Spasms, sleep disturbed by frightful dreams, distorted eyes, pale face, etc. If from worms, alternate with *Natr. Phos.*

Natr. Mur.—In chronic cases, *if caused by suppression of eruptions,* twitchings, jerkings of the limbs, etc. Note also the characteristic indications calling for this remedy.

Natr. Phos.—If due to worms or if acid symptoms are present. Note color of root of tongue.

CLINICAL CASES

Magnes. Phos. cured Chorea:

David P., æt. 12. This case was the most fearful I ever saw during the thirty years I have been practicing. Diagnosis: St. Vitus' dance (*Chorea*).

It was simply impossible for him to keep still a moment—limbs and features distorted; sometimes he would fall to the ground in convulsions and gasp for breath, frothing and snapping—a devil in human form. This boy inherited a nervous constitution from his father, who was an habitual smoker and drunkard.

The treatment was *Calc. Phos.,* as an intercurrent remedy, eight grains every morning, in a little water; *Magnes. Phos.* and *Kali Phos.,* fifteen grains each, in a glass two-thirds full of water, to be taken in alternation, by sips, until all was taken in one day; mixing and taking the same amount fresh every day. In six months was dismissed cured, and for the last eight months has not experienced anything of the above disease.
(Wm. Chapman, M. D.)

Magnes. Phos. in Chorea:

Case I.—Artie P., æt. 13, St. Vitus' dance (*Chorea*). He could not get his hand to his mouth; very nervous; in appearance, very pale and weak. Treatment: *Calc. Phos.,* as an intercurrent, in the morning; *Magnes. Phos.* and *Kali Phos.*, ten grains in two glasses half full of water, to be taken by sips, in alternation. In three months was dismissed, cured.
(Wm. Chapman, M. D.)

Case II.—Face and upper part of body affected; lateral and downward jerking of mouth; snapping of eyelids; sudden forward motion of head, and other irregular movements. Better during sleep; aggravated at stool and by emotions. *Magnes. Phos.,* for three months, produced gratifying results, but did not fully cure. Acting on Dr. Schuessler's advice, *Calc. Phos.*

was given alternately with the *Magnes. Phos.;* the former once daily; the latter twice. In one month the child was cured. (D. B. Whittier, M. D.)

COLDS

ETIOLOGY

A lack of ferrum molecules in the blood is the cause of "colds." When a deficiency of iron occurs, the blood is drawn away from the skin and the tissues beneath it in order that the process of life may be carried on more perfectly about the heart, lungs, liver, stomach, brain, etc.

A lack of blood in the minute blood-vessels of the skin allows the pores to close, and waste matter that should escape by this route is turned upon the inner organs. This causes an accumulation which, together with other organic matter, a deficiency in whose coefficient inorganic salts has thrown it out of the blood, forms the exudation of colds, catarrh, pneumonia, pleurisy, etc.

The cell-salt *potassium chloride* controls the fibrin in the circulation, and when the particles of this salt fall below the standard, a portion of fibrin, not having workmen to use it, becomes a disturbing element and leaves the vital circulation. If it is thrown off through the lungs a cough is produced (Nature's spasmodic effort to get rid of the heteroplasm). In some instances the quantity of fibrin thus produced is so great that the lungs are unable to throw it off and pneumonia results. If the fibrinous exudation is thrown off through the nasal passages, it is called catarrh.

BIOCHEMIC TREATMENT

Ferrum Phos.—First stage of cold in the head, with circulatory disturbances, *catarrhal fever,* congestion of nasal mucous membranes. Smarting in nasal passages; worse on inspiration;

excellent for a *predisposition to take cold;* alternately with *Calc. Phos.,* in pharyngeal catarrh, with characteristic white, albuminous expectoration.

Natr. Mur.—Catarrhs and colds, with *watery, transparent, frothy discharges.* Chronic catarrhs of bloodless patients. The mucus has sometimes a salty taste. Colds causing vesicular eruptions, with watery contents, which burst and leave thin crusts or scabs. Coryza, "running cold," with watery, clear, frothy discharge; worse on going into the cold or on exertion. Influenza. Epistaxis from stooping and from coughing. Posterior nares dry. *Loss of sense of smell.*

Kali Mur.—Stuffy colds in the head, with thick, white discharges and gray or white-coated tongue. Anterior nares inflamed and swollen

Kali Sulph.—In the first stage of colds, in alternation with *Ferrum Phos.*—frequent doses to promote perspiration. Colds, with dry, harsh skin to induce perspiration. Stuffy colds with large collections of greenish-yellow matter.

Calc. Sulph.—Cold in the head, with *thick, yellow, opaque, mattery secretions,* frequently *tinged with blood.* It clears up the condition of the mucous glands.

COLIC

ETIOLOGY

This trouble is characterized by a severe griping pain in the abdomen, the name colic being taken from the Latin word *colicus,* pertaining to the colon.

It may arise from gas caused by undigested food in the intestines, worms, suppression of chronic eruptions of the skin, gravel or organic derangements of the kidneys, acrid discharge of bile into the stomach and intestines, and other conditions originating from deficiencies in various cell-salts. The chief cause, however, is a lack of Magnes. Phos. occurring in the muscular fibres of the stomach and intestines, and setting up spasmodic contractions there.

BIOCHEMIC TREATMENT

Magnes. Phos.—*Colic of infants, with drawing up of the legs.* Pain causes the patient to bend double. Flatulent colic, eased by friction, heat or belching of gas. Remittent colic, with crampy pain. Colic of new-born infants, without indigestion.

Natr. Sulph.—Bilious colic, with vomiting of bile; *bitter taste in the mouth* and *brownish-green coating on root of tongue.* Flatulent colic caused by derangement of the liver. *Lead colic;* give the remedy quite frequently.

Calc. Phos.—Colic in teething children, greenish evacuations and undigested food (*Natr. Phos.*). Colic with indigestion, to promote assimilation of the food. Colics of any kind if *Magnes. Phos.* fails to relieve though indicated.

Natr. Mur.—In cases of bilious colic.

Natr. Phos.—Colic of *children, with worms* or symptoms of acidity, green, sour-smelling stools, vomiting of curdled milk, etc.

Kali Phos.—Colic in hypogastrium, with ineffectual urging to stool; better bending double. Abdomen distended with gas.

Kali Sulph.—Pains resemble those of *Magnes Phos.* Abdomen feels cold; pain sometimes caused by excitement and sudden coldness shortly after; gas from bowels smells like sulphur.

Ferrum Phos.—Colic at the menstrual periods, with heat, quickened pulse, etc.

CLINICAL CASES

Mag. Phos. in Colic:

W. E. A. Child two months old. Troubled with colic. Occurring at regular intervals after nursing. Any acid eaten

by mother would immediately, after nursing, produce violent colic. Relief from gas would relieve the colic. Child would draw up legs and suffer intense pain. This condition began when child was less than one month old. Many remedies had been tried. Used *Magnes. Phos.*, one tablet in two ounces of hot water, giving child one-third of teaspoonful every ten minutes. Relief would come before the third dose. This treatment only had to be kept up for about ten days, and there was no return of the colic. Many similar cases have reacted just as quickly, and the cure has been permanent.
(Dr. R. C. Wolcott.)

Natr. Sulph. in Colic:

One of the hard-working clergy of the metropolis was for several years subject to very frequent and very severe attacks of colic, always running into inflammatory character, violent vomiting, great tenderness of abdomen, restlessness, anxiety, misery. These attacks generally lasted from three days to one week.

More than a year ago it was ascertained that the *pain generally commenced in the right groin,* and thence spread over the whole abdomen. *Natr. Sulph.* was given, the attack yielded immediately, and though he has had several threatenings, he has had no colic since.
(Hering's "Materia Medica.")

Magnes. Phos. and Natr. Sulph. for bilious Colic:

Another case was that of a lady with bilious colic. I was sent for in the night, and for particular reasons did not go. However, I sent what I thought would relieve her. Early in the morning her husband was again at my office, saying she was no better, but suffering terribly. I gave him a different remedy, to be administered until I could get there. About half-past nine I arrived at the house and found her still suffering excruciating pains. Ascertaining that she had vomited bile and had a very bitter taste in her mouth all the time, I administered *Magnes. Phos.* and *Natr. Sulph.* in alternation.

In a short time after taking, she said she was considerably relieved for the first time since eleven o'clock in the night. In about five minutes she had a free movement of the bowels, and she continued to improve, and was up and about the next morning.

Natr. Phos. in Colic from oversecretion of lactic fluid:

Woman, æt. 50; suffered for two years from gastralgia and enteralgia, attacks lasting several days; at each attack vomiting of a fluid as sour as vinegar. Two physicians had treated her in vain, diagnosing the affection as cancer of the stomach and wandering kidney. My diagnosis was oversecretion of lactic acid. *Natr. Phos.;* improvement set in in two days, and in a few weeks was entirely cured.
(Schuessler.)

CONCUSSION OF THE BRAIN

BIOCHEMIC TREATMENT

Ferrum Phos.—For the febrile disturbances.

Kali Phos.—Dilated pupils. *Depression of function of the brain-cells.* Asthenic conditions.

Magnes. Phos.—Concussion of the brain *when optical illusions* follow.

Natr. Sulph.—Mental troubles after injuries to the head. To control the determination of blood to the head. Intense pain in occipital region.

Calc. Phos.—Intercurrently with the chief remedy or with numb sensations.

CONSTIPATION

ETIOLOGY

Constipation may be caused by a deficiency of sodium sulphate or sodium phosphate in the fluids of the liver causing an inspissation of bile, or a lack of potassium chloride causing a lack of bile or a deficiency of sodium chloride. which would cause an uneven distribution of water. A certain amount of water is required to carry on the process of eliminating the waste from the body through the alimentary canal, and there must be a proper balance of sodium chloride in order to properly distribute the water in the organism. Constipation is sometimes caused by a relaxation of the villi of the small intestines, or the mucous membrane of the colon, due to a relaxation of elastic fibre, which is due to a deficiency of calcium fluoride molecules.

The molecular action of this salt being disturbed, sagging of the mucous lining of the intestines results, thereby obstructing the canal and preventing a free passage of the feces.

BIOCHEMIC TREATMENT

Ferrum Phos.—Constipation, owing to heat in the lower bowel (rectum) causing a hardening of the feces. Piles, prolapsus of the rectum, or inflammation of the vagina or uterus often cause this condition. Stools very dry.

Kali Mur.—Costiveness, with light-colored stools, from torpidity of the liver and want of bile. *Constipation, with white or grayish-white coated tongue,* when fat or pastry disagrees.

Kali Phos.—*Stools dark-brown,* streaked with yellowish-green mucus. Paretic condition of rectum and colon.

Natr. Mur.—Constipation, when caused from lack of moisture in the intestinal tract. Dryness of the bowels, with watery secretions in other parts, watery eyes, excess of saliva, watery vomiting, etc. *Constipation, with water-brash* and dribbling of saliva during sleep. Dull, heavy headache; hard, dry stools, difficult to pass. *Torn, smarting feeling after stool.* Injections of hot water, with a little salt, will usually overcome this condition if persisted in.

Calc. Fluor.—*Inability to expel feces* requires *Calc. Fluor.* This is due to a relaxed condition of the rectum, allowing a too large accumulation of fecal matter. "This is frequently met with after confinement, when all the pelvic muscles are relaxed." (Chapman.)

Calc. Phos.—Hard stool, with occasional pieces of albuminous mucus.

Natr. Phos.—Constipation of infants, with occasional attacks of diarrhea; an excellent laxative when given in large doses.

Natr. Sulph.—Hard, knotty stools, sometimes streaked with blood. *Difficult to expel soft stools. Natr. Sulph.*, in massive doses, acts as a cathartic.

Silicea.—Loss of power of expulsion; *feces recede after being partly expelled.* Constipation of poorly-nourished children.

CLINICAL CASES

Kali Mur. in Constipation from sedentary habits:

Mr. K., æt. 30, had been constipated for several weeks, owing to sedentary habits; a movement of the bowels would not occur unless an injection or heavy cathartic was taken. Stools hard, small and difficult to expel. Diagnosed torpid liver and deficiency of bile; prescribed *Kali Mur.*, a ten-grain dose each evening; next morning there was a natural evacuation, and by continuing the remedy, satisfactory results were obtained. (J. B. Chapman.)

Silicea in Constipation following confinement:

Mrs. H., æt. 26; mother of three children; constipation since birth of last child, three months ago. Cathartics had failed. The stools were hard and dry, were partially expelled with much straining, and then receded into the rectum. *Silicea* cured in four doses, taken night and morning.

(I. P. Johnson.)

Natr. Mur. in congenital Constipation:

Dr. Gross relates a very remarkable case of chronic constipation cured with *Natr. Mur.* The patient, a boy, æt. 11, born of scrofulous parents, has an idiotic brother, patient himself mute and almost an idiot. The poor creature suffered with constipation from birth. Would go three to four weeks without stool. After a course of *Natr. Mur.*, the constipation was entirely cured.

CONSUMPTION

(See Cough.)

ETIOLOGY

WHILE the word consumption, in its true meaning, has a wide scope, it is generally used to denote consumption of the lungs. The pathology of this condition is not difficult to trace. Either from repeated injury to the cellular structure of the lungs, from sudden changes of temperature, or breathing dust or impure air, or inherited tendencies, the blood is unable to furnish lung tissue as fast as it decays. By inherited tendencies we do not mean to infer that consumption is an entity that may be transmitted from parent to offspring. But a person with poor digestive and assimilative powers, or who is deficient in chest development or breathing capacity, will sometimes (not always) beget offspring with the same weakness or imperfections.

This disease consists of a consuming of the lung tissues. It may primarily arise from repeated inflammations or congestions of the lungs, but very frequently it is insidious in its approach, and gives but little warning till too late. The greater number of consumptive cases are due to "poor blood," which is not sufficient to furnish lung tissue fast enough. It may also be caused by an imperfect expansion of the lungs, thereby failing to admit enough oxygen into the system. However, the disease itself is basically due to a deficiency of some of the organic salts in the blood which produces a condition in the lung tissues furnishing a breeding-place for the tuberculosis bacilli. This deficiency may arise from improper diet; bad air; sudden changes of temperature; repeated colds; insufficient exercise; improper exposure to the elements; bad ventilation in bed-rooms; incorrect position; non-expansion of the lungs; sagging beds, etc.; in fact, anything which will cause a deterioration of health. There are some climates which are conducive to this disease, viz.: damp or hot and moist climates. Some constitutions, also, are predisposed to consumption; not that they inherit the disease, but they inherit the tendency to the disease.

This disease is so general, and its symptoms so well known, that it is a waste of time to enumerate them here, further than to give a brief outline. The patient is usually thin, and in the later stages greatly emaciated; cheeks hollow; night-sweats; hectic flush on one or both cheeks; hollow chested; stoop-shouldered; constipation; poor digestion, and sometimes loss of appetite. There is generally a hollow or racking cough, which is worse in the morning; the mucus raised varies in color and consistency, according to the stage of the disease, at first being albuminous, but in the later stage assuming a thick, mattery or frothy form. There are frequent flashes of heat, and at times hemorrhage from the lungs, but this is not necessarily a symptom of consumption.

BIOCHEMIC TREATMENT

Ferrum Phos.—Consumption, with *febrile symptoms,* such as fever, flushed face, etc. Breathing short and oppressed. *Cough dry and tickling* from irritation of the bronchial tubes, with soreness and pain in the chest. *Hemorrhage from the lungs, blood bright-red and frothy.* Expectoration streaked with blood. *Ferrum Phos.* is an excellent remedy for bleeding from any part, if the blood be bright red.

Calc. Phos.—*In incipient consumption,* to lessen the emaciation (also give cream and carbonaceous food). Should be given intercurrently in all cases of phthisis, for its tonic effect. Chronic coughs of consumptives. Cough, with expectoration of albuminous mucus. *Excessive perspiration in phthisis.*

Calc. Sulph.—Sputa mattery, sanious, mixed with blood, raised without effort.

Natr. Mur.—In consumption, when the *expectoration* is *watery, clear* and *frothy,* also bloody sputa. *In large doses to check hemorrhage,* alternate with *Ferrum Phos.* General weakness and prostration after exertion. Mucus in the chest, loose and rattling. Patient worse in a salty atmosphere. Chronic cough in phthisis, with frothy sputa.

Silicea.—A most important remedy in phthisis, as it embraces most of the symptoms of this disease, especially those of the latter stages. Profuse easy expectoration of thick, greenish-yellow, fetid pus, with sweetish insipid taste in the mouth. *Profuse night-sweats,* burning of the soles of the feet, hectic fever, etc. Constipation. *Very offensive foot-sweat.* Cough is loose and rattling, with profuse expectoration.

Kali Sulph.—Consumption, with expectoration characteristic of this remedy; mucus slips back and is generally swallowed. *Skin is harsh and dry.* Evening aggravation.

Kali Mur.—*Thick, white expectoration, white* or *grayish-white coating on tongue.*

Kali Phos.—Shortness of breath, putrid sputa. *General weakness* and *prostration.* Sleeplessness.

Natr. Sulph.—Cough, with purulent, yellowish-green expectoration and general symptoms indicating this remedy. "All-gone" sensation in the chest.

CONVULSIONS

(See Spasms, Convulsions, etc.)

CORYZA

(See Catarrh.)

BIOCHEMIC TREATMENT

Kali Mur.—Catarrh, when there *is white phlegm,* thick, not transparent. Dry coryza. *Stuffy cold in the head, with a whitish-gray tongue.* Adherent crusts in the vault of the pharynx. In the purulent stage of acute nasal catarrh. *Kali Mur.* has proved to be the most satisfactory remedy in *acute inflammations of the nasopharynx* in which there is a decided *burning dryness.* The appearance is that of redness, with marked thickening, almost as though the mucous membrane were solidly infiltrated. Hawking of mucus from posterior nares.

Natr. Mur.—Coryza, "running cold," with clear, watery, frothy discharge; aggravation from going into a cold atmosphere and from exertion; relieved by cool applications.

CLINICAL CASES

Natr. Mur. in recurring Coryza:

Miss S., æt. 48, has suffered for the past ten years, following an accident, from a coryza that was peculiar and had regular periods of exacerbation. It appeared twice a week, lasted one or two days, and began with slight shuddering in the back and thirst. It was always worse from 10 to 12 a. m. The discharge was watery and so profuse that she was compelled to use a towel instead of a handkerchief. Everything cool brought relief. Wet weather, fog, wet feet, warmth and a warm room aggravated the condition. The attack was accompanied by sneezing that could be heard throughout the house.

On October 22, she received *Natr. Mur.,* five powders; one to be taken every third evening. On November 5th she reported that she was much better, the attacks only lasting about an hour. The same remedy was prescribed, a powder once a week. On January 15th, she stated that during the past ten weeks she had been better than at any time during the past ten years, no sign of the malady having shown itself until the day before. It had then occurred in a much milder form than usual, in consequence of a cold she had taken. The remedy was given again, with most satisfactory results.

COUGH

(See Pneumonia, Consumption and Whooping-Cough.)

ETIOLOGY

Cough is not, theoretically speaking, a "disease," but merely a symptom or sign of Nature, calling our attention to an abnormal condition. In another sense, too, it is an effort of Nature to throw off an accumulation of disorganized matter which, if not removed, might cause serious results. Coughs may arise from an irritation of the air passages, due to disease of the lungs, or from cold or other causes, or they may be sympathic, due to other diseased organs, such as the uterus, liver, etc.

BIOCHEMIC TREATMENT

Kali Mur.—Loud, noisy, stomach-cough, with white or grayish-white coating on the tongue. Cough, with *expectoration* of *thick, milky-white tenacious phlegm.* Short, acute cough, like whooping cough. Croupy, hard cough, with white-coated tongue; croup-like hoarseness. Hard cough, with protruded appearance of the eyes and corresponding tongue symptoms.

Ferrum Phos.—First stage of all coughs. Short, acute, *painful cough,* with *soreness in the lungs;* expectoration absent. Cough, tickling, from inflammation and irritation of the bronchi Hard and dry cough, with soreness from cold, without expectoration.

Magnes. Phos.—*Whooping cough, for the spasmodic symptoms;* alternate with *Kali Mur.* Spasmodic cough. Paroxysms of coughing, without expectoration; lungs feel sore and painful from the strain and exertion of coughing. Hot drinks give temporary relief. True spasmodic cough should not be confounded with the apparent spasmodic cough of *Kali Mur.;* the color of the tongue will usually be a safe guide.

Kali Sulph.—Cough in which the *expectoration is slimy, yellow or watery matter;* always worse in a warm room or in the evening; relieved in the cool, open air. (Sputa is tenacious and ropy.) Cough, when the mucus slips back and is generally swallowed. Hard, hoarse cough, like croup, with *weary feeling in the pharynx.*

Kali Phos.—Cough from irritation in the *trachea,* which *feels sore. Expectoration thick, yellow, salty and fetid.* Chest sore.

Natr. Sulph.—Cough, with a sensation of all-goneness in the chest. Mucus mixed with pus; *thick, ropy* and *yellowish-green expectoration;* must press upon chest to relieve soreness and weakness.

Silicea.—Cough in phthisis, with thick, yellowish-green, profuse expectoration of sweetish, greasy taste. Cough caused by cold drinks. Morning coughs of consumptives. *Cough* in consumption, *worse* on *lying down* or on rising in the morning. Sputa has offensive odor and falls to the bottom of vessel containing water.

Calc. Fluor.—Cough, with tickling in the throat from elongation of the uvula or mucus dropping from the posterior nares. Cough, with expectoration of tiny, yellow, tough lumps of mucus, sometimes smelling badly.

Natr. Mur.—Cough, with expectoration characteristic of this remedy; watery, tasting salty. Cough, with excess of watery secretions from the eyes, nose and mouth. Chronic coughs, with the above symptoms, often accompanied by dryness of other mucous membranes, constipation, etc.

Calc. Phos.—Cough, with albuminous expectoration like white of an egg. Intercurrently in all coughs of consumptives.

Calc. Sulph.—Cough, with sanious, watery sputa.

CLINICAL CASES

Calc. Phos. for Cough in malnutrition of infants:

Child, æt. 18 months; could not walk; fontanels open, and a short, irritating, troublesome cough; no expectoration. Had been under a good physician, but without relief. In despair, the parents decided to try the biochemic remedies. I believed the cough arose from a deficiency of lime phosphate, so prescribed *Calc. Phos.* In three weeks the cough had entirely disappeared, and the child began to walk.

(J. B. Chapman, M. D.)

Natr. Mur. in Coughs of Pneumonia:

In the short, dry, tickling, inflammatory cough, so often seen in pneumonia or fever cases, *Natr. Mur.* will often give relief after *Ferrum Phos. fails.* The action of the remedy, in many cases, was remarkable, the patient coughing but once or twice after taking it.

(J. B. Chapman, M. D.)

Kali Phos. for subacute Laryngitis:

Dr. J. A. Biegler reports a case of subacute laryngitis cured by *Kali Phos.* The prescription was given "as a forlorn hope," because the case came late under treatment, with weakness, pale, bluish face, etc.; speech slow, becoming inarticulate; creeping paralysis, and because Grauvogl says: "We know that the oxidation processes, the change of gases in the respiration, and other chemical transformations in the blood, are brought about by the presence of *Kali Phos.*"

Magnes. Phos. in spasmodic Cough:

Dr. F. W. Southworth reports two cases of spasmodic cough promptly relieved by *Magnes. Phos.*, the leading indications being its spasmodic character, worse on lying down and at night, and on breathing cold air; better on sitting up; tightness across the chest. The second case had spurting of urine when coughing.

Ferrum Phos. for Cough, with emissions of urine:

Dr. Fisher was consulted by a lady (*enceinte*) who was suffering from a cough which caused great inconvenience as with every cough there was emission of urine. *Ferrum Phos.* cured her very speedily. A short time ago the lady, under similar circumstances, was again troubled with a cough. *Ferrum Phos.* this time also cured her speedily.
(Schuessler.)

CRAMPS

(See Spasms, Convulsions, etc.)

CROUP

ETIOLOGY

The article on diphtheria will give the pathology of true croup. There is no difference in the cause of these two diseases.

But in false croup the fibrinous exudation accumulates in the mucous lining of the larynx and trachea. The biochemic treatment is the same in both cases.

Cut off the supply of organic matter that is causing the trouble, by furnishing the blood with the lacking material, Kali Mur., to take up the fibrin and diffuse it through the blood—carry it to the various tissues of the body, and thus prevent further accumulation at the seat of disease.

BIOCHEMIC TREATMENT

Kali Mur.—The *principal remedy in croup,* for the membraneous exudation; *frequent doses.* Alternate with *Ferr. Phos.*

Ferrum Phos.—Alternate with *Kali Mur.,* for the fever, hurried and oppressed breathing, etc

Calc. Fluor.—If *Ferrum Phos.* and *Kali Mur.* do not suffice, give *Calc. Fluor.;* also *Calc. Phos.*

Calc. Phos.—Intercurrently with the remedies indicated, or after them, if they fail to act.

Calc. Sulph.—*After* the *stage of exudation,* with cnaracteristic indications for the use of this remedy.

Kali Phos.—When treatment is delayed too long and there is danger of collapse; *nervous prostration;* pale, livid countenance. Alternate with *Kali Mur.*

CLINICAL CASES

Croup following Measles:

Was called about 10 p. m. to see boy, age 7 years, with violent attack of catarrhal croup following measles. I put a teaspoonful of *Ferrum Phos.* and *Kali Phos.* in half glass hot water. Ordered teaspoonful every fifteen minutes until relieved, then hourly. Prompt recovery.
(Dr. W. J. Grimes, East Liverpool, Ohio.)

Kali Mur. for the Exudation:

I have had occasion to treat quite a number of croup cases, and it has been my experience that, if taken in time, *Ferrum Phos.* and *Kali Mur.* is all that is required. *Ferrum Phos.* controls the febrile conditions, while *Kali Mur.* regulates the exudation. A gargle of *Kali Mur.* is very beneficial, when practicable.
(J. B. Chapman, M. D.)

Kali Mur. in spurious Croup:

D. R., a boy of seven years. A severe attack of spurious croup with fever and a loud, barking cough. He had had an attack of spurious croup a few years before, and whenever there was a sharp, keen northeast wind, he had since contracted cases of spurious croup.

Other remedies which have been recommended by many authors against croup, produced no change whatever, so I

accepted, in this case, the usual continuance of the affection for several days. The nights especially were very restless, with much coughing, rough and hard, so that his parents were very anxious. Dry heat and great oppression were present. I prescribed a full dose of *Kali Mur.* every two hours. After a few doses the cough became loose, completely lost the barking sound, and the whole of the following night my little patient slept quietly, and on the following morning was able to get up quite lively and well.
(Schuessler.)

CYSTITIS

ETIOLOGY

Cystitis, or inflammation of the bladder, is caused by bacterial infection, but this generally occurs only when the bladder has been put in a receptive condition by a lack of one or more of the cell salts. Other predisposing causes of cystitis exist, such as trauma from catheterization or instrumentation, congestion from exposure, pressure from tumors from without, or from growths or foreign bodies within the bladder, displacement of the bladder or anything causing retention, or lack of drainage. These other predisposing causes, however, always result in a loss of cell salts, and it is only after these invaluable constituents have been restored to the system, that a return to perfect health can be expected.

Cystitis may be either acute or chronic. The acute form may begin with or without pain and fever. Pain is usually felt persistently from the first, centered in the region of the bladder. Its acme is reached when the urine is voided, and there is usually some relief when this has occurred. There is a desire to pass urine every few minutes, the act being accompanied by intense vesical tenesmus or strangury, while only a small amount of urine is passed, often followed by a few drops of blood.

The urine is almost normal in amount during the twenty-four hours. It usually looks clear, but deposits considerable sediment containing pus, bladder epithelium, and bacteria; if the cystitis is diphtheritic or gangrenous there are also shreds of narcotic tissue, and blood corpuscles and blood clots if there has been hemorrhage. The urine is occasionally high-colored; it may be acid or alkaline, or even neutral, in reaction.

Fever ordinarily accompanies even a moderately severe cystitis. When there is extensive suppuration or necrosis, when the kidney is involved or when the inflammation extends into the pericystic tissues, the fever may become high and threatening. Such cases often show severe nervous symptoms, as headache, dizziness, nausea, and may terminate in delirium, somnolency, and stupor.

Chronic cystitis is characterized by increased frequency of urination and often pain. The urine looks cloudy, and contains some pus cells.

BIOCHEMIC TREATMENT

Ferrum Phos.—Cystitis, for the pain, heat and fever. Constant urging to urinate in the daytime.

Kali Mur.—Second stage of cystitis when swelling has set in. With discharge of thick, white mucus in the urine. Chronic cystitis, the chief remedy. Dark-colored urine.

Magnes. Phos.—Constant urging to urinate, with straining to pass a few more drops, from spasmodic conditions. All pains of the bladder where heat brings relief. Strangury.

Kali Phos.—Cystitis in asthenic conditions, with prostration. Hemorrhage of the kidney or bladder.

Natr. Mur.—Cutting pain after urinating. Cystitis, with symptoms characteristic of this remedy.

Calc. Phos.—Spasmodic retention of urine if *Magnes. Phos.* fails to bring relief.

Kali Sulph.—Cystitis with discharge of yellow, slimy pus.

Calc. Sulph.—Cystitis, with discharge of pus—third stage.

CLINICAL CASES

Calc. Fluor. in Cystitis:

A Mrs. E., Dallas, Texas, age 62, white. Under one of our leading physicians for several years for chronic cystitis, practically unable to do labor or walk. On close examination found a reflex cystitis, no bladder or urethral lesions, but a rigid bleeding cervix that I diagnosed as carcinoma of the cervix. After about eight months of *Calc. Fluor.*, three every two hours, she attends her house and spades in the garden and has no more symptoms of the trouble. She still continues her medicine.

(Dr. J. M. Jones, Dallas, Tex.)

DEAFNESS

(See Ears, Diseases of.)

DELAYED DEVELOPMENT

(See Marasmus.)

DELIRIUM

(See Brain, Meningitis.)

ETIOLOGY

It will only be necessary, under this head, to give the pathology of delirium tremens, as the remarks under the head of "Brain" will be sufficient for other purposes.

Delirium tremens, or *Mania a Potu,* is due to an uneven distribution of water. When any substance is taken into the human organism that is not needed in its economy, an effort is at once made to get rid of it.

Water is always used as the vehicle to carry off the waste from the system, or to eliminate intruders. When alcoholic drinks are taken, the water in the system is called upon to wash out the poison, as it has no place in the organization of man. Water itself is inert in the human body until it is vitalized with the molecules of sodium chloride; *i. e.*, without this salt, water would not act as a carrier.

A person, by the continual use of alcoholic drinks, breaks up the molecular action of sodium chloride, and thus disturbs the continuity of water in the tissue. A lack of water takes place along the spinal column, spinal cord, solar plexus and nape of the neck, and too much water accumulates at the base of the brain, and, by pressure on nerve centers, produces the hallucinations and delirium.

BIOCHEMIC TREATMENT

Kali Phos.—Delirium tremens; the horrors of drunkards; fear, sleeplessness, restlessness and *suspiciousness; rambling talk; endeavors to avoid imaginary objects.* Alternate with *Natr. Mur.*

Natr. Mur.—Delirium occurring at any time, with low muttering, starting of the body, wandering delirium, *frothy bubbles of saliva on the tongue.* Delirium tremens. Delirium occurring during a low run of fever. "*Natr. Mur.* must be given for the purpose of restoring the normal consistency of brain substance, which, in this disease, is disturbed." (Walker.) Alternate with *Kali Phos.*

Ferrum Phos.—If fever be present; intercurrently or alternately with the chief remedy.

CLINICAL CASES

Natr. Mur. in Delirium Tremens:

I was consulted by the relatives of a man suffering from delirium tremens. I ordered *Natr. Mur.* A complete cure followed speedily. *Natr. Mur.* is the principal remedy, as delirium tremens is caused by a disturbance of the balance of the molecules of sodium chloride and molecules of water in some portion of the brain.
(Schuessler.)

DENTITION

ETIOLOGY

So much has already been said about phosphate of lime in bone tissue, that it will hardly be necessary to urge its use in teething, or show how a deficiency of the salt causes most of the troubles arising from poor development of the teeth. The enamel of teeth is composed principally of the fluoride of lime, and when the edges of the teeth are ragged or the surface rough, this lime-salt should be administered.

BIOCHEMIC TREATMENT

Calc. Phos.—*Calc. Phos.* is the *chief remedy* in teething disorders, to supply material for the bony structure; it promotes the easy cutting of teeth. Do not give *lime water*, the molecules are entirely too coarse to be assimilated readily, and it frequently does harm. *Teething*, when *too late or retarded.* Associated with or without indigestion or non-assimilation of food. Troublesome ailments during teething; open fontanels; slow in learning to walk. If women are known to bear children deficient in the lime-salt, and subject to troublesome teething disorders, they should take occasional doses of *Calc. Phos.* during pregnancy, to overcome this tendency.

Magnes. Phos.—*Chief remedy for the convulsions and spasms of defective dentition.* Alternate with *Calc. Phos.*, to remove the cause. Give in *hot water;* frequent doses.

Ferrum Phos.—When fever is present. Gums swollen and hot.

Calc. Fluor.—Is sometimes necessary, especially when the enamel of the teeth is deficient. Teeth rough and crumble away.

Silicea.—In teething troubles, with *much sweat about the head,* alternately with *Calc. Phos.* Obstinate constipation.

Natr. Mur.—When there is dribbling of saliva from the mouth, when asleep or awake.

CLINICAL CASES

Calc. Phos. and Ferrum Phos. in Teething Infant:

I was called to see a baby seven months old who had been under the care of another physician for two months. I found it fretful, feverish, gums terribly swollen; didn't have a tooth. I gave the mother an ounce of *Calc. Phos.*, instructing her to give two celloids every two hours. I also left with her *Ferrum Phos.*, to be given in alternation for twenty-four to thirty-six hours. The mother called, as per instruction, in ten days and reported the baby had four teeth and had improved in every way. I gave her another supply of *Calc. Phos.* and told her to keep up the celloids, which she did. She now sends every mother, with a teething baby, to me.

(Dr. F. Gordon, Morrilton, Arkansas.)

Ferrum Phos. in Dental Irritation:

Child, 18 months old; hot skin; cheeks highly flushed; sparkling eyes; pupils dilated, and extreme restlessness and irritability. *Ferrum Phos.* in water every hour. The first dose had a decided quieting effect, the child going to sleep shortly after taking it, and the cheeks becoming much less flushed. A few repetitions of the remedy entirely removed all the dental irritations.

(Wilde.)

Calc. Phos. in Dentition:

Child, 18 months old, had cut but two lower lateral incisors, and the molars of lower and upper jaw. Thin, poorly nourished, "pigeon-breast" chest; difficulty in learning to walk; general lack of osseous development. Gave *Calc. Phos.*, three times a day, enough for ten days, corrected nourishment, prescribed cod liver oil. Did not see the case again for three months, when I hardly recognized my scrawny patient. Had now all the incisors, the molars and the "stomach" teeth were beginning to show. Continued treatment as before.

(C. R. Vogel, M. D.)

DIABETES

ETIOLOGY

DIABETES MELLITUS, or true diabetes, is a nutritional disorder characterized by a steady accumulation of sugar in the blood, which is excreted from the system through the urine. Its symptoms are inordinate thirst, ravenous hunger, a greatly increased output of urine containing a varying percentage of sugar, and progressive wasting of the body, with great exhaustion.

Diabetes is essentially a disease of middle adult life, a few cases only occurring among children and old people. It is found principally among the inhabitants of cities rather than in the country. Members of the Jewish race appear peculiarly susceptible to it. Heredity plays some part in creating a predisposition to the disease, although there must always be an exciting cause to bring on its active manifestations.

Overnutrition in persons of a nervous temperament seems the most general condition preceding the average case of diabetes. Josslyn has pointed this out recently, and warns strongly against obesity, as a most potent factor in the causation of diabetes. Autointoxication, the general accompaniment of obesity, undoubtedly has much to answer for in this connection, both by its general poisonous effect upon the system, and especially by its deleterious action on the nervous system. The results are seen in the typical pathological condition present in diabetes, the degeneration of the islands of Langerhans in the pancreas, with the consequent inability of the organism to assimilate sugar.

The nervous origin of diabetes is still further demonstrated by the fact that it may follow serious impairment of the nervous system by shock, overwork, the strain of great responsibility, anxiety, and worry, particularly when associated with close confinement and high living. Cases have also been traced to injuries of the brain and spinal cord, while pregnancy, with its depressing effect upon the nervous system, is often associated with diabetes.

The actual pathological changes occurring in diabetes consist in a degeneration of the islands of Langerhans in the pancreas, while in a very large percentage of cases, the structure of the kidneys is diseased. This results from the increased activity of the kidneys in excreting water and sugar, and by reason of the effect of toxic substances, such as diacetic acid and oxybutyric acid, which, as they are eliminated, damage the renal tissues. The liver, also, is frequently enlarged, sometimes slightly and again to two or three times its normal size. The liver cells are affected, swollen, granular, with a diminished amount or absence of the normal fat contents. The blood contains a large amount of sugar, and sufficient fat to give it a more or less milky appearance.

While the onset of the disease may be very sudden, as after an injury or following severe nervous shock, it usually develops gradually, the suspicions of the patient not being aroused until large amounts of urine are secreted, with insatiable thirst, ravenous hunger, and progressive and usually rapid emaciation.

The urine is pale, watery, acid in reaction, and of high specific gravity, averaging from 1.025 to 1.045. The amount passed in twenty-four hours varies from three or four quarts to several gallons in severe cases. It contains sugar running from one and one-half to two per cent. in mild cases to five, eight, or even ten per cent. in severe cases. There is an unquenchable thirst, worse after eating. The appetite is at first voracious, but may later, if indigestion sets in, become poor, with either constipation or diarrhea. Emaciation is marked and in proportion to the amount of sugar excreted.

As the disease progresses, pulmonary and renal complications are likely to occur, as well as gangrene, especially of the extremities. Death usually comes from one or more of these complications, or from diabetic coma.

DIET

In treating diabetes diet is of the utmost importance. On account of the inability of the system to utilize sugar, sugar and starch must be excluded, and fruits and vegetables containing them must be strictly avoided. Saccharine, if tolerated by the system, or glycerine, may be substituted. Insulin, a preparation of the islands of Langerhans discovered by Dr. Banting of Toronto, when given in proper dosage, will permit the use of sugar to a certain extent in the diet, but it must be administered under skilled medical supervision. Insulin is not curative in the strict sense of the word, but it supplies the missing pancreatic secretion, and gives the diseased islands of Langerhans an opportunity to recuperate.

In prescribing a diet for the diabetic, care must always be taken to watch the patient's general condition, and if rapid emaciation begins, to modify the rigidity of the diet. A suggestion along general lines as to diet follows.

Avoid: All starchy foods, sugar, potatoes and bread, except upon the advice of the physician; rice, tapioca, beans, peas, lentils, turnips, radishes, and all sweet and dried fruits, such as apples, grapes, pears, bananas, peaches, plums, pineapples, raspberries, etc.; wine, beer, brandy, cider, and all alcoholic and sweet drinks.

Allowed: Artichokes, cabbage, celery, cresses, cucumbers, olives, greens, lettuce, pickles, spinach, mushrooms, tomatoes, asparagus, onions; lemons, cherries, (sour) currants, gooseberries, strawberries and other acid fruits; beef, tongue, ham, bacon, mutton, poultry, fish, oysters and other shell-fish, cheese, eggs, butter and pure cream.

The biochemic remedies in diabetes vary with the condition present. Kali Phos. is practically always needed, as it is the lack of this salt which is the chief factor in bringing on the disease, and it is not until the nervous system has been restored to normal that the pancreas can be expected to function normally again. The deranged liver conditions and the excess of water in the system call for Natr. Sulph. Inflammation of the kidneys may cause a strain upon the blood supply that Ferrum Phos. and Calc. Phos. are required to meet. The fearful thirst and rapid emaciation show an unequal distribution of water in the system, for which Natr. Mur. is needed. Every case of diabetes is individual, but by careful superintendence of the diet and hygiene, and the prescription of the indicated biochemic remedies, the best results are to be anticipated.

BIOCHEMIC TREATMENT

Natr. Sulph.—An important remedy in all stages of diabetes. Excessive secretion of urine.

Kali Phos.—*Kali Phos.* is necessary to establish normal function of the medulla oblongata and pneumogastric nerve, which latter acts on the stomach and lungs; the symptoms arising from the disturbed action of these parts are nervous weakness, voracious hunger, sleeplessness, etc. Dr. Schuessler says that perhaps *Kali Sulph.* and *Calc. Sulph.* may also serve as diabetic remedies; while Dr. Walker gave *Ferrum Phos.* and *Natr. Phos.* as an additional tonic, with good results; *Natr. Sulph.* was also given as the chief remedy in each case.

Ferrum Phos.—Diabetes, when there is a *quickened pulse* or when there exist pain, heat or congestion in any part of the system, as an intercurrent or alternate remedy.

Calc. Phos.—Polyuria, with weakness, much thirst, dry mouth and tongue; flabby, sunken abdomen; craves bacon and salt. Glycosuria, when lungs are involved.

Kali Mur.—*Excessive and sugary urine. Great weakness and somnolence.* Note characteristic indications of this remedy.

Natr. Mur.—Polyuria; unquenchable thirst; emaciation; loss of sleep and appetite; *great debility and despondency.*

Diabetic Coma, treatment by Insulin:

In threatened or developed coma the stomach should be promptly emptied, preferably by lavage and liquids given at the rate of one liter every four hours, by mouth, if possible, otherwise normal saline with five per cent sodium bicarbonate rectally, by hypodermoclysis or intravenously in which case the amount should not exceed 1,500 c.c. in twenty-four hours. Glucose, twenty grams every four hours, and 20 to 50 units of Insulin should be administered until consciousness is regained unless sugar disappears from the urine when the amount of Insulin must be decreased. If the patient is unable to swallow, the Glucose five per cent with ten units of Insulin to the pint may be administered intravenously every third to fourth hour until the return of consciousness. The urine should be examined frequently and should continuously show the presence of a small amount of sugar to insure against a rapid fall in the blood sugar with a consequent hypoglycemia, any sign of which must be immediately combated by the further administration of glucose. Under this treatment, uncomplicated diabetic coma is rarely fatal.

DIARRHEA

ETIOLOGY

The cause of diarrhea is generally found in an imperfect digestion and assimilation of food. Or it may be due to climatic conditions, living in damp localities, the laxative properties of foods, or the frequent use of purgative medicines or any other irritative substances. The proper balance of the inorganic salts in the digestive fluids becomes disturbed, and non-assimilation is the result.

But diarrhea in typhoid fever may be caused by the decaying organic matter, together with the waste tissue finding an outlet through the intestines.

BIOCHEMIC TREATMENT

Ferrum Phos.—Diarrhea caused from a relaxed state of the villi or absorbents of the intestines, finds a remedy in *Ferrum*

Phos. Owing to this relaxed condition, the usual amount of moisture is not absorbed. Diarrhea, when the stools consist of undigested food. Diarrhea caused by a chill. *Diarrheas, with watery, frequent stools, fever and thirst;* alternate with remedies indicated by the color of stool. A copious injection of hot water, in the first stage of diarrhea, will cleanse the mucous membrane and greatly aid in a cure. If caused from relaxed state of the villi, it will often produce a cure without recourse to medication.

Natr. Phos.—Diarrhea caused from excessive acidity; *stools are sour-smelling and green. Diarrheas* of teething children, with the above symptoms; often *associated with worms;* note coating of tongue, which is yellow or creamy looking at the back part. Summer diarrheas, with lack of digestive power or *from eating unripe fruit.*

Calc. Phos.—One of the most valuable remedies for the diarrhea of teething children, due to non-assimilation of food; alternate with remedy indicated by color of stool. *Diarrhea of rachitic children. Calc. Phos., Ferrum Phos.* and *Natr. Phos.* cover nearly all the symptoms in diarrhea of infants and larger children, which are generally caused from non-assimilation of food, or from becoming chilled. *Stools are hot, watery, offensive, profuse and sputtering;* sometimes green or undigested.

Kali Mur.—*Diarrhea, with light-colored, pale-yellow, ochre or clay-colored stools,* denoting a deficiency of bile; also *Kali Sulph.* Diarrhea in typhoid fever, with stools as above. White or slimy stools in *diarrhea after eating rich, fatty food.* Diarrhea, with white-coated tongue and other characteristic symptoms. Bloody or slimy stools.

Kali Phos.—Diarrhea, with foul-smelling, putrid discharges from the bowels, to heal the underlying conditions. *Diarrhea, with evacuations like rice-water.* Diarrhea, with depression and exhaustion; offensive stools, with or without pain.

Kali Sulph.—Diarrhea, with yellow, watery, mattery stools; sometimes cramps in the bowels. If *Magnes. Phos.* does not relieve. Observe color of tongue, which should be light-yellow, especially at root.

Natr. Mur.—*Diarrhea, with watery, slimy, transparent stools,* or of glairy slime, caused frequently by an excessive use of salt. Diarrhea alternating with constipation. Stools cause soreness and smarting.

Natr. Sulph.—In diarrhea, with mattery, dark or green, bilious stools. *Chronic diarrhea,* with *loose, morning watery stools;* worse in cold, damp or wet weather. *Natr. Sulph.* controls the excess of water. Diarrhea in typhoid fever and bilious stools. Diarrheas of old people.

Calc. Sulph.—Evacuations mattery, or blood and matter.

Magnes. Phos.—Diarrhea, with cramp-like pain in the bowels, flatulent colic; relieved by hot applications. Alternate with remedies indicated by color of stools.

Silicea.—*Infantile diarrhea;* cadaverous-smelling; *after vaccination;* with much *acid perspiration on head,* and hard, hot, distended abdomen.

CLINICAL CASES

Magnes. Phos. and Calc. Phos. in Diarrhea:

Among the first cases in which I tried these remedies was a negro child, about two months old. The following are about the symptoms presented: Painful diarrhea; constant rolling of the head; eyes turned up; tongue brownish-yellow; no desire to nurse for some time. The mother said it had been sick for a week, and she had been giving it different things, but as it got worse, she called me. I told her I thought there was little chance for its recovery, but I would do what I could for it. Prescribed *Magnes. Phos.* and *Calc. Phos.*, in alternation, every fifteen minutes. This was about 9 or 10 o'clock a. m. I returned about 3 o'clock p. m., to see if it were still alive, and, to my astonishment, found it better. It had ceased rolling its head; eyes were natural; had nursed once or twice, and was sleeping. Ordered the medicine continued at longer intervals. The next morning it was considerably better. At this visit I found the tongue covered with a thick, *white* coating, and the mouth sore. I now prescribed *Kali Mur.*, the remedy for this condition, in place of the *Calc. Phos.*, to be alternated with the *Magnes. Phos. every hour.* The next day the tongue was clear, and after leaving a few more doses, to be continued for a day or two longer, the case was dismissed.

(E. H. H.)

Natr. Sulph. in morning Diarrhea:

Morning diarrhea on rising; sudden urging, gushing accompanied with flatulence. The stool splatters all over the vessel. *Natr. Sulph.* cured.

(C. Lippe.)

Calc. Sulph. in chronic Diarrhea:

Dr. Goullon relates a case of chronic diarrhea of two years' standing. Stools of mushy consistence; coated tongue; cured with *Calc. Sulph.*

Natr. Sulph. in chronic Diarrhea, morning aggravation:

Dr. T. F. Allen cured a case of chronic diarrhea in an old lady, with morning aggravation on beginning to move, with *Natr. Sulph.*

(N. A. J. H.)

Natr. Sulph. in chronic Diarrhea:

Natr. Sulph. has served me well in the treatment of chronic diarrhea of long standing; characterized by profuse gushing stools early in the morning; the character of stool found in a greater or less extent under all natrum salts. It seems as well to suit catarrhs generally of mucous membranes characterized by a tendency to profuse secretions of mucus. *Calc. Phos.*, if persisted in, seems generally sufficient to be alternated with other remedies as intercurrents for the ever-changing and shifting symptoms that are usually ingrafted upon these conditions.

DIPHTHERIA

ETIOLOGY

THIS disease occurs for the most part in children, although adults occasionally suffer from it. It is caused by the Klebs-Loeffler bacillus, and is very dangerous, the toxin created by the bacillus having a marked weakening effect upon the heart, in addition to the strain caused by difficulty in breathing, due to the diphtheritic membrane.

Like all other diseases due to germs, however, the real cause of diphtheria is found in a cell-salt deficiency. When for any reason the union between Kali Mur. and fibrin is broken down, the fibrin thus set free must be eliminated from the system. On occasions where this fibrin has been set free in the vicinity of the mucous membrane of the nose and throat, it is naturally eliminated there. This establishes a suitable breeding place for the Klebs-Loeffler bacillus, and a case of diphtheria is initiated.

The trouble will continue until the missing cell-salt Kali Mur. has been supplied, and the fibrin becoming united with it, has restored the mucous membrane to normal. The bacillus, losing its breeding place, will disappear, and the disease will go with it.

Biochemistry has no quarrel with the germ theory. It is a permanently established fact in medicine that germs do exist, and that they cause disease. But it is equally true, and as well proven, that a breeding place in the tissues must be found for them, before they can increase and multiply. This breeding place can only be provided when the tissues are weakened by a lack of cell-salts and, in consequence, the organic substances with which they are united.

Nor can a return to health be expected until the integrity of the tissues has been restored by providing the lacking cell-salts, establishing their union with the organic substances with which they work, and thus depriving the invading germs of their breeding place.

Furthermore, biochemistry has no argument against the administration of antitoxin in diphtheria. It is recognized that this is only a means of introducing from outside an antidote to the toxins which the bacillus is forming in the blood, and which may otherwise destroy the body before the cell-salts have had time to unite with their organic material.

But in no way does this lessen the necessity of supplying the cell-salts, nor can a complete, permanent cure be expected until this is done.

DIET

Ordinary precautions should be observed in regard to diet, but to set any special rule would be absurd; as each patient is a law unto himself in this respect. During an acute attack of disease, the diet should be light and generally unstimulating. A good general rule is to *never* overload the stomach; a *true* appetite or craving will be found a cry of nature and should be satisfied—but in moderation. Common sense should always govern the diet during disease.

BIOCHEMIC TREATMENT

Ferrum Phos.—In the first stage of diphtheria, for the febrile symptoms, in alternation with *Kali Mur.*

Kail Mur.—Should be given early in alternation with *Ferrum Phos.*, in a majority of cases. A gargle of *Kali Mur.* (ten or fifteen grains in a glass of water) should be used very frequently, to control the plastic exudation.

Natr. Mur.—When vomiting of watery fluids or watery diarrhea sets in. When the face is puffy and pale, associated with drowsiness or excessive flow of saliva from the mouth. Dryness of tongue, stertorous breathing.

Natr. Sulph.—If the *fluids vomited are green* or *with bitter taste, Natr. Sulph.* is the remedy, and should be given in alternation with the chief remedy. Welling-up of mucus in the throat.

Kail Phos.—For *exhaustion* or *prostration* in any stage of the disease, also the well-marked malignant conditions of the latter stages; *after-effects of diphtheria,* weakness of sight, loss of speech or paralysis in any part of the body, require this remedy.

Calc. Fluor.—If from mismanagement the disease has gone to the trachea, this remedy will be needed in alternation with *Calc. Phos.* "Such a complication is very rare when the biochemic remedies are used." (B. & D.)

Calc. Phos.—Diphtheric exudation spreading to the trachea. Such a complication is very rare when the tissue remedies are used exclusively. A white speck or patch remains after the main exudation has come off. (B. & D.) After diphtheria, also as an intercurrent remedy during the disease.

Natr. Phos.—Diphtheritic throat, falsely so-called, when the *roof of mouth, tonsils and back part of tongue are covered with a moist, creamy, yellow coating.* In speaking of diphtheria Dr. Schuessler says: "Under no circumstances should other remedies, such as lime-water, carbolic acid, iced water, etc., be used along with these remedies, because they may interfere with the proper action of these salts."

CLINICAL CASES

After Effects from Diphtheria:

Mrs. C., age 41, developed a case of diphtheria the second day after her return from a hospital, where she had been for treatment. The family physician was called, who administered 1,000 units of antitoxin. The following day 5,000 more units were administered, after which the patient made a good recovery. About three weeks later she returned to her family physician complaining of a numbness in all of her extremities. Various remedies were prescribed with no effect. She again returned to her physician, and again received no relief. After three or four weeks of treatment, with no results, she called at my office. Her condition was such that when walking across the floor she was not conscious of her feet touching the floor, or upon picking up an object she could not tell if she had the object in her hand unless she looked to see.

I prescribed for her *Calc. Phos.*, three grain celloids, and *Kali Phos.*, three grain celloids, alternately, every two hours. At the end of one week she returned to my office much improved. I continued the above treatment for another week, and to the satisfaction of both the patient and myself, she had made a complete recovery, none of the symptoms ever having returned.

(Dr. John W. Purdy, Long Rapids, Michigan.)

The prophylaxis and antitoxin treatment of Diphtheria:

The immunization against diphtheria by toxin-antitoxin has been proved to be a positive factor in preventive medicine. In New York City with an estimated population of over seven million, the annual death rate per thousand population for the last quarter of 1931 shows .03 with an annual case rate of .56. Among thirteen thousand exposed persons receiving immunization injections only three-tenths in one per cent had a subsequent mild grade of diphtheria with only one death.

Recent advances in the procedure of diphtheria immunization have been made, the immunization agent has been improved upon as has the method of administration. Toxoid, which is more active in immunization than toxin-antitoxin, contains no serum and its use eliminates any sensitization to the protein of serum. Toxoid is given in doses of ½ c.c. for three injections, one week apart.

If toxin-antitoxin is used the first dose will determine susceptibility and so serves the purpose of the Schick test, whereas if toxoid be used an initial Schick test would be necessary.

The figures above quoted are far below the average incidence of diphtheria among children not immunized, hence it would seem that this disease might well be placed among the conditions classed as preventable, and that such measures of prevention should be universally adopted, diphtheria being one of the great communicable scourges of childhood.

The low mortality of diphtheria treated early with antitoxin has made its therapeutic use almost universal in the medical profession. It is recommended that it be given as early as possible as the results are better the sooner after the onset of the disease the antitoxin is administered. In its improved form there are no contra-indications to its use. In suspicious cases antitoxin should be given without waiting for a report on the cultures from the nose and throat. Two thousand units should be given in mild cases of faucial or nasal diphtheria, increasing from three to five thousand units in more severe cases. In laryngeal diphtheria from five to ten thousand units should be given at the first dose and this may be repeated in twelve hours in stenosis if the respiratory difficulty is not ameliorated. The later in the disease antitoxin treatment is started the larger the initial dose should be.

The injection of antitoxin should be made into the loose subcuticular tissues in the pectoral or the iliac regions through skin made surgically clean and the wound sealed with collodion. The pseudomembrane, after the injection of antitoxin, slowly tends to become detached. In laryngeal cases where the membrane is below the range of visibility, the decreasing symptoms of obstruction give evidences of its good effect. The hypertrophied lymph nodes decrease in size and the general symptoms are all improved.

Locally, in children old enough to gargle, the use of a common salt solution, one gram to the pint, will assist in removing the loosened membrane. In nasal cases an irrigation of the saline solution will keep the nose clear and clean. Sometimes the mouth and throat may be irrigated with the same solution if gargling is not sufficient or in the case of younger children. The solution used for this purpose should be at a temperature between 105° and 110° F.

Intubation:

A life saving measure in laryngeal diphtheria with obstruction of breathing is available in O'Dwyer's tubes, which should be within immediate reach of anyone caring for cases of this serious disease, as often when they are needed the time is short. Intubation should be performed when there is marked dyspnea, restlessness, retraction of the epigastric and supraclavicular spaces with evidence of cyanosis.

The tube should be left in the larynx until there is marked improvement in general symptoms and decrease in the laryngeal obstruction. If cyanosis should follow the removal of the tube it must be replaced at once. Intubated cases are best fed in the prone position with the head lower than the body.

Tracheotomy:

Tracheotomy should be performed only when intubation is unsuccessful in relieving the laryngeal obstruction. This is most often when the tube forces the membrane lower down in the larynx, where the membranes form below the end of the tube or in edema of the glottis. An emergency tracheotomy may be performed in a few minutes with few instruments and the edges of the trachea retracted with small wire hooks until a suitable tracheotomy tube and cannula are obtained. When either intubation or tracheotomy is done but particularly with the latter, moist air should be made available for the patient to breathe as dry air is exceedingly irritating to the larynx and bronchi. As in the cases of intubation, removal of the tracheotomy cannula must be experimental with preparations made for replacement if the breathing is not satisfactory without it.

An exceedingly important but often neglected precaution in the care of all diphtheria cases is enforced rest in bed. Even in mild cases this program must be rigidly followed as the paralyzing effect of the toxin of diphtheria on the heart is not always apparent while the patient lies quiet but becomes suddenly evident when any effort is made to get up. Paralysis of the heart is sometimes the result of neglect of this precaution and frequently with fatal results. Post-diphtheritic paralysis of other muscles occurs in a small percentage of cases but there is a tendency to spontaneous recovery in a large majority of such instances.

DIZZINESS

(See Vertigo.)

Kali Phos.—Especially indicated in *cases of nervous character,* without any marked dyspeptic symptoms. Best effects derived if given immediately after meals.

DROPSY

(See Kidneys, Affections of.)

ETIOLOGY

The origin of dropsy is a deficiency of calcium phosphate and sodium chloride in the blood and blood-serum.

Then, the water and albumen, not having the needed workmen to properly diffuse them, accumulate in the connective tissue.

Other salts become deficient as the disease progresses. One peculiarity of this condition is that the pores of the skin become chronically closed and the patient rarely perspires. The closed pores, of course, cause a large amount of waste to remain in the body, and unless removed by artificial means, adds to the accumulation in the tissues.

BIOCHEMIC TREATMENT

Kali Mur.—*Dropsy* arising *from heart, liver or kidney disease,* when the characteristic symptoms are present. When the liquid drawn off is whitish or white mucus in the urine; also *white coating of tongue.* Dropsy arising from weakness of the heart, with palpitation; this remedy in alternation with *Kali Phos. Dropsy from obstruction of the bile-ducts,* indicated by a white or grayish-white coated tongue.

Natr. Sulph.—Simple dropsy invading any of the areolar tissues of the body. Dropsy, internal or external. Hydrocele. Alternating or intercurrently with other remedies to eliminate the water in the tissues.

Natr. Mur.—To be given in alternation with *Natr. Sulph.* in a majority of cases of simple dropsy or dropsical swellings. Hydrocele. Post-scarlatinal dropsy.

Calc. Phos.—Ferrum Phos.—*Dropsy* arising *from loss of blood,* anemia, non-assimilation, etc., requires these remedies in alternation.

Calc. Fluor.—Dropsy arising from heart disease; dilation of any of the cavities. Hydrocele, when from a strain.

Kali Sulph.—Post-scarlatinal dropsy.

CLINICAL CASES

Natr. Mur. in post-scarlatinal Dropsy:

A little girl, æt. 9, had recovered from diphtheria and scarlatina rather easily, and was allowed to be in the convalescent room. Suddenly she began to swell without any apparent cause. Her face became puffy; the feet also edematous to above the ankle. Urine somewhat decreased, containing no albumen. No pain over the kidneys on pressure. Pulse somewhat feverish, but appetite, sleep and stools natural. I gave three different medicines without success. Dropsy (*Anasarca et Ascites*) was increasing rapidly; urine became scanty; only very small quantities occasionally, being slightly turbid and containing much albumen. Whether any epithelial sheathings were

present was not ascertained. Kidneys were now more sensitive to pressure. Occasionally delirious. *Natr. Mur.* alone cured this case in about a fortnight.
(Dr. Cohn. From Schuessler.)

Natr. Mur. in Scarlatinal Dropsy:

Scarlatinal dropsy in a child, æt. 4. Quantity of urine voided in twenty-four hours was very scanty, and during the past forty-eight hours had ceased entirely. The patient was fearfully anasarcous. Reclining position was impossible. *Natr. Mur.* every two hours. In twenty-four hours the child voided two quarts of urine and a speedy recovery followed.

Kali Mur. in chronic Swelling of Feet:

Dr. Goullon, Jr., who used *Kali Mur.* with much success in a swelling of the feet and lower extremities, adds the following particular indications for its use: The remedy in question appears indicated in chronic persistent swelling of the feet and lower limbs, when the swelling is soft at first; afterwards becoming hard to the touch, without pain or redness. It is, however, itchy; and at one stage may be termed snowy-white and shining. Lastly, the swelling becomes less perceptible in the morning than in the evening, but may acquire such dimensions as to cause great tension, with a feeling as if it would burst.

DROWSINESS

(See Sleep.)

DYSENTERY

ETIOLOGY

The same general causes as for diarrhea are applicable to dysentery, except that dysentery is an exaggerated form of diarrhea in which certain germs have found a breeding ground in the diseased membranes of the intestines. In this case there is a deficiency of iron molecules in the walls of the blood-vessels, giving rise to hemorrhage, inflammation, etc. The water in the system is either in excess or is unevenly distributed, allowing watery stools. As a secondary symptom, the Magnes. Phos. molecules become disturbed, giving rise to cramps, spasms, etc., in the bowels and abdomen. The exciting causes are: suddenly checked perspiration, especially during or just after a spell of warm weather. Becoming chilled in the evening after perspiring heavily through the day. Suppression of piles; local irritation, such as worms; living in marshy places; and in infants cutting teeth.

Symptoms are: Constant urging to empty the bowels; straining; cramp-like pains in the abdomen; fever, stools of either mucus or blood, or both. The attack sometimes appears suddenly, but is frequently preceded by loss of appetite, costiveness, sickness of the stomach, fever, pain in the bowels. The discharges are increased and soon nothing is discharged but white mucus, which may change to blood; very frequent and foul-smelling stools. Ulceration or gangrene of the bowels may result if it is not checked in time; but under the proper biochemic treatment it loses its terrors.

BIOCHEMIC TREATMENT

Kali Mur.—This remedy, in alternation with *Ferr. Phos.*, is generally sufficient to cure this disease if taken in time. Intense (steady) pain in the abdomen, or cutting pain, with almost *constant urging to stool, tenesmus and purging. Stools are slimy, pale-yellow, sanious.*

Ferrum Phos.—In alternation with *Kali Mur.*, for the febrile disturbance, fever, inflammatory pain, etc. *Stools hot and watery.*

Kali Phos.—Dysentery, with *putrid, offensive stools,* dry tongue, etc. *Evacuations* consist *of pure blood;* patient becomes delirious, abdomen swells and the discharges have a putrid smell.

Calc. Sulph.—*Mattery, sanious stools,* or stools of matter mixed with blood. After *Kali Mur.*

CLINICAL CASES

Calc. Sulph. in Dysentery:

Dr. E. H. Holbrook reports a case of dysentery which was greatly relieved by *Calc. Sulph.* Turning into a bilious diarrhea, *Natr. Sulph.*, cured.

Magnes. Phos. for Tenesmus and Tormina:

Lady complaining of extreme tenesmus and tormina, and constant desire to pass water and go to stool. Every time this pain came on, must rise and bend forward, and the only relief obtained was from hot water. *Magnes. Phos.*, every fifteen minutes, cured in third dose.

(Dr. Reed.)

Magnes. Phos. in Dysentery:

In treating a case of dysentery lately, I was at my wits' end to control the terrible pain in defecation. The stools were growing less frequent, but the pain was increasing, being so severe as to cause fainting. Something had to be done if I held my case. The pain in rectum and abdomen was very severe; more in rectum than abdomen. The tenesmus was like prolonged spasm of the muscles employed in defecation. I gave *Magnes. Phos.* in hot water. A hypodermic of morphia could hardly have acted more quickly. The pain was almost entirely relieved by the first dose. The whole condition changed for the better, and I discharged my case the next day. In all my experience I never had a more prompt or pleasing result. *Magnes. Phos.* is a wonderful antispasmodic, and fully as reliable as our more frequently used remedies. I was led to think of it for my case of dysentery by a statement made to me by Dr. E. E. Snyder, of Binghamton, New York. He gave it with equally as prompt results in spasmodic tenesmus vesicæ occurring in a case of cystitis resulting from gonorrhea. It certainly did me great service.

(H. K. Leonard, M. D.)

DYSMENORRHEA

ETIOLOGY

Dysmenorrhea, or painful menstruation, may be due to several causes. *First,* a mechanical obstruction of the uterus; *second,* a contraction of the muscular fibers of the womb, causing a hardened condition; and, *third,* an excessive congestion of blood to the womb. There are several other causes, but they are rarely met with. By far the greatest number of cases are due to the last two named causes.

Owing to taking frequent colds, lack of proper exercise, improper diet, etc., there results a determination of blood to the uterus; the veins, becoming engorged, press upon the sensory nerves, which, in turn, cause the muscular fibers to contract and close the mouth of the womb. In order for the menstrual discharge to pass, it is necessary for Nature to force the way—which becomes a very painful proceeding.

These consist principally of sharp cramp or labor-like pains over the region of the womb and in the lower part of the abdomen. These pains usually come several hours before the discharge appears, but at times they are present during the flow. The menstrual discharge varies from a bright red to a deep black. At times a membrane is thrown off, which is an indication of the amount of inflammation.

The pains are usually described as colicky, bearing-down, dragging, griping, etc. At times severe nausea and headache are present, but they are secondary symptoms. The disease reappears at each succeeding month, and frequently increases in severity till the pains become almost unbearable.

BIOCHEMIC TREATMENT

Ferrum Phos.—*Painful menstruation,* with *bright, red flow,* flushed face and quick pulse; sometimes with vomiting of undigested food. *Membraneous dysmenorrhea.* Excessive congestion at the periods; the vagina is dry and very sensitive.

Ferrum Phos. should be taken before the periods as a preventive, if the case be chronic. This remedy, alternated with *Kali Phos.,* and occasional doses of *Calc. Phos.,* if taken steadily, is almost a specific for this disease. *Magnes. Phos.* should be used for the excessive crampy pain. "The intense pain is due to a spasm of the muscular fibres, caused by the excessive congestion of the parts. *Magnes. Phos.* relieves the spasm, while *Ferrum Phos.,* given before the period, prevents the congestion. (Chapman.)

Magnes. Phos.—Is the *chief remedy for* the excessive *crampy pain* in dysmenorrhea. Pains just before the flow begins, or coming on after it has begun, and are slightly checked. Warmth is soothing. A small quantity of the remedy should be dissolved in hot water, and applied with cloths (as hot as can be borne) immediately over the uterus; also internally in hot water.

Kali Phos.—Menstrual colic in *pale, lachrymose, irritable, sensitive females* from lack of proper nerve power; alternate with *Ferr. Phos.* Flow deep red, or dark red.

CLINICAL CASES

Magnes. Phos. in Dysmenorrhea:

Miss S., æt. 22; brunette; short, plump, round body; large, active brain; intellectual; was since puberty troubled every month with dysmenorrhea, beginning several hours previous, and during the first day of flow, with severe pains in the uterus, back and lower limbs, and these so severe that they seemed unbearable and hysteria seemed threatening. In one of these attacks I was sent for. Found the patient in bed; the feet had been bathed in hot water and hot cloths applied for hours to the lower abdomen; pains no better. I immediately gave her a large dose of *Magnes. Phos.* In less than half an hour the pain lessened; I repeated the dose; in a few moments the patient was easy, the flow began, and went on the usual time. Next month I advised the patient to begin

the day before period, and take three doses, and on the day period was to come on take a dose every two hours. No pains this month. This process was repeated the third month; no more trouble; patient is now well, and no return of pain for over three years.
(*Med. Advance.*)

Magnes. Phos. in Dysmenorrhea:

At each menstrual period a membrane, varying in size from one to two inches in length, was discharged. Her symptoms were: After the flow began, severe, sharp, shooting pains low down in the abdomen. Relieved by lying curled up in bed with a hot water bag on the abdomen. When the severe pains ceased, a dull aching for a day or two followed, and the next, or the following day, a membrane passed. With this exception was in very good health. After one of her periods I gave her *Magnes. Phos.* in water, a dose night and morning, for two days. The next menstrual period was nearly free from pain, and the succeeding ones were painless, but the usual membrane was passed. Before this she had always remained in bed. Painless menstruation went on for six or eight months, when she got her feet wet just before her menses, and received *Magnes. Phos.* It relieved her, and she has had no trouble since.
(S. A. Kimball.)

Kali Phos. cured her Dysmenorrhea after all else failed:

Dr. D. B. Whittier reports the cure of a dysmenorrhea of fifteen years' standing (in a highly neurotic and hysterical woman) by a course of *Kali Phos.* continuing over six months, after other medicines had failed. Some of the symptoms were: The mammæ were so painful that the touch of her clothing was unbearable. The menstrual pains were cramp-like, with severe bearing-down in the hypogastrium, and most severe after the flow commenced. When the suffering was most intense, a sharp, shooting pain would extend from hypogastrium to the epigastrium, followed by a sensation as if something were flowing up to the stomach, and immediately succeeded by a vomiting of bile or frothy acid substances, sometimes streaked with blood. The vomiting would relieve the painful distress of the stomach, when the uterine pains would be increased and sometimes continue for twenty-four hours. A headache, at first general, soon settled over the left eye. When the headache was severe the pains elsewhere were lessened, and *vice versa*. The first menstrual period following the administration of the *Kali Phos.* was comparatively comfortable, and her condition continued to improve with further treatment along these lines.

Magnes. Phos. in Dysmenorrhea with intra-uterine exfoliations:

Dysmenorrhea that had lasted for some time: in each menstrual period a membrane was discharged, varying in size from one to two inches long. The pains came on after the flow began, low down, in the abdomen, and were relieved by lying curled up in bed with a hot water bag on the abdomen. The pains would last for a day—dull, aching—and next day, or day after, a membrane would be passed. I gave her, after one of her menstrual periods, *Magnes. Phos.*, one dose dry. The next menstruation was somewhat easier. *Magnes. Phos.* in water for two days, night and morning, and the next menstrual period was painless, though she passed the membrane, as before. After that the menses were perfectly painless.

(Dr. Campbell.)

Magnes. Phos. in pains centered in pit of Stomach:

I had a patient with very severe, shooting, neuralgic pains during the menstrual period. The pains were in the stomach, and lasted the first day or two. Commenced in the back and came directly around and centered in the pit of the stomach. They were relieved by heat and pressure. *Magnes. Phos.*, given frequently in hot water, relieved the pain and after a few months' treatment at the menstrual periods, she was cured.

(T. J. Kent, M. D.)

DYSPEPSIA

(See Gastric Derangements.)

EAR, DISEASES OF

ETIOLOGY

The pathology of diseases of the ear is very similar to that of other mucous membranes. A deficiency of Kali Mur. causes an excess of fibrin which endeavors to make its way out of the system through the mucous membranes of the ear, and thus causes clogging of the eustachian tubes, trouble in the labyrinth and mastoid cells. A deficiency of Ferr. Phos., occurring at the same time, may cause inflammation and fever. Deficiencies in other cell-salts may result in characteristic symptoms.

BIOCHEMIC TREATMENT

Ferrum Phos.—Diseases of the ear in the inflammatory stage, with fever, pain, congestion, etc. Inflammatory earache; pain is burning and throbbing. *Earache, with sharp stitching pains,* due to inflammation; hot outward applications relieve by making counter-irritation; but cold, directly on the seat of pain (in the ear), relieves by reducing the congestion. Noises in the ears through blood pressure from relaxed condition of the veins not returning the blood properly; noises in the ears simliar to those which arise after taking quinine. "Noticeable pulsation in the ear, every impulse of the heart is felt here, beating in the ear and head, the pulse can be counted." (Houghton.)

Chronic inflammation of the ear and eustachian tubes, *causing deafness* (*Kali Mur.*). A ringing in the ears from engorgement of blood.

Kali Mur.—A very important remedy in treatment of disease of the ear when, *after* inflammation, the *membranes become thickened,* causing deafness. *Deafness* caused *from* *swelling of the eustachian tubes.* Can hear better when there is confusion, such as in a street car, or in a mill. Deafness, with swelling of the glands of the ear; cracking noises in the ear on blowing the nose or when swallowing. Earache, with swelling of the glands or membranes of the throat or ear; the tongue generally has a white or grayish-white coating. *Catarrh of the middle ear,* with *white discharge.* Chronic inflammations of the internal or external ear.

Kali Phos.—*Deafness,* with noises in the ear *from nervous exhaustion.* Deafness from want of nervous perception; noises in the head, with weakness and confusion; confused noises make hearing worse. *Ulceration* of the ear, with suppuration, *pus* being *dirty, foul* and *ichorous,* with very *offensive odor.* Atrophic conditions of the ear, especially in old people.

Magnes. Phos.—Deafness or dullness of hearing from weakness of the auditory nerves. Follows *Kali Phos.,* where that remedy is indicated, but does not give relief. *Earache* purely *nervous in character.* Neuralgic pains in and around the ear.

Kali Sulph.—*Earache, with thin, yellow, watery matter.* Catarrh of the ears, with discharge of thin, yellow, greenish matter (also daily injections of the same, in tepid water). Sharp pains under the ear; cutting and stitching pain. Deafness from swelling of the tympanic cavity. Catarrhal conditions, with swelling of the membranes, if discharging a thin, yellow matter; the tongue has a yellow, slimy coating.

Calc. Phos.—*Cold feeling of outer ears.* The bones around the ear hurt and ache. Earache, with rheumatic complaints, associated with swollen glands in *scrofulous children.* Chronic otorrheas in children, associated with painful dentition.

Natr. Mur.—Deafness from swelling of the cavities, with watery discharges and watery condition of the tongue; tongue covered with bubbles and excessive flow of saliva.

Calc. Sulph.—Deafness, with discharge of thick matter, sometimes mixed with blood; to control suppuration. Compare with *Silicea*.

Silicea.—Inflammatory swelling of the external meatus. *Foul, purulent discharges from the ear.* Gatherings of the ear, to promote suppuration. Dullness of hearing, with swelling and catarrh of the eustachian tubes, with characteristic discharge indicating this remedy.

Natr. Phos.—External ear sore; outer part covered with thin, cream-like scabs. Note also color of tongue. "One ear red, hot and frequently itchy, accompanied by gastric derangement and acidity." (Walker.)

CLINICAL CASES

Kali Mur., Magnes. Phos. in Deafness:

Edna R., æt. 9 years; deafness. The history of this case is as follows: Five years ago she commenced to have frequent spells of high fever and severe pain in head and ears, followed by swelling of the muscles of the neck and stiffness of the neck. These spells would last, at first, for two or three days, but increase in length of time and intensity, so that when I took the case they lasted from one to three weeks, and kept her confined to her bed. Three years ago her hearing was almost gone, and remained so until I took the case, when I had to speak loudly to make her hear me. Flushing the ears with hot water, quite frequently, was suggested, which did no good. For the first three months I gave her *Kali Mur.* and *Magnes. Phos.*, three small powders of each daily; after that only two of each a day. Improvement set in at once and the pain and sick spells ceased and her hearing improved, until at present it is almost as good as ever. I also gave, for the first few weeks, *Ferrum Phos.*, for the fever symptoms.

Ferrum Phos. in Otitis Media:

Dr. Wanstall reports three cases cured by the use of *Ferrum Phos.*, with results the most gratifying, controlling the high fever, delirium and pain accompanying the acute middle ear inflammation.

Kali Sulph. in Polypoid Growths producing Deafness:

Case of a young girl, light complexioned, scrofulous, with brown, offensive discharges from right ear. Polypoid growth, or excrescence, closed the meatus near the opening. For eight weeks she had been entirely deaf in this ear, the deafness having gradually increased for four months. *Kali Sulph.* given. In two weeks the offensiveness had entirely disappeared. On examination, found polypus shriveled to a hard, black mass. The hearing had entirely returned. Every third day two doses were taken. This case was entirely cured. (W. P. Wesselhoeft, M. D.)

Kali Mur. in Otitis Externa and Otorrhea:

Dr. Stanley Wilde reports a case of otitis externa, with subsequent otorrhea and deafness, the latter resisting several remedies. The case presented a thickening and narrowing of the meatus, with a thin, flaky discharge therefrom, watch-hearing four inches. *Kali Mur.* stopped the discharge, and the hearing became normal. Dr. Wilde has used this remedy with good effect in eustachian deafness in children from chronic enlargement of the tonsils.

Kali Phos. in Tinnitus Aurium:

Dr. Goullon reports a case of an old gentleman who suffered greatly with a buzzing in the ears, which was made much worse in the noisy street. The patient had repeated attacks of inflammatory rheumatism, and the tinnitus was probably of a rheumatic origin. Mentally, much depressed. Difficult hearing. After a few days' use of *Kali Phos.*, all symptoms, including the mental condition and difficult hearing, permanently disappeared.

Silicea in Mastoid Periostitis:

Dr. A. T. Sherman, of Minnesota, reports a case of a man who had suffered for six days with pain in mastoid region. On examination, found the tympanic membrane highly injected; tuning-fork was heard indifferently on each side when pressed against parietal bones; hearing impaired on the affected side. Temperature 102. Very weak; nervous; complete muscular paralysis of right side of face. The condition of the sense of hearing precluded brain disease. There was no difficulty in swallowing, or other evidence of paralysis of the muscles of the fauces, which placed the trouble beyond the origin of the petrosal nerve. There was no disturbance of taste or of the salivary glands, which placed the trouble beyond the origin of the chorda tympani. He diagnosed mastoid periostitis, with pressure on the seventh nerve immediately on its exit from the duct of Fallopius. Gave *Silicea,* a dose every three hours. In forty-eight hours all pain had ceased, and temperature normal.

Kali Phos. and Silicea in Otitis:

A gentleman wrote me the symptoms of otitis of a little child, æt. four months, who had a discharge from one ear of an ichorous, thin, offensive character, producing an eruption wherever the pus came in contact with the integument. I at once sent *Kali Phos.,* ordering it given every six hours. In three months the running had all ceased, and the hearing was perfect. I frequently use *Silicea* in alternation with *Kali Phos.,* when the connective tissue is involved.
(A. P. Davis, M. D.)

Silicea in Suppuration of Mastoid:

A patient with a case of "otitis catarrhalis internus" came into my office to see me. This case was the most remarkable that I have ever witnessed or treated. The man was a tall, slim, sanguine, nervous specimen of the *genus homo.* There was an enormous protuberance involving the whole mastoid region, the skin red and glistening, soft, pappy, showing signs of an induration, and broken-down connective tissue, the whole mass filled with pus, and emitting an odor that was as sickening as carrion. I at once plunged a knife into the mastoid process, out of which ran about half a pint of blood and pus.

After cleansing the tumor with a local antiseptic, I bound up the wound, leaving in it a drainage-tube. I treated the wound every day, putting him under the influence of *Silicea,* a dose every two hours. Under the treatment, I had the satisfaction of seeing him improve from day to day, and in four weeks the whole trouble ceased. He had no relapse, but the cure advanced steadily until he was well.
(A. P. Davis, M. D.)

Ferrum Phos. in deafness from chronic Catarrh of Middle Ear:

Wm. McKee, æt. 27, suffers from deafness, due to chronic non-suppurative catarrh of the middle ear. This was caused by contracting one cold after another, until he found himself a sufferer from chronic catarrh of the nose and throat, the discharge being continual and very annoying. At this time (about six years ago) he noticed a noise commencing in his ears, and it gradually increased until he became aware of the fact that his hearing was damaged. He then commenced treatment, and not getting immediate relief from his first doctor he changed, and soon changed again, in this way going to several doctors, a few of them specialists, and then gave up, discouraged, and let the disease run its course unhindered. When he came to me (last March) he said he had been unable to hear anything but confused noises, even when the loudest tones were used to accost him, for five years. He is of medium height, rather slender, with inclination to red hair; has blue eyes, a fair complexion, and has a slightly anemic appearance. He describes the noise in his ears as dull and rumbling, if he pays no particular heed to it; but if he concentrates his thoughts on it, he can imagine that it resembles almost any kind of a noise. One thing I wish to mention, which was quite prominent and quickly disappeared under the remedy, viz., he would be awakened in the night by a loud bombing noise and afterward be unable to sleep "for the racket in his ears." There were a number of nervous symptoms in the case that led me to show him to Dr. Bartlett: *First,* Slight melancholia; would go off alone and brood over his troubles for hours. *Second,*

He would stagger while he walked. I found his tendo-patella reflex much decreased, and on standing with his eyes closed he would fall over in my arms; could not manage, at best, to take three steps forward with his eyes closed without falling. I have kept him pretty steadily on *Ferrum Phos.*, and the improvement is remarkable. He can hear every word of the longest sentence, by slightly raising the voice when accosting him, at several feet away. The noises are greatly lessened, he sleeps well, and the nervous symptoms are fast disappearing. I have continually inflated the middle ear by Politzer method once a week.
(Dr. F. W. Messerve.)

Kali Mur. in Deafness:

Mrs. ——, æt. 45. About three years ago began to be troubled with pain and noises in the left ear; aggravated greatly at the time of the menses; the pain severe and neuralgic in character, extending over the left side of the head. The noises seem to get their character from some pronounced sound which is heard, and this persists sometimes for hours. For the last six months there has been no pain on the left side, but deafness is constant. The right side is now beginning to become deaf, but with no pain and no noises. This has been going on, on the right side, for several months. General health excellent, with the exception of redness, fullness and desire to rub and pull the skin about the neck for a few days after the menses, with marked swelling of the glands of the neck at the same time. This has been noticed only during the time that the ears have been troublesome. The fork is heard best on the left side by bone conduction, and best on the right side by air conduction. Meatus tympani dry and depressed. Eustachian tube on the left almost occluded, on the right more free. Frequent burning of the auricle on the left side. *Kali Mur.*, cured.
(H. P. Bellows, M. D.)

ECZEMA

(See Skin, Affections of the.)

EDEMA OF THE LUNGS

(See Consumption.)

BIOCHEMIC TREATMENT

Natr. Mur.—Acute edema of the lungs, with excessive serous, frothy secretions. Excessive *accumulation of mucus in the lungs and bronchi,* causing great rattling in the chest.

Kali Phos.—"Edema pulmonarium, spasmodic cough, threatening suffocation; for dyspnea and livid countenance." (Walker.) Alternate with *Natr. Mur.*

ENDOCARDITIS

(See Heart Affections.)

ENURESIS

(See Urinary Disorders.)

BIOCHEMIC TREATMENT

Ferrum Phos.—Incontinence of urine, if from weakness of the sphincter muscle. *Wetting of the bed, especially in children.* Enuresis nocturna from weakness of the muscles, often seen in women, when every cough causes the urine to spurt. Diurnal enuresis depending on irritation of neck of the bladder and end of the penis.

Calc. Phos.—Enuresis in young children and in old people.

Kali Phos.—Wetting of the bed, due to nervous debility. Incontinence from partial paralysis of the sphincter.

CLINICAL CASES

Kali Phos. in Incontinence of Urine:

Dr. Cruwell reports on incontinence of urine: When I became acquainted with Dr. Schuessler's preparations I was very anxious to test the effects of *Kali Phos.,* as Dr. Schuessler recommends this against paralysis and paralytic conditions. Whoever has been occupied with the study of psychology is naturally ready to suspect paralysis everywhere. I acknowledge I may have given *Kali Phos.* too frequently, as I was desirous to find out what it could do. For various reasons it led me to give it for incontinence. I gave it three or four times daily in a little water. In five cases, two of which I treated with good results, *Kali Phos.* brought about amazingly rapid improvement. With a young girl, æt. 7, I had until lately to repeat the remedy every time it was given up, as the incontinence always returned when it was discontinued. The most successful case was that of an old gentleman, æt. 60. No doubt, in this case there existed a subparalytic condition of the sphincter muscle. Some months after the treatment he called back to say that he was perfectly cured.

Enuresis:

Boy, age 5, was troubled with nocturnal bed wetting, urine alkali in reaction. I prescribed *Natr. Phos.* and *Kali Phos.*, two tablets three times daily. Urine soon changed to slightly acid reaction. In two months child was entirely cured.
(Dr. S. W. Jones, Wilbur, Washington.)

Ferrum Phos. in Incontinence of Urine:

Lady, æt. 35, had had trouble for three years, and could assign no cause thereto; was able to retain the urine at night, but not in the day-time, when she passed large quantities of water involuntarily. General health good. *Ferrum Phos.*, four times a day. A week later she reported that she could now retain her urine much better during the day. The medicine was continued for three weeks longer, when she informed me that the power over the bladder was now complete, and that she was better than she had been for two years. Nine months afterwards the patient came to me again with a return of the same malady, and although she was then *enceinte*, *Ferrum Phos.* again completely stopped the incontinence.
(Wilde.)

EPILEPSY

(See Spasms, Convulsions, etc.)

ETIOLOGY

Epilepsy is characterized by sudden loss of consciousness and power of co-ordination of motion, with convulsions. It is sometimes caused by vicious habits, which drain the vital system of its fluids, leaving a deficiency in the molecules of certain phosphates in nerve tissue and muscle fibre.

The physician should spare no pains to ascertain the cause, and he will then be in a position to intelligently prescribe the lacking salts.

BIOCHEMIC TREATMENT

Kali Mur.—The *chief remedy in epilepsy;* tongue coated white or grayish-white. *Epilepsy after suppression of eczema,* with characteristic tongue symptoms.

Ferrum Phos.—In epileptic fits, with rush of blood to the head, in alternation with *Kali Mur.,* the chief remedy.

Magnes. Phos.—For the spasms and contortions of epilepsy; stiffness of limbs, drawing back of head, clenched fists and teeth, etc. *Epilepsy from vicious habits,* which must be restrained. Give *Magnes. Phos.* in hot water, frequent doses, till the spasms are relieved.

Calc. Phos.—Epileptic fits, usually the result of vicious habits, masturbations, etc.

Natr. Phos.—If with intestinal irritation from worms, *Natr. Phos.* should be alternated with the chief remedy, *Kali Mur.*

Silicea.—Epilepsy, with the spasms coming on at night (intercurrently).

Kali Phos.—Epilepsy, for the sunken countenance, coldness and palpitation, after the fit.

CLINICAL CASES

Jacksonian Epilepsy from Menopause:

Mrs. T., Dallas, Texas. Age 65, white. Jacksonian epilepsy, so diagnosed by several competent physicians. From history, it developed at menopause and seemed to be accompanied by chronic pelvic inflammation that I believe to be malignant. Now, three months since I began with *Calc. Fluor.,* three tablets every two hours, with an occasional dose of *Magnes. Phos.,* she has no more attacks and feels better than she has for several years; but I shall insist on *Calc. Fluor.,* every day during this year, after which I expect her to be as well as anyone her age.
(Dr. J. M. Jones, Dallas, Texas.)

Kali Mur. in Epilepsy from suppressed eruptions:

Dr. C. C. J. Wachendorf reports the case of a man 45 years old, who had an eruption in September, which disappeared until August of the next year. In November, the eruption was suppressed and he began to have irregular attacks of "fainting fits." He would grow pale, a warm feeling following, then spasm, with pain in the cerebellum and burning in the region of the stomach. Attacks nearly always proceeded from a fright or fear. *Kali Mur.* was prescribed on the indication: "Epilepsy from suppressed eruptions." After the sixth day he had no attack. He still takes occasional doses of the medicine to keep up its action.

The care and management of the Epileptic:

The epileptic patient must be carefully examined for any possible source of focal irritation. The points most often at fault are the eyes, ears, teeth, nose including obstruction from adenoids, the colon and the external genitalia. Do not, however, depend upon relief of irritation at these points to complete the cure but merely as a preliminary step toward that end.

The hygiene of the patient must be regulated. Assure plenty of fresh air and exercise with regular habits as to sleeping and particularly as to eating. The diet should be largely vegetable with a minimum of meat and with emphasis on regular meals and no overeating.

In the case of children mental training is important and if the heredity be bad from a neurotic tendency, institutional training may be the best solution of this problem.

For the purpose of lessening the frequency and violence of the attacks it is often advisable to attempt medicinal control by the use of the bromides or phenobarbital given in sufficient amounts to prevent the occurrence of spasms. This may be continued for such period of time as to allow other corrective measures to be effective. In any case the treatment should be continued for several years after the cessation of attacks as recurrences are very common.

ERUPTIONS

(See "Skin, Affections of," also "Exudations.")

EPISTAXIS

(See Hemorrhage.)

BIOCHEMIC TREATMENT

Ferrum Phos.—Epistaxis, especially in children, of bright, red blood.

Kail Phos.—*Epistaxis* in weak, delicate constitution, *from old age,* debility, weakness, with a predisposition to bleeding of the nose. *Blood* dark, thin, *like coffee-grounds;* putrid.

ERYSIPELAS

ETIOLOGY

"Erysipelas is an acute infectious disease due to the entrance into the skin in its deeper layers of the Streptococcus pyogenes, sometimes called the Streptococcus erysipelatis. The skin of the part affected becomes dusky red and swollen. A peculiarity of the area of redness is that it has a sharp line of demarcation separating it from the surrounding healthy tissue, which is usually of its natural color and appearance. The line of demarcation can be not only seen but can be felt by the finger-tip, and if the affected area be punctured and the serum which then exudes stained with methylene blue the chains of streptococci can readily be found under the microscope. Erysipelas is sometimes called 'St. Anthony's Fire.'

"Two additional factors are nearly always active in the production of the disease, namely, a break in the skin or in a neighboring mucous membrane, so that the streptococcus gains access to the tissues, and, secondly, some cause, local or general, which diminishes vital resistance to such a degree that the tissues afford a favorable site for the growth of the micro-organism." (Hare.) These two factors are both due to the same cause, a deficiency in cell-salts which so act upon the tissues that a favorable breeding place is provided for the micro-organisms to grow.

The first noticeable symptoms are: heat, shining redness, tingling pains, swelling, and tension of the parts. This is followed by burning, and sometimes tearing or shooting pains, worse from movement. Other symptoms generally present are: shiverings, followed by flushes of heat; sleepiness; wandering pains; dry tongue; nausea and headache; blisters frequently arise on the affected parts. In a few days the color changes to a yellowish hue. The disease, when it attacks the face or head, assumes a serious aspect, and great care should be taken. Sometimes quite severe bilious symptoms are present.

An external application of flexible collodion to the affected area is suggested, as the staphylococcus is aerobic and in this way its supply of air is shut off.

BIOCHEMIC TREATMENT

Ferrum Phos.—*Chief remedy in the first or inflammatory stage,* for the heat, redness, fever and pain. Rose erysipelas, externally and internally. Alternate with *Natr. Sulph.* for the bilious symptoms.

Natr. Sulph.—*Chief remedy for erysipelas,* with or without vomiting of bile, with smooth, red, shiny, tingling or painful swelling of the skin.

Kali Mur.—For the *vesicular form, chief remedy*, in alternation with *Ferr. Phos.*

Kali Sulph.—Erysipelas, in the blistering forms, to aid in desquamation.

Natr. Phos.—Erysipelas; smooth, red, shiny, tingling or painful swelling of the skin.

CLINICAL CASES

Kali Mur. and Ferrum Phos. in Erysipelas:

I was called to see Mrs. D., aet. 38, on November 30, 1914, at 4 p. m. I found her in a highly nervous state, with a temperature of 102° There was a shining red saddle over the nose, extending over both cheeks. I diagnosed the case erysipelas. I had very similar cases in the past, and prescribed the same remedies, *Ferrum Phos.* and *Kali Mur. celloids,* to be taken in alternation, and a saturated solution of *Ferrum Phos.* on an absorbent cotton mask applied to the face.

Next day the nurse's chart showed a restless night, temperature 103°, also the patient complained of backache, and both eyes were nearly swollen shut. I calmly continued with the same treatment, and an occasional dose of *Kali Phos.* Third day, temperature 101 2/5°, patient more comfortable, same treatment continued.

Fourth day, temperature normal, patient comfortable, swelling and redness subsiding. Today, the eighth day, I saw the patient, prescribed the same remedies, and told her that further consultations were not necessary.

In uncomplicated cases of erysipelas, *Ferrum Phos.* and *Kali Mur.* celloids are the only remedies necessary, and the trouble will be of short duration.

(Dr. P. T. Johnson, Erie, Pennsylvania.)

Natr. Sulph. in facial Erysipelas:

Mr. J., æt. 56; erysipelas of the face; face much swollen, shiny, smooth and tingling; high fever and distressing pain. *Ferrum Phos.*, alternated with *Natr. Sulph.*, with local applications of *Ferrum Phos.*, and occasional doses of *Kali Mur.*, soon cured the case.

(J. B. Chapman.)

Natr. Sulph. and Ferrum Phos. in Erysipelas accompanied by prostration and delirium:

Mrs. Forbes, a widow, was lying very ill with erysipelas; high fever and quite prostrate. The members of her family thought her dying, as she had become delirious. Her head and face so swollen tnat her eyes were literally closed, suffering intense pain. *Natr. Sulph.* and *Ferrum Phos.*, alternately, a dose every hour and oftener, were given. After the second dose of the former she ejected a great quantity of bile. The severe symptoms subsided. This was on Saturday night. The medicine was continued; *Ferrum Phos.* now only intercurrently, as the pulse had become less frequent. To the astonishment of all her friends, on Wednesday morning she was so well that she went out to her work as usual. Statistics show a death rate of 2,000 per annum from this disease. In a similar case of erysipelas in a lady, æt. 87, these two remedies and a few doses of *Kali Phos.* cured her, when the usual treatment, painting with iodine, brandy, etc., had no effect in arresting the disease.

(M. D. W. From Schuessler.)

EXOPHTHALMIC GOITRE

(See Goitre.)

BIOCHEMIC TREATMENT

Natr. Mur.—Vision not clear, the eyes seem misty all day; cervical glands swollen and painful, chokes easily when swallowing; changed voice; eccentric; dilatation of the heart, with systolic bellows sound; difficulty of breathing, even when keeping quiet, on standing or walking, with trembling of hands and feet; sensation of violent constriction in the heart, with intermitting pulse and feeling of oppression in lower part of the chest fluttering of the heart; intermitting pulse; short breathed from least exertion. (Lillienthal.)

EXPECTORATIONS

(See Exudations.)

EXUDATIONS

ETIOLOGY

It is important for the student of Biochemistry to fully understand the real cause of exudations, swellings, inflammations, eruptions, and all accumulations of morbid matter that accompany disease.

Heteroplasm is defined by Virchow as a substance foreign to the normal constituent parts of the organism. It therefore follows that the normal constituent parts of the body have become abnormal for some reason, as this heteroplastic accumulation must have its origin in the organism of man and not outside.

The fluids of the body, containing sugar, oil, fibrin, and other albuminous substances, could not so combine as to render them non-functional or form vitiated compounds causing exudations, eruptions, etc., if the vitalizers, the workers, called inorganic cell-salts, were present in proper quantity.

There is a small per cent. of muriatic acid in gastric fluids, and a deficiency of the same causes indigestion, and possibly catarrh of the stomach, which means exudations of certain organic matter from the blood; but this abnormal state could not exist unless there first arise a deficiency in some one or more of the inorganic or mineral cell-salts. Muriatic acid is formed by the union of certain dissimilar substances which conjoin and form new compounds.

Any breaking up of the chain, or continuity of the cell-salts, of course, disturbs the process of assimilating new organic material to replace that cast off as worn out and useless.

In health all the organic substances of the body are controlled entirely by the mineral salts of the blood, and oxygen. They are thus held in proper solution, diffused through the system, ready to be used to rebuild the human structure, that is continually crumbling away. Any deficiency in the inorganic salts must of necessity cause a disturbance in the organism, *i. e.*, cause organic matter to become non-functional and thrown off through the skin or some orifice or membrane of the body. A large amount of this vitiated matter at a given point will, of course, produce swellings or inflammations.

According to Schuessler, the following secretions or discharges are characteristic of the remedies set opposite to them. It matters not whether the exudation be from the skin, deep-seated tissues or mucous membrane in any part of the body the remedy will be the same.

Secretions when white and fibrinous indicate a deficiency in *Kali Mur.*

When albuminous, *Calc. Phos.*

When yellow, with small tough lumps, *Calc. Fluor.*

When yellow, like gold, *Natr. Phos.*

When yellowish and slimy or watery, *Kali Sulph.*

When greenish, thin, *Kali Sulph.*

When clear, transparent, thin like water, *Natr. Mur.*

When pus, or streaked with blood, *Calc. Sulph.*

When pus, *thick* yellow, *Silicea.*

When very offensive smelling, *Kali Phos.*

When causing soreness and chafing, *Natr. Mur.* and *Kali Phos.*

In coughs, with expectoration, colds in the head, leucorrhea, bronchial catarrh, etc., the above distinctions in color and consistency of secretions must decide the choice of the remedy.

EYE DISEASES

The pathology of the greater proportion of all diseases of the eyes will be found under the pathology of exudation. There are also eye troubles due to deficiencies of *Kali Phos.* and *Ferrum Phos.*

BIOCHEMIC TREATMENT

Ferrum Phos.—*Inflammations of the eyes,* with pain and redness, *in the first stage,* before pus-secretion has commenced. Burning sensation in the eyes. Acute pain in the eyeballs, aggravated by movement, and relieved by bathing in cold water. Dry inflammation, bloodshot, sometimes sore and watery. First stage of retinitis, abscess of the cornea for the pain, and inflammation. Granulations of the eyelids, for the inflammation and pain, feeling of sand in the eyes. Local applications.

Kali Mur.—*Inflammations of the eye, in the second stage,* when there is a discharge of white mucus or of yellow-greenish pus; alternate with *Kali Sulph.* Sore eyes, with specks of white matter or yellowish scabs on the lids (*Kali Sulph.*). Retinitis, second stage. Granulated eyelids, with *feeling of sand in the eyes;* alternate with *Ferrum Phos.* Superficial flat ulcer, arising from a vesicle.

Kali Sulph.—*Third stage of inflammations,* with *discharge* of *yellow* or *greenish* pus, *slimy yellow* or *watery* secretions (*Kali Mur.*). Yellow crusts on the eyelids. Cataract, dimness of the crystalline lens; alternate with *Natr. Mur.* Inflammation of the conjunctiva, with characteristic exudations.

Kali Phos.—Weak eyesight from an exhausted condition of the system after disease. Blindness from partial decay of the optic nerve. Excited, staring appearance of the eyes, with dilated pupils, indicating a nervous disturbance, during the course of the disease. Drooping of the eyelids from partial paralysis of the muscles. Squinting after diphtheria, from asthenic conditions.

Magnes. Phos.—Drooping of the eyelids; in alternation with *Kali Phos.* Affections of the eyes in which there is *great sensitiveness to light,* contracted pupils. Vision affected, *sees sparks* and *colors before eyes.* Dullness of sight from weakness of the optic nerve. Neuralgia of the eye, pain is relieved by warmth and aggravated by cold. Spasmodic squinting and twitching of the eyelids.

Natr. Mur.—Discharge of clear, watery mucus from the eyes or flow of tears, with obstruction of the tear-ducts; alternate *Ferrum Phos.* Frequently mechanical interference is necessary. *Discharges from the eyes causing soreness of the skin,* or eruption of small vesicles. Granulated eyelids, with or without secretion of tears, to absorb the vesicles. White spots on the cornea; also syringe the eyes daily with a solution of the same. Muscular asthenopia. Neuralgic pains recurring periodically, with flow of tears. Blisters on the cornea.

Calc. Sulph.—Inflammation of the eyes, with *discharge* of *thick, yellow matter.* Deep ulcers of the cornea, with characteristic discharge of pus. Abscess of the cornea. Hypopyum, to absorb the pus. Retinitis, pustular keratitis and conjunctivitis, when there is a discharge of characteristic pus. Compare *Silicea*

Silicea.—Deep-seated ulcers of the eye. *Inflammations, with thick, yellow discharges* (*Calc. Sulph.*). Styes on the eyelids; also as a lotion. Hypopyum. Weakness of the sight after suppressed foot-sweats. Little boils and tumors around the eyelids.

Natr. Phos.—Inflammation of eyes (*Conjunctivitis*), with *discharge of golden-yellow, creamy matter,* the *lids* are *glued together in the morning;* note also coating of tongue, palate, presence of acid conditions, etc. Squinting from intestinal irritation, worms, etc. Scrofulous ophthalmia (also local application).

Natr. Sulph.—Yellowness of the eyeballs from derangement of the liver. Burning of the edges of the lids, with tears, chronic conjunctivitis, with blister-like granulations on the lids.

Calc. Phos.—Spasmodic affections of the eyelids, after *Magnes. Phos.,* if that remedy fails to give relief. Neuralgia of the eyes, when *Magnes. Phos.* fails. Photophobia, parenchymatous keratitis in scrofulous diathesis. Diplopia (also *Magnes. Phos.*).

Calc. Fluor.—Flickering and sparks before the eyes, spots on the cornea, conjunctivitis. Cataract.

CLINICAL CASES

Kali Mur. in Parenchymatous Keratitis:

Inflammation of right cornea, extending over the whole of its surface, of three months' duration; patient could only count fingers; some pain, slight photophobia and redness, pupil dilates slowly under *Atrop.* but quickly contracts again. *Kali Mur.* cured. Cases of choroidoretinitis cured by *Kali Mur.*
(Allen and Norton, Ophthalmic Therapeutics, p. 106.)

The following cases by George S. Norton, M. D., show the action of *Kali Mur.* in ulceration of the cornea:
Kali Mur. in Corneal Ulcer:

CASE I.—Case of ulcer of the cornea, large in size, steadily increasing in extent, vascular base, moderate redness, no pain, slight photophobia, profuse lachrymation, nose sore, corners ulcerated. *Kali Mur.* Improvement set in at once, and ulcer commenced to heal; within five days the vascularity disappeared, and in ten days the eye was perfectly well.

CASE II.—Case of ulcer of the cornea, with elevated edges and vascular base, resulting from phlyctenular keratitis; in spite of all treatment it had steadily increased; cornea hazy around ulcer. *Kali Mur.* The ulcer began at once to heal, and in two weeks all inflammatory symptoms had disappeared.

CASE III.—Ulcer of cornea from the same cause as the above; also a rapidly-increasing purulent infiltration between the corneal layers. Photophobia well marked; moderate redness and no pain. Several remedies were administered with no benefit. *Kali Mur.* was prescribed, and a rapid cure followed.

CASE IV.—Child, with ulcer near center of cornea, which was deep; infiltration considerable. Pus in the anterior chamber; moderately red, no pain. *Atrop.* instillation. Hypopyum disappeared, and in twenty-four hours a rapid recovery followed under *Kali Mur.*

Natr. Mur. in excessive Lachrymal Secretions:

Dr. Kock writes: An old woman came to me, æt. 72. She had worn a green shade over her eyes, to my recollection, since my younger days, when, as a student, I spent my holidays at Simbach with my grandparents. This person complained of a constant burning sensation in her eyes, causing a continual flow of smarting tears. This commenced at 8 o'clock in the morning and lasted until sunset. During the night it was better. She had much thirst, but little appetite. Externally, the conjunctivæ palpebrarum was in a chronic state of inflammation. On each side of the nose there were excoriation and eczema of the skin, caused by the flow of acrid tears. The punctæ lachrymosæ were dilated, but the tear-ducts were unobstructed. Dr. Schuessler's special mention of *Natr. Mur.* in regard to the excessive lachrymal secretions quickly determined my choice of remedies, and I gave *Natr. Mur.* in water, one teaspoonful three times a day. In three weeks the

symptoms all greatly subsided and shortly after entirely disappeared.
(From Schuessler.)

Natr. Phos. in Conjunctivitis:

One case was particularly striking on account of its being cured so rapidly. In May last, a little girl, æt. 8, was brought to me, who suffered from severe conjunctivitis, with great dread of light. She had been treated for some time by an another practitioner, but without effect. I ascertained that her eye affection dated from the time she had had the measles, some years before. The enlargement of the glands of the neck, and the creamy secretion of the eyelids, led me to try *Natr. Phos.* of which I administered a dose three times daily. A week later and the child was brought to me, her eyes bright and perfectly cured.
(From Schuessler.)

Ferrum Phos. and Calc. Sulph. in Hypopyum and Conjunctivitis:

Dr. Kock informed us that a farm-servant came to him and said he could not see. Some time before this a piece of wood had struck him in the eye. He had been treated for it; had had purgative leeches and cold water applications, and now his sight was quite gone. The particulars of the case were these: The bulbus was infiltrated, with vascular engorgement. The conjunctiva was swollen, and the eyelids also in an irritated condition. The cornea was dim, with a smoky appearance of the anterior chamber (*i. e.,* between the cornea and iris), and some matter could be seen floating, quite distinctly. I found no foreign body. The subjective results were: severe burning pain in the eyes, as if from a foreign body, and a continuous flow of tears. The man had to keep his eye tied up. His appetite was good and pulse normal. As to the therapeutic treatment, I had evidently to deal with two different affections—hypopyum (matter in the eye) and conjunctivitis. First of all, I gave *Ferrum Phos.*, a dose every two hours; and in a

week the burning pain and water in the eye were less. One week after this the man complained that his sight had not improved. Now I had the task of absorption of the matter before me, as well as the clearing of the cornea. Remembering an expression of Dr. Quagleo, that he considered Schuessler's *Calc. Sulph.* a powerful medicine, I gave some *Calc. Sulph.*, to be taken in water in three doses. Scarcely a week after, the man came to me greatly delighted, saying he could see gleams of light in the right eye. Positively, I found the cornea less cloudy, and could observe that some of the matter had been absorbed. I now gave him a dose only night and morning. In three weeks the absorption was complete and dimness of the cornea quite removed and his sight restored. Besides all this, all the inflammation of the conjunctiva was cured.
(From Schuessler.)

Calc. Phos. in Recurring Keratitis:

Girl, æt. 16; recurring keratitis. Left eye much inflamed, photophobia, slight haziness of the cornea, and traversed with red vessels; zonular redness. *Calc. Phos.* completely restored the patient. I have never found it of any use where the palpebral conjunctiva was much engorged.
(R. T. Cooper.)

Natr. Mur. in Overstrained Eyes:

Bookkeeper, æt. 28; overstrained eyes. "Feel like chilblains," must wipe them often, and pull at the lashes. Is emmetropic, though can read No. 15 at fifteen feet with difficulty, from blurring of the letters; not improved by glasses. A candle held twelve inches seems double, and the left image is seen with the right eye, hence he has asthenopia from paresis of the internal recti muscles. *Natr. Mur.* cured.
(T. F. Allen.)

FAINTING

BIOCHEMIC TREATMENT

Kali Phos.—Predisposition to fainting in weak and nervous subjects.

Calc. Phos.—To tone up the general system; alternate with *Kali Phos.*

FELON

(See Abscess.)

BIOCHEMIC TREATMENT

Ferrum Phos.—In the first or inflammatory stage of felons, for the heat, pain congestion and fever. Will frequently abort pus formation if given early.

Silicea.—In felons, this remedy is indispensable, to control the formation of pus, and promote the growth of new nails, which are largely composed of this salt.

CLINICAL CASES

Ferrum Phos. for Felons:

A dressmaker, in her busiest season, to her dismay, got a felon on the right thumb. *Ferrum Phos.,* in water, every three hours, promptly relieved and, as she supposed, cured it. She used it vigorously, and within three days it reappeared, with greatly increased pain and hard swelling. *Kali Mur.,* finished the cure at once, a single drop of pus appearing beneath the cuticle and escaped when snipped with the scissors.
(J. C. Morgan, M. D.)

FEVERS—[Simple]

ETIOLOGY

Webster defines *fever* as a disease marked by heat, thirst and accelerated pulse. This is quite right, but is too meagre a definition. Fever is the result of nature's effort to throw off non-functional matter or the disorganization of the inorganic cell-salt phosphate of iron. Fever is not always the disease itself, but the result of disease.

Iron is a carrier of oxygen and when there is a deficiency or molecular disturbance in the phosphate of iron, the blood endeavors to carry enough oxygen to all parts of the body, with the limited supply of iron at hand. In order to do this, the circulation is increased and the resulting friction is called *Fever.* The molecular disturbance of *phosphate of iron* will soon extend to other of the cell-salts (notably potassium chloride) and various symptoms will appear. The biochemic procedure is to increase the oxygen carriers (*Ferrum Phos.*) and by so doing decrease the rapidity of the circulation. But should the disturbance have extended to the others of the cell-salts, thev will need to be supplied as indicated.

BIOCHEMIC TREATMENT

Ferrum Phos.—This is the *chief remedy in all fevers;* as first remedy for quickened pulse, rise of temperature, heat, etc. Inflammatory, catarrhal or rheumatic fevers, for the febrile symptoms, *Ferrum Phos.* is the remedy, in alternation with other indicated remedies. Feverishness in all stages.

Kali Mur.—*Second remedy in fevers,* with *thick, white coating on the tongue,* or with constipation. To restore the integrity of the affected tissue. Alternate with *Ferrum Phos.*

Kali Phos.—In purely nervous fevers, with high temperature, quick and irregular pulse, nervous excitement and weakness; alternate with *Ferrum Phos.*

Kali Sulph.—When the *temperature rises in the evening.* To promote perspiration, if not produced by *Ferrum Phos.* In fevers from blood-poisoning.

Natr. Mur.—*Hay fever, with watery discharges* from the eyes or nose. Alternate with *Ferrum Phos.* when there is a considerable dryness of the tongue in the commencement of all fevers.

CLINICAL CASES

Kali Mur. in simple Fevers:

Mr. L., a gentleman, æt. 38, took a chill while in a state of perspiration. He suffered in consequence from tearing pains in the limbs, noises in the ears, with dullness of hearing and frontal headache. The pains were accompanied by fever; and although he induced sweating at night, it brought no relief. The appetite was poor and the tongue covered with a white coating. I gave a small quantity of *Kali Mur.*, in water every two hours. A rapid general improvement set in, but pain and numbness in the feet were still present. Also the habitual perspiration of the feet was still absent. At this stage the patient received *Silicea,* two doses daily for a week. Perspiration of feet was re-established, and on the appearance of this, the rest of the ailments left him and health was quite restored. (From Schuessler.)

Ferrum Phos. in Fevers:

Dr. G. H. Martin reports a case of high fever (104 degrees), general exhaustion, lameness in muscles, headache and diminished appetite, in which he prescribed *Ferrum Phos.*, which caused an immediate improvement.

FISTULA IN ANO

BIOCHEMIC TREATMENT

Calc. Phos.—After surgical interference for the fistula. Fistula in ano alternating with chest symptoms, or in persons who have pains in joints with every spell of cold, stormy weather, especially in tall, slim persons; burning and pulsating in anus; bearing down toward anus; sore feeling in anus when getting up in the morning.
(Lillienthal.)

Silicea.—Fistula in ano, with chest symptoms; sharp stitches in rectum while walking; abdominal pains, relieved by warmth; suppuration of abscess; purulent sputa.
(Lillienthal.)

FITS

(See Epilepsy.)

FLATULENCE

(See Gastric Derangements.)

FLOODING

(See Hemorrhage.)

GALL-STONES

ETIOLOGY

A calcareous deposit, *i. e.*, a deposit of lime found in the gall-bladder or in its ducts. The cause is, first, a deficiency of sodium sulphate molecules, which cause an inspissation (thickening) of bile. The gastric juice then parts with molecules of calcium phosphate, to make up the deficiency, by the albumen which is carried with the lime to again thin the bile to its normal consistency. In some instances it fails, and the lime and albumen become non-functional and by the action of vitiated bile form the stone.

BIOCHEMIC TREATMENT

Calc. Phos.—To prevent the formation of the stone; in alternation with *Natr. Sulph.* in bilious subjects with gouty diathesis.

Magnes. Phos.—For the excessive pain and *spasms from gall-stones.*

GASTRIC DERANGEMENTS

ETIOLOGY

Disorders in the gastric region are largely due to a lack of certain inorganic salts in the cells of the digestive fluids or in the membranes that line these organs. The underlying cause of such deficiency may be from exposure, over- or under-eating, eating of poisonous foods, or from any of the many abuses to which these organs are subjected.

Diet is a very important item in dealing with the disorders of this region of the body, and great care must be taken to give the stomach, liver and intestines as much rest as possible by supplying them with only the simplest and most easily digestible foods. Then, by supplying the deficient cell-salts in the form of the biochemic remedies, a normal, healthy condition can again be attained.

The process of cure may in some cases be slow—especially where the disease is one of long standing; but if the proper cell-salts are regularly supplied and a judicious diet maintained, a steady improvement will unquestionably take place.

BIOCHEMIC TREATMENT

Ferrum Phos.—Gastritis, with much pain, swelling and tenderness of the stomach, accompanied with vomiting of undigested food. Pain is relieved by hot applications over the region of the stomach, causing a counter-inflammation, or by cold drinks. *First stage of gastric fever.* Flatulence, bringing back the taste of the food. *Dyspepsia, with hot, flushed face;* stomach is tender to the touch; alternate with remedy indicated by coating of the tongue. Dyspepsia, with beating or throbbing pain, tongue clean, or with vomiting of undigested food.

Indigestion from relaxed condition of the muscular walls of blood-vessels of the stomach, with tenderness, burning, flushed face, etc. Stomachache from chill, with loose evacuations. Loss of appetite, with feverish conditions.

Kali Mur.—All gastric or bilious derangements, when the *tongue has a white or grayish-white coating,* especially noticeable *in the morning.* Indigestion, with pain or heavy feeling in region of liver, or under right shoulder-blade, with white-coated tongue and protruding eyeballs. Gastritis, when from taking too hot drinks, this remedy should be given at once to heal the scalded membrane.

Flatulence, with inactivity of the liver; *sick feeling after eating fat or rich food.* Gastritis, for the second stage. Dyspepsia, with constipation.

Natr. Phos.—Gastric derangements, with excess of lactic acid; acidity of the stomach, sour risings, and thin, moist, *creamy golden-yellow coating on the back part of tongue, tonsils and palate.* Acid taste in the mouth. Belching of wind tasting acid. Gastric ulceration. Severe pain in stomach after eating, with acid risings. "Heart-burn" alternate *Ferrum Phos.* Stomachache, with symptoms of acidity of stomach, or from worms. Loss of appetite, with acid conditions.

Natr. Mur.—Indigestion, with water-brash. Pain in stomach, with water gathering in the mouth or *vomiting of clear, frothy water,* not acid. Indigestion, with the above symptoms, frequently accompanied with constipation.

Calc. Phos.—Useful, if given intercurrently in all cases of indigestion, immediately after each meal. Indigestion is frequently from non-assimilation of the food; therefore, *Calc. Phos.* is a most important remedy to aid in digestion, as it has the power of breaking up the particles of food. *Pain after eating* even the *smallest quantity of food or drinking cold water,* if there are no acid conditions present. "A valuable remedy for excessive accumulation of gas in the stomach." (Foster.) After gastric fever, a course of this remedy is useful to rebuild wasted tissue and promote digestion of food.

Kali Phos.—Indigestion, with *"gone feeling" in the stomach,* from nervous disturbance. Hungry feeling after taking food. *Voracious appetite after* typhoid fever or other *wasting diseases.* Flatulence, with weary pain in left side, gas gathers about heart, causing distress, pain and weakness of heart. Gastritis, if it comes too late under treatment, with asthenic conditions. Stomachache from fright or excitement.

Kali Sulph.—Indigestion, with slimy, golden-yellow coated tongue. Dyspepsia, with sensation of pressure and fullness at pit of stomach. Indigestion, with pain in stomach and water gathering in the mouth, if *Natr. Mur.* or *Kali Mur.* does not give relief. Colicky pains in the stomach (if *Magnes. Phos.* fails). "Pain in the intestines, fixed in the abdomen, just above the angle of the crest of the ileum, in a line toward the umbilicus, deep within, beside the right hip." (Walker.) Chronic catarrh of the stomach, with characteristic slimy, yellow coating of the tongue.

Magnes. Phos.—*Spasms and cramping of the stomach, with clean tongue.* Indigestion, with nipping, griping pains in stomach, belching of gas gives no relief. *Gnawing pains in the stomach.* "Pains, with crampy, tight, drawing, lacing sensation." (Schuessler.) Convulsive hiccough. Neuralgia of the stomach, relieved by hot drinks.

Natr. Sulph.—Gastric derangements, with biliousness, bitter taste in the mouth, excess of bile, vomiting of bitter fluid. *Tongue* is generally *covered with a greenish-brown or greenish-gray coating;* mouth full of slime, tenacious and thick, greenish-white; dark bilious stools. Derangement of the stomach, with bitter taste in mouth in morning; headache, vertigo and lassitude. Stitching pains in the liver, with bilious symptoms, vomiting of bile or greenish matter.

CLINICAL CASES

Kali Phos. in Unnatural Appetite:

A young man complained of an unnatural appetite. He had to eat almost every hour, feeling such an intense craving for food, yet he felt exhausted and languid. There were no secondary symptoms present. The tongue was clean, the urine was not increased, evacuations normal. *Kali Phos.* cured the patient in the course of two days.

(From Schuessler.)

Natr. Mur. cured Chill caused by acid food:

Farmer B. consulted me for a singular affection. All acid food caused an attack beginning with a strong chill, followed by fever and profuse weakening sweat. *Natr. Mur.* After fourteen days he informed me that the attacks had entirely ceased, and the partaking of acid foods did not cause him the least discomfort.
(From Schuessler.)

Natr. Phos. for Burning in Stomach after meals:

Patient, with troublesome burning in the stomach after eating and continuing until next meal-time; pain develops one or two hours after meals; tongue light-gray; no bad taste, no tenderness; bowels regular; stools normal; no thirst; the burning was so troublesome as to keep him awake at night. *Natr. Phos.* cured.
(*Med. Era.*)

Natr. Phos. in indigestion after Typhoid:

Child, with indigestion after typhoid fever. Everything soured on his stomach; breath sour; vomited curdled milk and sour-smelling fluids; green stool alternating with constipation; was troubled with colic; white coated tongue and white around mouth; fretful, cross and restless. *Natr. Phos.* cured
(*Med. Era.*)

Natr. Sulph. cured him as if by magic:

A gentleman, æt. 44, wrote to me a few weeks ago:

"The medicine I have taken very steadily, and for a long time attended strictly to my diet. In spite of this, my trouble is no better; I may almost say it has become worse. The conditions are these: 1. I feel almost constantly a taste as of bile. 2. My tongue is covered with a curdy, bitter coating. 3. During the day, especially after food, I suffer from eructations of gases, which have either bitter taste or are tasteless. 4. My complexion is rather yellow. 5. The appetite very slight; no thirst. My favorite beverage, beer, is distasteful to me. 6. I incline to shiver, and am somewhat faint. 7.

My head is but little involved, but feel a constant pressure over one eye. 8. Stools are normal, but scanty, on account of spare diet. The whole condition discloses that I have bile in the stomach."

Thus far, the patient's own report. To this I may add that the patient in question had already taken, by my orders, several remedies. He had used the waters of Marienbad the previous summer, on recommendation of another medical man. I sent him now *Natr. Sulph.*, with the request to take daily three doses of this salt. The gentleman came, six or seven days later, to my consulting rooms to thank me for the valuable medicine.

"The remedy," he said, "has really worked wonders. All my ailments have disappeared as if by magic, and I feel at last perfectly well."
(From Schuessler.)

Ferrum Phos. in Gastralgia:

Dr. Mossa, Bamberg, reports: Toward the end of last year I received a letter with the following details, asking me to forward some medicine:

"My boy, a child æt. 7, hitherto healthy and strong, has been suffering from pains in the stomach for some weeks. Latterly, he has vomited all his food, sometimes immediately after taking it, and at other times, not until during the night. The child has now become emaciated. Last week he was frequently feverish. This has, however, not returned since taking the medicine our doctor here has given him. The boy complains of much exhaustion."

To form a scientific diagnosis of the case on such information was clearly impossible. But, as it was convenient for me personally to examine the case, I had to do my best with the details furnished. The nature of the abdominal pains pointed to swelling and enlargement of the organs of the viscera, liver, spleen, etc., also the feverish attacks, probably subdued by quinine, and the vomiting of food, all coincided with my surmises. As to the selection of the medicine, I hesitated considerably, and then decided to give *Ferrum Phos.* night and morning. The report was favorable, some time after. The fever had not returned; the vomiting of food and pains in the stomach had quite ceased soon after taking the medicine. The little fellow was so much stronger that he attended school again.

(From Schuessler.)

Prompt cure in Gastric Ulceration:

Miss A., age 35. Ailing for thirteen years. Very emaciated. Continual vomiting when food was taken. Severe pains in stomach, also in umbilical region. Very depressed condition. Advised, as a last resort, immediate surgical operation. I diagnosed chronic gastric ulceration. Sclerotic condition of the preaortic lymphatic nodes and vessels in the umbilical region. The Biochemic Remedies used were *Ferrum Phos.*, *Kali Phos.* and, intercurrently, *Calc. Fluor.* A non-irritating and fat free diet was maintained. Length of treatment was from November 5, 1923, to January 16, 1924. The condition at the end of the treatment was as follows: No pain in stomach or umbilical region. Sclerotic condition softened. Abdominal pulsations hardly perceptible. Emaciation rapidly disappearing.

(Dr. Ford Wilson, Vancouver, B. C., Canada.)

Ferrum Phos. in Gastric Ulceration:

W. Watson, æt. 40; ulceration of stomach; vomited all his food, and, latterly, the egesta had the appearance of coffee-grounds. He had suffered from vomiting and indigestion, more or less, for fourteen years, and had seen many doctors and taken much medicine without avail. I advised him to take *Ferrum Phos.* and *Natr. Phos.* every two hours alternately for a fortnight. On his second visit he was free from vomiting, and had little pain, and felt greatly better. He continued another ten days with the same remedies, and returned quite well. On making special inquiry if he had nothing troubling him, he said: "No, the only thing I sometimes trouble myself

about is thinking, after taking any kind of food, whether it will trouble me, but it never does." His cure has proved permanent, as it is now nearly two years since, and he is keeping well.
(M. D. W. From Schuessler.)

Ferrum Phos. in loss of Appetite:

Sudden attacks of deathly sickness at the stomach, coming on at no particular time, even in sleep, and lasting one-half or one hour; appetite poor. *Ferrum Phos.* cured, and appetite became ravenous.
(Raue.)

Natr. Phos. in chronic Dyspepsia:

A young man with chronic dyspepsia. After trying several remedies without effect, I discovered in the mouth a thin, yellow, creamy coating on the soft palate. This induced me to give the patient *Natr. Phos.*, which cured him in a short space of time.
(C. Hg.)

Natr. Sulph. in Non-Assimilation:

An old man, some 60 years of age, came to see me; he had "dyspepsia," the doctors said. Emaciated, pale, swarthy; no appetite; restless; bowels inactive, stools sometimes light-colored and at times costive; tongue thickly coated with a brownish-yellow tinge, bitter taste; conjunctiva bluish-white; skin wrinkled and abdomen retracted and shrunken, shriveled; and a pain in the stomach of a burning character after eating; and from the general character of the case, assimilation was greatly at fault. After surveying the situation and taking all conditions, I at once put him on *Natr. Sulph.*, three doses a day before meals, and *Kali Phos.*, as a nerve remedy. These two remedies perfectly cured the "dyspepsia" and all the other troubles, so that in about three weeks he was a well man, the *Natr. Sulph.* correcting all the liver and stomach troubles, and the *Kali Phos.* building up the nerve forces.
(A. P. Davis, M. D.)

GLANDULAR AFFECTIONS

BIOCHEMIC TREATMENT

Kali Mur.—Is the *chief remedy in glandular swellings,* when the gland is not excessively hard. Scrofulous enlargement of glands. Swelling of the glands of the throat and neck. *Mumps.* In all swellings, where practicable, the remedy should be used externally as well as internally; apply with vaseline, well rubbed in, or a solution on lint.

Calc. Fluor.—Glandular swellings, if of stony hardness; alternate with *Kali Mur.* *Hardened glands in the female breast.* Chronic inflammation of glands, when very hard.

Natr. Mur.—Glandular swellings, with characteristic watery symptoms, excessive secretion of saliva, etc. Chronic swelling of lymphatic glands, with watery symptoms. *Enlargement of sebaceous glands.* Mumps, with watery symptoms. Exophthalmic goitre.

Ferrum Phos.—Acute swelling of the glands, for the fever and pain. In alternation with other remedies.

Calc. Phos.—*Chronic enlargement of the glands, chief remedy.* Bronchocele, goitre, requires *Calc. Phos.,* the chief remedy. Scrofulous enlargement of the glands.

Silicea.—Swollen glands which are inclined to suppurate require *Silicea,* to facilitate the formation of pus. *Scrofulous glands.*

Calc. Sulph.—When the glands are discharging pus, to control suppuration. See under Abscess, for nature of discharge. If the edges around the suppurating parts are hard and callous, *Calc. Fluor.* will be required.

Natr. Phos.—In goitre, with tongue and acid symptoms indicating this remedy.

CLINICAL CASES

Natr. Sulph. in chronic swelling of Cervical Glands:

Grauvogl, in his *Text-Book,* page 360, gives a remarkable result from six weeks' use of *Natr. Sulph.* in case of chronic swelling of the cervical glands, so extensive as to practically obliterate the neck. All known treatment at the universities failed, but *Natr. Sulph.*, every two hours, produced rapid improvement in the swelling and general health of the patient.

Kali Mur. reduced the Swelling:

A swelling under the chin, the size of a pigeon's egg, was considerably reduced by *Kali Mur.*, but still there was induration (hardness), with an uneven surface. *Calc. Fluor.*, taken for a few days, caused it to disappear altogether. Shortly after its disappearance, the patient had slight conjunctivitis, with swelling, which *Kali Mur.* soon cured.
(Dr. K. From Schuessler.)

GLEET

(See Gonorrhea.)

GONORRHEA

ETIOLOGY

The basic cause of gonorrhea is the same as that of diseases affecting the other mucous membranes of the body. A deficiency of the cell-salt Kali Mur. causes an excess of fibrin which seeks to find an exit from the body through the mucous membrane of the urethra. In this way the mucous membrane is weakened, and a suitable breeding place is provided for the gonococcus. This may result in still more cell-salt deficiencies, which will require replacement. Whatever local treatment may be given for the gonococci, no permanent return to health can be expected until the deficiency of Kali Mur. and other lacking cell salts has been overcome.

BIOCHEMIC TREATMENT

Kali Mur.—This is the *principal remedy in gonorrhea.* Almost a specific in cases where swelling of any of the parts exists. Discharge of thick, white or yellowish-white pus. Avoid pressing along the urethra to bring out pus, as it produces an inflammation and greatly retards the cure. Walking and other exercise should also be avoided.

Ferrum Phos.—For the inflammatory conditions accompanying gonorrhea. In alternation with *Kali Mur.*, the chief remedy.

Kali Phos.—Gonorrhea glans penis, balanitis, requires *Kali Phos.* internally and externally. *Gonorrhea, with discharge of blood.*

Calc. Sulph.—When the discharge consists of blood and pus or purulent matter.

Natr. Mur.—*Gonorrhea,* when *chronic, with* characteristic *watery, transparent discharges.* Gonorrhea, with watery, scalding discharges, also *Calc. Phos.* Gleet, alternate with *Calc. Phos. After injections of nitrate of silver,* to destroy the injurious effects of the drug.

Calc. Phos.—Gonorrhea, with anemic conditions. Gleet, in alternation with *Natr. Mur.* Slimy, transparent, albuminous discharges.

Kali Sulph.—Gonorrhea, with slimy, yellow or greenish discharge. Gleet, with characteristic discharge of yellow matter.

Natr. Sulph.—Chronic *gonorrhea, with yellowish-green discharge,* which keeps up, of thick consistence. Very little pain. (Grauvogl.) *Enlarged prostate. Fig-warts.*

Silicea.—Gonorrhea cases of long standing, with thick, fetid pus. *Constant feeling of chilliness,* even during exercise. Balanitis.

Magnes. Phos.—For stricture accompanying gonorrhea. Gonorrhea with sharp, sticking pains—in alternation with the remedy indicated by the nature of the discharge.

CLINICAL CASES

Magnes. Phos. in chronic Gonorrhea:

A man, æt. 70, suffered for three years from discharge from the urethra; secretion small in quantity; clear mucus; on urinating violent, burning, sticking pains. *Kali Sulph.*, *Kali Mur.* and *Natr. Mur.* did no good. *Magnes. Phos.* cured the case in four weeks. The character of the pains was the prominent indication.
(Schuessler.)

Natr. Mur. in chronic Gonorrhea:

Mr. M., a prominent business man, consulted me regarding a chronic gonorrheal discharge of some two years' duration. The characteristic symptom of his case was the discharge of a bland, transparent, watery nature. He had been treated with the nitrate of silver; used almost everything that had been advised him, in fact. I prescribed an injection of olive oil, every two or three days, and gave *Natr. Mur.*, internally, every two hours. In three weeks' time discharge had completely disappeared.
(C. R. Vogel, M. D.)

Kali Mur. for thick, yellowish-white Discharges:

Have been asked to prescribe quite frequently in pharmacy for cases of gonorrhea. The cases presented marked characteristics of *Kali Mur.*, swelling of prepuce, with thick, yellowish-white pus discharges from the urethra, considerable pain along the urethra, especially back of the glans penis. Prescribed *Kali Mur.*, with plenty of hot water locally, and an injection of the permanganate of potash, grain one to aqua pura ounces eight, once a day. All have reported favorably.
(R. Meyer.)

GOUT

(See Rheumatism.)

BIOCHEMIC TREATMENT

Ferrum Phos.—First stage of gout and for the inflammatory conditions.

Natr. Phos.—Acute gout; chronic gout; profuse sour-smelling sweat.

Natr. Sulph.—In acute attacks of gout, should be given in alternation with *Ferrum Phos.* Chronic gout; gout in feet, both acute and chronic. This is the ***principal remedy*** in this affection.

GUMBOIL

BIOCHEMIC TREATMENT

Ferrum Phos.—For the inflammatory conditions, internal and locally.

Kali Mur.—For the swelling, before matter begins to form.

Silicea.—When pus is forming.

Calc. Sulph.—Given early will abort suppuration, but should be followed by *Silicea* when suppuration has commenced.

HEMOPTYSIS

(See Hemorrhage.)

HEADACHE

Nothing need be said under this head, as the intelligent reader will see at a glance that a deficiency in any one or more of the inorganic salts may produce a headache.

BIOCHEMIC TREATMENT

Kali Phos.—*Kali Phos.* is indicated in those purely *nervous headaches* resulting *from overstrain of* the *mental faculties* or great exertion of the mind. Headaches of pale, irritable or excitable persons. Headache followed by exhaustion. *Headaches of students and those worn-out by fatigue,* when no gastric symptoms are present; the *tongue* is frequently *coated brownish-yellow, like stale mustard;* bad breath. Pains and sensation of weight in back of head, with weariness and exhaustion (after *Ferrum Phos.*). Note *Natr. Sulph.* Nervous headaches, with inability for thought, loss of strength, sleeplessness, etc.; better under cheerful excitement; gentle motion relieves. *Headache, with weary, empty feeling at pit of stomach,* associated with or the precursor of bilious trouble (*Natr. Sulph.*). Neuralgic headache, with nervous symptoms, humming in the ears, etc.

Ferrum Phos.—Headaches which can be traced to an inflammatory state or a relaxation of the muscular walls of the blood-vessels of the head, allowing an engorgement to take place. *Headache, with bruising, pressing, stitching pains,* worse on movement or by stooping; *congestive headache;* red face and suffused redness of eyes. Throbbing headache from rush of blood to the head; cold applications and pressure relieve by reducing the congestion. Blind, sick headache, with vomiting of undigested food. Scalp sore and tender to the touch. Headaches from gouty predisposition (alternate *Natr. Sulph.*). Effects of sun-heat or excessive cold. If the tongue is coated, alternate with the remedy indicated by the color.

Kali Mur.—Headaches, with *sluggish action of the liver, white or grayish-white coating of the tongue,* vomiting or hawking of milk-white mucus, etc., requires *Kali Mur.*

Natr. Mur.—Dull, heavy headaches, with profusion of tears, caused by a derangement of the sodium chloride molecules; watery discharges from eyes and nose; excessive secretion of saliva, frequently associated with constipation and torpor of the bowels. *Headache, with drowsiness,* unrefreshing sleep, or vomiting of watery, transparent fluids. *Headaches of girls at puberty,* or with irregular menstruation, with characteristic symptoms of this remedy, such as *drowsiness, stupor and watery secretions.* Headaches which are generally worse in the morning or disappearing with the sun.

Kali Sulph.—Headaches which grow worse in a heated room, and in the evening, and are better in cool open air. (Schuessler.)

Magnes. Phos.—*Neuralgic headache, with excruciating, stinging, shooting, darting pains;* intermittent or paroxysmal in character. Headache, when heat relieves and cold aggravates. Rheumatic headache, when very severe. *Nervous headache,* with *sparks before the eyes* and other optical defects. Headache, with spasmodic crampy pains, worse from draughts of cold air.

Calc. Phos.—Headache, with cold feelings in the head, and the head feels cold to the touch (alternate with *Ferr. Phos.*); pains are worse from hot or cold applications. *Headache, with creeping coldness and numbness on the head.* Neuralgic headache, if *Magnes. Phos.* fails to give relief.

Natr. Sulph.—*Headaches* when they are caused or *accompanied by bilious symptoms,* vomiting of bile, bitter taste, greenish-gray coated tongue, etc. Sick headache, with any of the above symptoms or colicky pains and bilious diarrhea. Headaches, with giddiness, vertigo and dullness. Violent pains at base of brain or on top of the head; note also color of tongue and bilious symptoms.

Natr. Phos.—*Headache on the crown of the head, on awakening in the morning, with moist yellow, creamy coating on the back part of the tongue, roof of mouth.* Headache, with acid, sour risings or vomiting of sour, watery transparent fluids. Frontal or occipital headaches; very severe pain, as if the skull were too full, after *Ferrum Phos.*

Silicea.—Headaches accompanied with small lumps the size of a pea, upon the scalp.

CLINICAL CASES

Kali Phos. in partial insanity from Headache:

A very interesting case came under my treatment. A lady, 55 years old, had such excruciating headache that she was partially insane; she claimed her brain was ruptured and running out of her eyes; a yellow-gray curd was exuding from her eyes. She had been suffering for some days. I gave her *Kali Phos.*, which acted like a charm. In two hours the dose was repeated, and the result was perfect relief.

Natr. Sulph. in periodic Headache:

M. H., æt. 16, has suffered for years from periodically returning headaches. The pain is concentrated in the right temple, and of a boring nature, as if a screw were being driven in— as the patient expresses herself. Preceding this pain there are burning sensations at the pit of the stomach, bitter taste in the mouth and lassitude. These symptoms are only felt at night or in the morning. When the attack comes on, the patient is quite unable to attend to any ordinary duties. Generally, vomiting of bile follows, and then improvement sets in. *Natr. Sulph.*, dissolved in water, and taken several times daily, cured the young lady entirely.
(From Schuessler.)

Kali Phos. in nervous Headache:

Case of a young lady with excruciating nervous headache, with great sensitiveness to noise, during the second day of menstruation. *Kali Phos.* produced, immediately after taking it, a great increase of the menstrual flow, with sudden relief of the headache.
(W. P. Wesselhoeft, M. D.)

Kali Phos. in Headache of students:

While attending college I was troubled with a very severe headache, due to biliousness and overstrain of the mind, from too close application to study. The pains, of a neuralgic character, were accompanied by roaring and buzzing in the ears, dimness of vision, specks before the eyes; could not think properly, everything seemed to be confused; there was also a nasty, disagreeable, brownish-yellow coating on my tongue. Consulted one of the professors, who prescribed twelve powders of *Kali Phos.*, one every three hours. Began to get better at once; continued the medicine for about three weeks, less often daily, and now, three years afterward, am troubled only occasionally with the headache, and then it is no comparison to what it was.

(Dr. H. H. Hawkins.)

HEART AFFECTIONS

ETIOLOGY

It was shown under Abscess, that before the organic matter was thrown out of the blood that afterwards commenced to decay and caused the condition called abscess, it might form clots and thus disturb the vascular action of the heart. This is the pathology of embolus and, in some instances, palpitation. Pericarditis is caused by a lack of the proper balance of the mineral salts in the blood, but particularly in the tissue of the pericardium.

A lack of iron molecules in the tissue of any membrane causes an inflammatory condition or excess of heat, in the following manner: Iron molecules are carriers of oxygen, and when the number is reduced, from any cause, the circulation is increased by nature's effort to carry sufficient oxygen through the organism, with the limited amount of iron at hand; the increased motion produces heat. The extra amount of blood flowing through the minute vessels of the membrane (pericardium) also causes more or less engorgement and thickening of the tissue.

The action of the heart is frequently interfered with by pressure through the diaphragm of gas in the stomach caused by indigestion.

BIOCHEMIC TREATMENT

Kali Phos.—Heart complaint, functional, intermittent, with palpitation. Intermittent action of the heart, with nervousness, sensitiveness or exhaustion. *Palpitation of the heart after rheumatic fever; weak action of the heart. Kali Phos.* is a most valuable heart stimulant in wasting fevers, when, after the fever is broken, sinking spells occur and the pulse becomes imperceptible. Palpitation, with anxiety, melancholia, sleeplessness or general depression of the nervous system. Fainting, from any cause whatever.

Ferrum Phos.—*Dilation of heart or of blood-vessels,* in alternation with *Calc. Fluor., the principal remedy.* Inflammatory condition of the heart, in the congestive stage. Carditis, pericarditis, endocarditis, etc. Palpitation of the heart, in alternation with *Kali Phos.*

Calc. Fluor.—*Dilation* of the heart or blood-vessels *from a relaxed condition of the muscular fibres; Calc. Fluor.* is the *chief remedy* to restore contractility of these fibres; alternate with *Ferr. Phos.* Weak action of the heart from over-engorgement of that organ.

Kali Mur.—Embolus; for that condition of blood which favors the formation of clots (*fibrinous*) which act as plugs (alternate with *Ferrum Phos.* for the circulatory disturbance). Second remedy in inflammatory conditions of the heart. Palpitation and weakness of the heart from excessive flow of blood to the heart. Hypertrophy of the heart (alternate with *Calc. Fluor.*)

Calc. Phos.—Weak heart-action, as an intercurrent remedy. Palpitation of the heart, followed by weakness. Poor circulation, coldness of the extremities. Palpitation when caused by an accumulation of gas on the stomach.

Kali Sulph.—"Pulse quick, with slow, throbbing, boring pain over crest of ileum, disinclination to speak, pallid face." (Walker.) Alternate with *Ferrum Phos.*

Magnes. Phos.—Palpitation of the heart, when of purely spasmodic character. Sharp, shooting, darting pains in heart or in the region of heart.

Natr. Mur.—*Palpitation in anemic subjects,* watery blood, dropsical swellings, etc. Palpitation, with sadness, anxiety and watery conditions characteristic of this remedy.—Note condition of tongue.

HEART-BURN

(See Gastric Derangements.)

HEMORRHAGE

ETIOLOGY

Hemorrhages are caused by a deficiency of certain cell-salts in the circular walls of the blood-vessels. Iron gives strength, toughness and elasticity to the vascular system, while sodium chloride, the water-carrier, furnishes moisture.

A lack of one or both of these salts causes brittleness and weakness of the muscular tissue composing the walls of veins and arteries, and when they are subjected to a strain—(1) from an excess of heat; (2) or too much food or matter in intestines; (3) or non-functional organic matter in the circulation—fibrin, albumen, etc.—there may be a breaking down of the vascular walls, especially of the capillaries or minute blood-vessels, and, consequently, hemorrhage. (See article on Dysentery.)

BIOCHEMIC TREATMENT

Ferrum Phos.—This is the *principal remedy* for hemorrhage in any part of the body, when the *blood* is *bright-red* and *coagulates quickly.* Epistaxis, from any cause; the remedy should be given internally, and applied locally where practical. In bad cases apply dry powder thickly on bleeding vessel. Hemorrhage from lungs. *Vomiting of bright-red blood. Predisposition to bleeding, especially* from the nose, *in anemic subjects,* alternate with *Calc. Phos.* and *Kali Phos.*

Kali Phos.—Bleeding in weak, delicate constitutions, from debility; blood is dark, blackish, red and thin, not coagulating. Predisposition to bleed in anemic subjects, alternate *Ferrum Phos.* and *Calc. Phos.* Putrid blood, with symptoms of decomposition. *Uterine hemorrhage.*

Kali Mur.—Hemorrhage, with dark, black, dotted or tough blood.

Natr. Mur.—Hemorrhage, when the blood is thin, pale-red and watery, not coagulating readily.

Calc. Fluor.—*Uterine hemorrhage,* alternate with *Kali Phos.* Flooding, to tone up the contractile powers of the uterus. Hemorrhoidal hemorrhage.

CLINICAL CASES

Ferrum Phos. in Epistaxis:

Willie N., æt. 16; troubled for years with frequent hemorrhage from the nose, caused by a sun-stroke; blood bright-red; very anemic countenance. After taking *Ferrum Phos.* for two months, the bleeding entirely ceased, with but one return during the last year, and then it was during an attack of inflammatory rheumatism.

(Dr. Chapman.)

Ferrum Phos. in Apoplexy:

Lady, æt. 72; large and corpulent; dark hair and eyes; subject to attacks of apoplectiform cerebral congestion; was found

in apoplectic state, with cold extremities, clammy sweat on forehead and face; head hot and livid; unconscious; low, stertorous breathing. *Ferrum Phos.*, teaspoonful every half hour; consciousness returned in two hours. Was up the next day. The same remedy has been used in subsequent attacks, with the same results. Patient states that never before had she been relieved so soon and effectually.
(F. A. Rockwith, M. D.)

Kali Mur. in Hemorrhage of the Bowels:

Dr. E. B. Rankin reports a case of hemorrhage of the bowels, of dark, black blood, viscid and profuse, cured by *Kali Mur.*

Ferrum Phos. in Epistaxis:

Dwight H., æt. 12, has been subject to nose-bleed for past few years. During this time he became very anemic. He has taken different remedies from the family physician without permanently arresting the trouble. I was called to see him after a very severe attack, and found him much prostrated and blanched from loss of blood. Gave him at once *Ferrum Phos.*, which he took in solution for some weeks, a few doses each day, with result of permanently arresting the hemorrhage.
(C. T. M.)

Ferrum Phos. in Hemorrhage of Lungs:

Have received good results in a case of hemorrhage from the lungs, with *Ferrum Phos.*, five-grain doses every half-hour. The blood was of a bright-red color and coagulated almost as soon as it was vomited. The Ferrum Phos. was also prescribed with marked benefit in same case about two months later.
(C. R. Vogel, M. D.)

HEMORRHOIDS

ETIOLOGY

The cause of hemorrhoids is dependent upon three factors:

First: A lack of the proper balance of certain tissue or cell-salts in the fluids of the liver—probably sodium sulphate or potassium chloride—either causes a thickening of the bile or a lack of same.

Second: For this reason undigested food and abnormal or vitiated feces reach the sigmoid flexure.

Third: This vitiated, fermented and acrid matter interferes with the peristalsis of the intestines, creating a greater or less amount of constipation, which still further increases the fecal contents of the bowels.

On being forced down through the colon, the weight of the fecal mass, as well as the pressure of the gas created by it, irritates and inflames the anorectal veins, either internal or external.

This irritation causes a disturbance of the molecular action of the calcium fluoride in the elastic fibre of the veins, with a consequent varicose condition known as hemorrhoids.

BIOCHEMIC TREATMENT

Calc. Fluor.—Is the *principal remedy* in this disease, in alternation with remedies indicated by the color of the blood and coating of the tongue. *Bleeding piles, with pressure of blood to the head.* Piles, internal or blind piles, frequently with pains low down in the back; note also the tongue symptoms. *Piles, with chronic constipation. Itching piles. Calc. Fluor.* should also be used externally with vaseline or with a compress. Chief remedy for prolapsus recti.

Ferrum Phos.—*Hemorrhoids, with discharge of bright-red blood,* coagulating easily. Local applications will relieve the soreness and inflammation. Prolapsus recti.

Kali Mur.—When the blood is dark and thick, alternate with *Calc. Fluor.*, for relaxation of the elastic fibres.

Kali Sulph.—Frequently indicated in piles, as an alternate remedy with *Calc. Fluor.*, with characteristic yellow, slimy coating on the tongue.

Natr. Sulph.—Hemorrhoids, with heat in the lower bowel and bilious conditions; note also color of the tongue. An alternate remedy with *Calc. Fluor.*

Kali Phos.—Prolapsus recti, in alternation with *Calc. Fluor.*, the chief remedy.

Calc. Phos.—As an intercurrent remedy in hemorrhoids of anemic persons. Has, also, the power of working with muscular fibre.

Natr. Mur.—As an alternating remedy with *Calc. Fluor.*, for the bowel conditions; *stools are hard, dry and crumbling,* with *excess of saliva in the mouth.*

Magnes. Phos.—*Pains in hemorrhoids,* cutting, darting, very acute, often like lightning, in external piles. (Also as tepid lotion.) "As a rule, besides the local hemorrhoids, there are disturbances in the functions of the liver, the digestive organs, etc., present; these stand in close connection with the former; attention must be paid to those, if a radical cure of hemorrhoids is to be insured." (Schuessler.)

CLINICAL CASES

Calc. Fluor. in Chronic Hemorrhoids:

I have in mind a patient who came to me to be treated for itching hemorrhoids of long standing. He said the itching was almost intolerable; said that he had been treated by a number of good physicians with no relief. He was cured with *Calc. Fluor. in a few weeks.* It is now more than two years and there has never been any return of the trouble. (Dr. I. M. Howard, Cross Plains, Texas.)

Calc. Fluor. in Hemorrhoids:

Mr. F. A.; hemorrhoids, external; were cured, after using almost every local application, by *Calc. Fluor.*, taken every night.

Calc. Fluor. in Hemorrhoids:

Mrs. K. had been in bed with hemorrhoids, sore, bleeding, painful. Three weeks under other medical treatment. *Calc. Fluor.*, three tablets every three hours, relieved her in a very short time.

(Dr. Wm. B. Deffendall, Washington, Indiana.)

Kali Mur. in Hemorrhoids:

I have prescribed *Kali Mur.* in many cases of hemorrhoids of the bleeding variety, when the blood is dark and thick, in alternation with *Calc. Fluor.*, with much benefit. I have found, though, that *Calc. Fluor.*, from the fact that the lack of it is one of the principal causes of hemorrhoidal conditions, serves me better in the majority of cases, no matter what variety—internal, external, bleeding, etc. Have also used *Natr. Sulph.* and *Kali Sulph.*, when the characteristic color of the tongue of those remedies was present.

(Chas. F. Wright, M. D.)

Calc. Fluor. in Hemorrhoids:

Wm. S., æt. 28, has been troubled with hemorrhoids for some years. Bleeding piles, accompanied by chronic constipation, with much straining at stool; great pressure of blood to the head, and flushes of heat; tongue mapped or covered with a grayish-white coating. I prescribed *Calc. Fluor.* and *Kali Mur.* in alternation, every four hours, corrected the diet, and in a few weeks he was completely cured, with no return of the trouble. I might also add that I had an ointment of one-half ounce of *Calc. Fluor.* to two of vaseline made and had it applied locally up into the rectum every night, which greatly assisted the internal medicine.

(C. R. Vogel, M. D.)

HEPATITIS

(See Liver, Affections of.)

HICCOUGH

ETIOLOGY

A spasmodic contraction of the diaphragm, causing inspiration and sudden closure of the glottis. It is wholly due to a lack of the inorganic salt magnesia phosphate in the muscular fibres of the tissue at the part affected.

BIOCHEMIC TREATMENT

Magnes. Phos.—*Principal remedy* in this affection, *for the spasmodic and convulsive symptoms;* acts quicker in hot water; frequent doses.

Natr. Mur.—"Hiccough, after abuse and in consequence of quinine." (Dr. Burnett.)

CLINICAL CASES

Natr. Mur. cures Hiccough of ten years' standing:

Dr. Burnett, in his work on "Natrum Muriaticum," relates a case of singultus of ten years' standing brought about by abuse of quinine, and renewed after every dose, cured permanently by *Natr. Mur.*

Magnes. Phos. in Hiccough in Typhoid Fever:

Obstinate case of singultus in a patient suffering from typhoid fever; almost continued; so violent in character that the patient was sore for three days. Other remedies were tried without effect; prescribed *Magnes. Phos.* The result was remarkable; within an hour the difficulty was modified, and next day it was very much improved, and speedily yielded to the continued use of the remedy.
(John Fearn, M. D., *California Med. Journal.*)

HIP-JOINT DISEASE

BIOCHEMIC TREATMENT

Ferrum Phos.—In the first or inflammatory stage of hip-joint disease, for fever, pain, throbbing and inflammation; also local application of the same.

Kali Mur.—In the second stage, when there is swelling of the parts, but before pus has begun to form.

Silicea.—To prevent or control suppuration and heal the parts. It limits the destruction of bone.

Calc. Sulph.—For the discharge of pus and matter, alternate with *Ferrum Phos.* to effect a cure. Complete rest is also necessary.

CLINICAL CASES

Tuberculosis of the Hip:

A young man, age 19. Father and older sister died of tuberculosis. First symptom, a limp favoring right hip. X-ray showed affection of hip joint. He moved to Muncie, Indiana, and I did not see him for six months. He had been in plaster cast for weeks, he told me; and when I saw him again he was on crutches with a tubercular abscess of right hip joint. On removing dressing the discharge was very profuse. Emaciated, night sweats. *Silicea* (no other medicine) was given with little hope and no encouragement to anxious mother. But improvement was noticed in three or four weeks. The boy was faithful with his "tablets" and at the end of seven months laid aside *one crutch* and at the end of a year *both* crutches. Favored hip for a while by using a cane, then no cane. Saw him recently; walks without limp; hip is well; no night sweats; gained in weight, etc.

(Dr. I. N. Agenbroad, Dayton, Ohio.)

HIVES

(See Skin, Affections of.)

HOARSENESS

(See Throat and Aphonia.)

BIOCHEMIC TREATMENT

Ferrum Phos.—*Painful hoarseness of speakers and singers,* due to a slight inflammation of the throat, from overexertion of the voice or from taking cold. Aphonia.

Kali Mur.—Loss of voice, hoarseness, and huskiness from cold. If obstinate and not yielding to this remedy, alternate with *Kali Sulph.*

Kali Phos.—After *Ferrum Phos.,* if there is exhaustion or nervous depression; also a tired, weary feeling in throat, from a rheumatic affection.

Kali Sulph.—When *Kali Mur.* fails to give relief, though seeming to be indicated.

Calc. Phos.—Constant, chronic hoarseness, with much hemming and scraping of the throat.

HYDROCELE

BIOCHEMIC TREATMENT

Natr. Mur.—Hydrocele, scrotal edema, with serous infiltration.

Natr. Sulph.—With erysipelatous conditions, alternate with *Natr. Mur.*

Calc. Phos.—Intercurrent with other remedies, or if *Natr. Mur.* fails.

Calc. Fluor.—Hydrocele, to contract the relaxed muscles of the testicle and force out the infiltration.

Silicea.—As an intercurrent remedy in scrofulous conditions or improperly nourished children.

CLINICAL CASES

Silicea in Hydrocele of Children:

Silicea cured two cases of hydrocele: one left-sided, in a babe four days old; the other right-sided, in a child. (Dr. Guernsey.)

Silicea for Sarco-Hydrocele:

A man suffering from a herpetic eruption, for the cure of which *Silicea* was taken. But at the same time a sarco-hydrocele of large dimensions, which he had carried about four years, was reduced to a minimum.

HYDROCEPHALUS

(See Meningitis.)

HYSTERIA

BIOCHEMIC TREATMENT

Kali Phos.—The *principal remedy* in this nervous disease. Nervous attacks from sudden and intense emotion. Hysteria, from passion, in the highly nervous. Hysterical fits of laughter and crying. *Hysteria, with a feeling as of a ball rising in the throat.* Look to the primary cause.

Natr. Mur.—Hysteria, if associated with sadness, moody spells or irregular menstruation. Alternate with *Kali Phos.*, the chief remedy.

CLINICAL CASES

Kali Phos. in Hysteria from non-occurring Menstruation:

Miss R., æt. 16; menstruated once when thirteen years old, and not since. Was a remarkably healthy and well-nourished girl, until three months before she consulted me, when she began to decline. She lost flesh, became pale, languid and weak, and suffered much with her stomach. When I was called to see her she was not able to retain her food, and it would be vomited as soon as taken; complained of great pain in the stomach immediately after eating even the lightest food; on several occasions the pain caused severe hysterical convulsions. The tongue was but slightly coated white; bowels constipated; abdomen tympanitic and very sensitive to the slightest pressure; no fever, but much thirst; water, like food, was ejected as soon as swallowed. At first I thought that I had a case of nervous

dyspepsia to deal with, but finally concluded that I had a case of true hysteria, as she was so extremely nervous and hyperesthetic all over, and much given to tears when anyone was around I also found that she had the convulsions whenever her plans were thwarted in any way, but upon my threatening to put her in cold water if she had another, she stopped them. *Ferrum Phos.* relieved the stomach trouble in one week, and *Kali Phos.* relieved all the other symptoms in two weeks more, and my patient was soon as strong and healthy as before her illness. Menstruation returned two months after, and she has been all right since.
(Geo. H. Martin, M. D.)

Kali Phos. cured in ten days:

Miss B., æt. 50, tall, slender and dark, had been suffering for many years from an excessively nervous condition, and would become hysterical upon the slightest provocation. She also suffered much from spasmodic retention of urine, and often had to use the catheter. One day she came to me, saying that the end of the catheter had been broken off while she was using it, and the end was still in the bladder. I dilated the urethra with my forefinger, and soon recovered it, the bladder at the time being well filled with urine. She would not take an anesthetic, although I advised it, as the pain was intense. That evening, six hours after the removal of the catheter, she sent for me, saying that she was in great pain and very ill. When I saw her I found her very nervous and suffering much from pain in the bladder and abdomen, with a great desire to urinate. The abdomen was enormously distended and very sensitive. There was no fever. I gave her a prescription and returned next morning. Symptoms all worse, but still no fever. Attempted to drain urine, but could not introduce the soft rubber catheter, as the spasm of the urethra was so great. Two hours later, returned with silver catheter; introduced it, but only got a few drops of urine. Thinking there might be some uterine trouble, I determined to examine and find out As she was so sensitive, I gave her a little chloroform. She

had taken but a few inhalations when the tympanitis disappeared. I examined uterus and bladder, and found nothing abnormal, so concluded she was suffering from hysteria. Gave *Magnes. Phos.*, which very shortly relieved bladder symptoms, and *Kali Phos.* cured the case in about ten days. She has had no more return of the trouble since, and the other symptoms of hysteria were also much modified.
(Geo. H. Martin, M. D.)

INCONTINENCE OF URINE

(See Enuresis; Urinary Disorders.)

INDIGESTION

(See Also Gastric Derangements.)

ETIOLOGY

Some of the principal underlying causes of indigestion are: irregularities in diet, such as overeating; eating too rich or indigestible food; highly-seasoned and stimulating soups; excessive use of wine, liquors, tea, coffee and other stimulants; too long fasting or irregularity of meals; imperfect chewing of food; keeping late hours; sedentary habits; exhaustion from study; mental emotions; irregularity of the bowels, etc., etc.

All these causes or irregularities create a disturbance in the tissues of the digestive organs—as well as in the digestive fluids—causing a breaking up of the union between the organic and inorganic matter in certain cells rendering them biologically inert, so that the digestive fluids are unable to complete the process of digestion.

CLINICAL CASES

Ferrum Phos. in Indigestion from drinking cold water while overheated:

A lady, 29 years of age, of sanguine temperament, with rather high color of face, has been suffering the last five years

from the following digestive troubles, which she contracted by a draught of very cold water whilst in a stage of heat and perspiration: She has no desire to eat; great dislike to milk. After food, nausea and vomiting of food, which is so acid that it sets her teeth on edge. She can take nothing sour. Meat, and also salt herring, causes much pain, and so do cake and coffee. The sickness and retching occasionally come on before breakfast; otherwise only after food. To this is added cephalalgia. She feels a beating pain in her forehead and temples—formerly on the left, now more on the right side. This pain is most violent. Catamenia appears every three weeks. with much loss; dragging pain in lower abdomen and lumbar region. The *bowels* are normal, the sleep is disturbed by anxious dreams, and feels in the morning as though she had been beaten. In the evening she feels oppressed and swelled, so that she has to loosen her dress; she cannot wear it in the least tight. Her pulse is accelerated, being 100 per minute. As a girl she was quite healthy and had never suffered from anemia. On the whole, the lady was not much emaciated, in spite of her ailing so long. This was the description the patient gave of her case. The leading symptoms of this case led me to choose iron. I ordered her a dose of *Ferr. Phos.*—to be taken before meals, three times daily. When I saw her again, she was able to give me the very satisfactory report that her ailments were cured.
(Dr. Mossa.)

INFLUENZA

(See La Grippe.)

BIOCHEMIC TREATMENT

Ferrum Phos.—For the inflammatory conditions, fever, heat, pain, etc.

Natr. Sulph.—*Chief remedy* to increase secretion of urine and diminish the excess of intercellular fluids.

Kali Mur.—For the rheumatic pains, and *when the tongue is coated white or gray;* for the depression, *Kali Phos.* in alternation.

INFLAMMATIONS

(See Fever, Simple.)

BIOCHEMIC TREATMENT

Ferrum Phos.—In the first or hyperemic stage, always *before exudation has taken place.* The principal symptoms are heat, redness, pain, etc. Given internally and applied locally, it will, in the majority of cases, prevent exudation.

Kali Mur.—In the second stage of inflammations, of any part, *when exudation has taken place*—indicated by recent swelling or discharge of opaque white mucus.

Kali Sulph.—When the exudation has changed to a *ripe yellow, or yellow, slimy discharges.*

Calc. Sulph.—Third stage of inflammations, with *profuse discharges of thick, yellow, purulent matter,* sometimes streaked with blood.

Silicea.—When, after inflammation, pus has begun to form, *Silicea* will greatly assist in promoting suppuration. NOTE: It matters not where the inflammation may be located, internal or external, the treatment will be the same. In the hyperemic stage, local applications of the remedy should always be used where practicable.

INJURIES

(See Mechanical Injuries.)

INTERMITTENT FEVER [Malaria]

ETIOLOGY

THE predisposing cause of intermittent fever, or malaria, as it is frequently called, is found in an excess of water in the system due to the following facts.

Hot weather causes a rapid evaporation of water, especially in low, marshy districts, and regions where there are many ponds and other small bodies of water. This water is held in solution in the atmosphere, and is, of course, taken into the blood through the lungs by the act of breathing; thus the blood becomes overcharged with water.

The cell-salt Natr. Sulph. has an affinity for oxygen, and oxygen has an affinity for water, and thus, in health, Natr. Sulph. is able to eliminate this excess of water from the system. If, however, from any cause, a deficiency of Natr. Sulph. exists in the system, this surplus water cannot be carried off.

Thus a suitable breeding place in the blood is supplied for the plasmodium malariae or haematozoa of Laveran, a vegetable micro-organism to which the active manifestations of malarial fever are due. The plasmodium is introduced into the human system by a species of mosquito, the anopheles, which carries the organism in its blood, and transmits it through its bite.

When once established in the blood, the plasmodium causes a series of paroxysms, nearly always occurring with remarkable regularity either at the end of 24, 48 or 72 hours. If occurring at the expiration of 24 hours from the beginning of the preceding paroxysms, the fever is said to be of the quotidian type. If the interval between paroxysms is 48 hours, the paroxysm occurring every third day, the fever is of the tertian type. If the interval is 72 hours, the paroxysm recurring on the fourth day, it is a quartan fever. The quotidian and tertian type of intermittent fever are the most common, the quartan being comparatively rare.

Each paroxysm usually consists of three stages. The first is known as the *cold* stage, or chill. This may come on suddenly, or be preceded by headache and a general feeling of lassitude. The chilly sensation usually begins in the back and loins, and spreads over the entire body. There is yawning, stretching, bitter taste in the mouth, pale-coated tongue, and increasing headache. Finally, the chill becomes so severe that the muscular rigors shake the entire body. The tips of fingers, ears and nose are livid; the voice is husky and faint; respiration is rapid and often labored; the pulse is quick, small and hard. In severe cases symptoms of collapse may appear. The cold stage continues for ten or fifteen minutes to an hour, and even longer.

As the *hot stage* begins, the sensation of chilliness is gradually replaced by a comfortable feeling of heat. The blood returns to the surface, and the face flushes. The surface of the body becomes burning hot, dry, red. The patient is extremely thirsty, and drinks water in large quantities. There is severe frontal headache, and the pulse is full and bounding, running as high as 120 to the minute, or more. The temperature may reach 106° or more, although occasionally there is only a slight increase over the temperature reached during the cold stage. This stage lasts from one to several hours, rarely more than five or six.

The *sweating* stage begins with moisture on the head and face, gradually and often rapidly involving the entire surface of the body This culminates in a profuse, drenching sweat, with a disappearance of all other symptoms, the patient, in a majority of cases, falling into a quiet, natural sleep. This stage lasts from two to four hours or longer.

During the interval between the paroxysms the patient may be about as usual, but slightly indisposed.

There is also a form of malarial fever known as remittent fever, in which the temperature varies, but never gets as low as normal. This fever ranges from mild to severe, and lasts from one to two weeks.

Quinine seems to possess a specific action against the plasmodium malariæ, but as its maximum effect is not obtained from four to six hours after its administration, it should be given in the quotidian type eight hours, in the tertian twelve hours, and in the quartan type fifteen to eighteen hours before the expected chill, and repeated. Ten to 15-grains doses are usually sufficient in the milder types, while in the more severe types 30 to 60 grains are often required. The quinine should be given in powder in soft capsules easily dissolved.

Quinine is not, however, the only nor the most important remedy in malarial fever. The basic cause of the trouble is an excess of water in the blood, which has provided a suitable breeding place for the plasmodium malariæ, and this excess of water must be removed, so that a recurrence of the disease may be prevented, and a permanent restoration to health assured.

This excess of water is due to a deficiency of the cell-salt Natr. Sulph., and it is only by supplying this lacking salt that the condition can be overcome. Natr. Sulph. is thus the chief remedy in malarial fevers. When the trouble has continued for some time, the nervous system is frequently affected by a lack of Kali Phos., and this salt is also needed. The fever, too, always calls for Ferrum Phos.

BIOCHEMIC TREATMENT

Natr. Sulph.—Intermittent fever, in all its stages, requires this, the *chief remedy for the bilious conditions,* and to eliminate the excess of water in the tissues. See article in relation to its pathological action. Ague patients must abstain from a rich diet. Eggs, milk, buttermilk, fats and fish should be avoided.

Ferrum Phos.—For the febrile conditions and when vomiting undigested food; in alternation with the chief remedy, *Natr.*

Sulph., in all cases of intermittent fever. *Ferrum Phos.* attracts oxygen which is essential for the cure of this disease.

Kali Phos.—When there is debility and profuse perspiration.

Kali Mur.—As an intercurrent or alternate remedy if the tongue has a thick white or grayish-white coating.

Natr. Mur.—In intermittent fever, when the characteristic watery symptoms are present. Great thirst and *fever-blisters around the lips. After the abuse of quinine,* to eliminate the drug from the system.

Magnes. Phos.—Intermittent fever, with cramps in the calves, intercurrently with *Natr. Sulph.*

Natr. Phos.—Intermittent fever, with acid conditions; vomiting of acid, sour fluids.

Calc. Phos.—Chronic intermittent fever of children (intercurrently).

CLINICAL CASES

Natr. Sulph. in Chills and Fever:

Allow me to report a case of chills and fever, cured with one of the Biochemic remedies. May 3, Mr. S. called to consult me in regard to chills and fever. In May, the year before, was taken with chills, which always began between 9 and 11 o'clock every other day. He consulted a physician, who dosed him heavily with quinine, blue mass and Fowler's solution for six weeks, when the chills came only once a week, and in three weeks more ceased entirely. Last October, he was again taken, and in the same way, and received the same drugging. April 30, he was again taken and was advised to come to me for treatment. Patient is a light-haired, blue-eyed slender-built young man, and presented the following symptoms: Appetite good, but has lost fifteen pounds in six weeks. Takes cold easily; has headache daily, of a bursting nature, and mostly left-sided. The skin of face looks rough and as if patient had taken a salt bath and the water had dried on, leaving a crusty white look in folds of skin and wrinkles. Said his hair was falling out. Constipated most of the time. Has vivid dreams nightly—mostly of trouble and danger. Chills come at 10 a. m. Great thirst, much heat, bursting headache and thirst, and much aching. Sweat, with thirst, which relieved all pains. Yellowish-white coating on tongue. Some vomiting during fever. Gave him *Natr. Sulph.* four times a day. No return of chills to date, and is gaining in weight.

Natr. Sulph. and Natr. Mur. in Chills and Fever:

Mr. P. W., age 21. Had a severe chill at 11 a. m. He had had chills for three days before he came to me. I put him on *Natr. Mur.*, four tablets every three hours, and *Natr. Sulph.*, five tablets three times a day. The next chill was very light and there were no others.
(Dr. H. Whisler, Tingley, Iowa.)

Natr. Mur. after Quinine:

Mr. L.; chills and fever for three months. Had quinine and other remedies. Paroxysms every other day at 11 a. m., with severe pain in limbs and small of back; chill lasted nearly two hours, with no thirst during chill. Fever all the afternoon, with bursting headache and intense thirst for large quantities of cold water. Little or no perspiration; eats and sleeps well, and next day resumes his occupation. *Natr. Mur.* every four hours during the apyrexia. Next chill light and no return.
(H. C. Allen.)

Natr. Mur. in Chills:

Was called to see Mr. H., æt. 27, living about four miles in the country, in a low, marshy district. I found that he had been having chills every third day, coming on at 9 a. m. and lasting until 11 o'clock, sometimes till noon. Chill began in the small of the back, creeping over the entire body; dreads chills; could feel spell coming on, on account of headache, which began before chill and gradually grew worse. Constant desire for water, which tastes salty to him. Headache becomes so violent during chill that he must hold head with his hands. Fever comes on about 1 p. m. and lasts all afternoon, accompanied by much lassitude, increased headache, increased thirst; profuse sour-smelling sweat, which seems to relieve him; lips covered with hydroa; no appetite. Twelve doses of *Natr. Mur.* were left to be given, one every four hours. Reported much better after taking them. Continued treatment for two weeks, and now, more than eight months afterward, no return of chills.

(C. R. Vogel, M. D.)

Natr. Sulph. in Malaria:

Mrs. M., æt. 32; of sanguine temperament; easily excited; nervous and irritable. Thinks she caught the chills from taking her shoes off while feet were perspiring; symptoms ill defined. Complains of being chilly all the time, but always worse about 3 o'clock in the morning. Compelled to go to bed early in the evening, because she cannot keep warm. Limbs, feet and face especially chilly; dreads getting up for fear of being more chilled. Feels chilly all morning; great hunger; can eat anything. Fever comes on and increases gradually; at its highest about 2 p. m. Thirst intense; difficult breathing. Profuse perspiration, mostly on face and chest; sweat rolls down face. Offensive foot-sweat. *Natr. Sulph.* and *Silicea* were prescribed every three hours, for one week, with a complete cure of chills and fever; the foot-sweats still continue, but less profuse and not so offensive.

(C. R. Vogel, M. D.)

JAUNDICE

(See Liver, Affections of.)

KIDNEYS, AFFECTIONS OF

(See Bright's Disease, Diabetes Mellitus.)

ETIOLOGY

Kidney troubles may arise from numerous causes and may be due to a deficiency of several cell-salts. Little may be said, therefore, to cover in a general way the entire subject of disorders of this region.

The excessive use of intoxicating liquors is frequently the cause of most diseases of this region, the excretory organs being unable to cope with the constant presence of alcohol in the system. The use of alcoholic drinks should, therefore, be strictly abstained from by the patient whose kidneys or bladder have become diseased.

If Biochemic treatment is begun and a careful diet observed soon after the inception of the disease, a complete and early recovery may be hoped for. If, however, the disease has become chronic, improvement of the condition will necessarily be slow. For this reason it is obviously far better that treatment be begun as soon as possible.

Biochemistry does not conflict with any other recognized system of combating disease and the Biochemic remedies will in no way interfere with the action of any other remedies that may be found efficacious. The Biochemic remedies supply the body's deficiencies, and until those deficiencies are supplied the body cannot get well. Drugs may be taken to relieve pain or stimulate the resistive forces of the body; serums may be given to combat germs and bacilli; diet and proper nursing may overcome the exciting causes of the disease; but health cannot be restored until the deficiencies have been overcome and the tissues brought back to a normal condition.

BIOCHEMIC TREATMENT

Ferrum Phos.—All affections of the kidneys, when there is inflammation, fever, heat or pain. Nephritis, Bright's disease, etc., in the first or inflammatory stage, to reduce the congestion.

Kali Mur.—Second stage of inflammatory diseases of the kidneys, for the swelling and recent cell-proliferation.

Kali Phos.—For the disturbance of the nervous system as alternate remedy.

Calc. Phos.—Kidney disease, with albumen in the urine, in alternation with *Kali Phos.,* for the nervous symptoms. Principal remedy for Bright's disease.

CLINICAL CASES

Calc. Phos. in "laziness of the kidneys".

G. S., an old man of 77, consulted me for what he called a "laziness of his kidneys." Urine was, in fact, very scanty and loaded with albumen. The case seemed, at first sight, to be a hopeless one; he was also forgetful and quite nervous. I gave him *Calc. Phos.,* a dose every two hours in alternation with *Kali Phos.* After six weeks' treatment, urine was normal, his memory was somewhat restored, and for six months he has not complained. As to diet, I only recommended to him to eat just as much asparagus as he could at his meals, and continue the use of the afore-mentioned medicines.
(E. A. de Cailhol, M. D.)

Biochemic Remedies to abort Nephritis:

A male, aged 40, who had, according to his history, both typhoid fever and scarlet fever when younger. He came to me complaining of a hurting in the region of the kidneys. specks before the eyes, and a frequent desire to urinate. The pulse, temperature, and respiration were normal. Blood pressure normal. The analysis showed very low specific gravity, no albumen, no sugar, neutral in reaction. The nervous system showed a minus condition by the phosphate test of Dr. Henry Doud of New York State. The patient was anemic, constipated, poor appetite, slept fairly well, and was in a general weakened condition all over and had a yellowish tint of the skin, sclera, etc., although no tenderness over the gall-bladder.

After a careful study of the case I decided he was in a prenephritic condition and would develop into nephritis if something was not done for him at once. I treated him with the ordinary regular remedies with no influence on the specific gravity, although I bettered his general condition. I then decided to try Biochemic Remedies, and after a careful survey of the symptoms, I decided to give him as follows:

Ferrum Phos., 5-gr. celloid.

Magnes. Phos., 5-gr. celloid.

Kali Phos., 5-gr. celloid.

Calc. Phos., 5-gr. celloid.

Natr. Mur., 5-gr. celloid.

Silicea, 5-gr. celloid.

M. S.: One celloid each, four times a day.

At the present writing the specific gravity has climbed up to 1010 and the general condition has improved beyond belief. I have only been treating him about a month and have hopes of a complete cure.
(Dr. J. H. Stevens, St. Jacob. Illinois.)

LABOR AND PREGNANCY

ETIOLOGY

BOTH pregnancy and labor are physiological processes, and as such should theoretically not require medical intervention. Among the American Indian tribes, the pregnant woman followed the trail with the others, dropped out of line for an hour or two, while delivery took place, and then took up the march again. The pioneer American women were almost equally hardy. Among the mountaineers of Kentucky as recently as fifty years ago, it was customary for the mother to arise and prepare dinner for the doctor as soon as the baby arrived.

These halcyon days have now departed, however, possibly forever, perchance to be brought back by the sensible methods of dress, hygiene, exercise and diet to which the modern woman is happily becoming addicted.

At the present day, both pregnancy and labor, even under the best conditions, cause a terrific drain upon the female system, particularly the nerves, and it is rarely, indeed, that the supply of Kali Phos. does not fall below the normal. For this reason the routine administration of Kali Phos. during the entire period of pregnancy, and especially during the last six weeks, will be found to accomplish much towards overcoming morning sickness, with the typical malaise which so often accompanies it, as well as strengthening the nervous system for the shock and strain of labor, and thus helping to insure a normal, uneventful delivery.

During labor itself, especially with primaparae, Kali Phos. is very useful. Child-birth is a natural process, and no pain should be experienced during its occurrence. The muscles of the uterus must, however, have the proper amount of nerve force, or they cannot properly contract and produce expulsive force. As the Biochemic pathology teaches, pain is a call for reinforcements—the greater the deficiency the louder the call, or the greater the pain. Kali Phos. is therefore the chief remedy in labor pains, but when cramps are present, Magnesia Phos. should also be prescribed.

When miscarriage threatens, the patient should be kept quiet, preferably in bed, and Kali Phos. should be administered in hourly doses, as there is always a lack of this cell-salt under those circumstances. If miscarriage has actually occurred, Ferrum Phos. is called for, as well as Calcarea Fluor., to tone up the contractile power of the uterus. Later Calcarea Phos. should be given as a constitutional tonic. This cell-salt should also be given where the mother complains of indigestion before confinement, as otherwise the child will suffer from Calcarea Phos. deficiency.

When puerperal eclampsia occurs, which is seldom, fortunately, when biochemic methods of treatment are pursued throughout the course of pregnancy, the patient should be given chloroform, and the uterus emptied immediately. Free sweating should then be induced, and normal salt solution injected, either by hypodermic, in a vein, or by the rectum. Ferrum Phos. and Kali Phos. are usually the cell-salts called for in this condition.

The prophylactic treatment for puerperal eclampsia is the strict observance of proper diet, hygiene and exercise during the period of pregnancy; regulation of all the organs of excretion, with frequent examination of the urine for albumen; regular administration of Kali Phos., as suggested above. If an attack is feared, the patient should be put on a strict milk diet.

Post-partum hemorrhage should be dealt with along the general lines described in the article on Hemorrhage (page 257).

Puerperal sepsis differs much in its manifestations, the most common form, however, being sapremia, from infection by saprophytes, which usually appear in the first three days after delivery. Its symptoms are a rise in temperature; rapid pulse; enlarged uterus; and foul lochia.

This should be treated by immediate curettement, followed by irrigation with mercury bichloride (1:4,000). In case it becomes necessary to control hemorrhage an iodoform gauze pack should be employed. Ferrum Phos., Kali Phos. and Kali Mur. are the cell-salts indicated here.

BIOCHEMIC TREATMENT

Kali Phos.—"*Kali Phos.* is the most wonderful remedy known in the hands of the accoucheur. Occasional doses for a month previous to labor will give vigor and tone to the system and insure a safe, easy confinement. In labor, *Kali*

Phos. takes the place of ergot, and leaves the patient in better condition." (Dr. Chapman.)

Weak, annoying, ineffectual labor-pains are met by this remedy. Rigid os, patient is restless, tearful and intolerant of her pains. Dr. Rozas, in the *Pop. Zeit.*, says: "For three years I have employed *Kali Phos.*, in 10-grain doses, dry on the tongue, every ten or fifteen minutes, as a remedy to excite labor-pains. It has never failed me, and I seldom have to give the third dose. My practice is extensive; have had over ninety cases in six years. *Magnes. Phos.*, in spasmodic pains and eclampsia, has done well for me. I give generally after the birth, *Ferrum Phos.*, a dose daily to avoid inflammation."

"From my own experience and the reports of other physicians and midwives, I am led to believe the testimony of Dr. Rozas is not overdrawn." (Dr. Chapman.) *Chief remedy in puerperal mania,* for the brain symptoms and blood-poisoning; also *Kali Sulph.* Threatened miscarriage in nervous subjects.

Ferrum Phos.—After labor, for the relief of after-pains and to heal small lacerations (internally and externally). Milk fever, first stage of mastitis. *In pregnancy, for sickness of stomach,* with vomiting of undigested food. First remedy in puerperal fever in alternation with *Kali Phos.*, the chief remedy.

Magnes. Phos.—Spasmodic labor-pains and eclampsia; excessive expulsive efforts. *Puerperal convulsions;* frequent doses in hot water.

Kali Mur.—*Chief remedy in the commencement of puerperal fever.* Inflammation of the breasts, to control the swelling, before suppuration forms. *Morning sickness in pregnancy,* with vomiting of white phlegm.

Calc. Phos.—Decline before or after child-birth. Spoiled milk, salty and bluish; child refuses to nurse. *Menstruation during lactation.*

Calc. Sulph.—Inflammation of the breasts, when matter is discharging; to be given after *Silicea,* to control suppuration.

Silicea.—In mastitis, after *Kali Mur.,* when pus-formation has taken place. Ulceration of nipples. Hard lumps in the breast (if *Kali Mur.* fails).

Calc. Fluor.—When the after-pains are weak and contractions too feeble. If there has existed prolapsus of the uterus, injections of this remedy will be beneficial to correct the malposition. Knots and kernels in the breast, if of stony hardness. Miscarriage, flooding, to tone up the contractile power of the uterus. "In the treatment of agalactia (failure or scanty supply of milk), *Calc. Fluor.* stands prĕ-eminently at the head in a majority of cases." (P. W. Pearsall.)

Natr. Mur.—Morning sickness of pregnancy, with watery, frothy vomiting.

Natr. Phos.—Morning sickness, with vomiting of sour, acid fluids.

Natr. Sulph.—Vomiting in pregnancy of bilious matter, and with bitter taste in the mouth.

CLINICAL CASES

Magnes. Phos. in Labor-Pains:

The better acquainted I become with this system, the more pleased I am with it. In labor, when the pains are too weak and irregular, I have seen nothing act more promptly and effectually than *Kali Phos.* For spasmodic, crampy pains, *Magnes. Phos.* is a gem. After a delivery, I gave *Ferrum Phos.* to be followed or accompanied by whatever may be indicated. I also use a wash to the vulva and abdomen, and for syringing the vagina, morning and night. The parts heal quickly under this treatment, and with the use of other remedies, as indicated, the patient makes a good recovery.
(E. H. Holbrook, M. D.)

Ferrum Phos. in Vomiting of Pregnancy:

Mrs. W.; two weeks pregnant; had been vomiting nearly everything that she had eaten for these two weeks. Only food was vomited, and that soon after eating. Gave *Ferrum Phos.*, four times a day, a small powder, dry. What I wish to say of the case is this: Mrs. W. has had four children, and with everyone had commenced vomiting almost at the moment of conception, and would continue all through pregnancy. The last four or five months of the time she would have to remain in bed, being so weak that she could not get about. She commenced the same way this time, but after giving the *Ferrum Phos.* a few days, the vomiting was very much controlled, and in a month had ceased entirely, and she went to term in splendid condition. While we cannot absolutely say that she would have been the same as at other times, yet ditions and to arrest them should they occur."
(Private letters; C. R. Vogel, M. D.)

Magnificent results from the Biochemic Remedies:

"The efficacy of the Biochemic remedies has been demonstrated to me, especially in the magnificent results I have observed from their administration during and after parturition. For weak labor-pains, *Kali Phos.* brings effectual pains and hastens delivery; *Magnes. Phos.*, when the pains are crampy in character; *Ferrum Phos.*, to prevent any inflammatory conditions and to arrest them should they occur." (Private letters; C. R. Vogel, M. D.)

LA GRIPPE (Influenza)

ETIOLOGY

THIS disease, while always with us to some extent, appears periodically in epidemic form, sweeping like wildfire through whole communities, and being followed in successive years by increasingly milder outbreaks.

La grippe, or epidemic influenza, as it is more properly termed, is extremely virulent when an epidemic of it first appears, and the mortality from it is high. Later, on the symptoms become milder, and deaths are not so frequent.

Its chief danger to the patient, however, lies in its after-effects. The sufferer from la grippe usually recovers very slowly, and is apt to suffer from sequelae of various sorts. A large percentage of tuberculosis cases give a previous history of la grippe. Heart and kidney troubles often follow it, while pneumonia, frequently fatal, may also result. Severe middle ear inflammation is a frequent complication in both children and adults.

The onset of la grippe is nearly always sudden. A sense of chilliness or a severe rigor followed by severe, aching pains in the back and legs is the first symptom with a feeling like a cold in the head, caused by congestion of the nasal mucous membrane.

The initial chill is quickly followed by fever, which may rapidly rise as high as 105°, although 103° is more ordinarily the maximum. A sense of severe illness, mental depression, and a feeling of great wretchedness is also present, making the patient believe himself much sicker that he really is.

If convalescence is not soon established, a pulmonary congestion resembling pneumonia may become established, and this may later develop into true pneumonia, which with heart failure is the most frequent cause of death in la grippe epidemics.

In many cases the chief symptoms are gastro-intestinal or nervous.

Severe diarrhea and vomiting frequently mark the onset of the gastro-intestinal form, with collapse and violent abdominal pain. In some cases the pain is entirely absent, while the stools are profuse and watery. There may be jaundice also, due to an extension of the gastro-intestinal catarrh to the common biliary duct.

In the nervous form of la grippe the symptoms present consist of profound nervous and mental depression, or in severe neuralgia pains. Mental disturbances, also, are by no means rare in the course of this disease.

The exciting cause of la grippe is found in the bacillus of Pfeiffer, which is usually received by contact with another patient, or through the air. In order for the bacillus to thrive and multiply, however, and thus cause an attack of la grippe, a breeding place must be provided for it in the mucous membrane of the respiratory tract. This can only occur when through a lack of Kali Mur. an excess of fibrin has arisen in the mucous membrane, and its power of resistance has been weakened.

Not until the mucous membrane of the respiratory tract has been restored to normal, and the breeding place of the bacillus of Pfeiffer been made uninhabitable, can a return to health be expected. Kali Mur., therefore, with Ferrum Phos. for the needed extra hemoglobin, as evidenced by the fever present, are therefore the first and most logical remedies.

If nervous symptoms predominate, Ferrum Phos. and Kali Phos. should be given in alternation, with a dose of Kali Mur. four times a day.

In the gastro-intestinal form of this trouble, Natrum Mur. and Natrum Sulph., according to the symptoms present, should be alternated with Ferrum Phos.

Rest is a great essential in la grippe. The patient should be put to bed at once, however mild the attack. The diet should be nourishing but easily digestible. During convalescence, the patient should be carefully watched for possible sequelae, and Kali Phos. alternated with Calcarea Phos. for their tonic effect.

BIOCHEMIC TREATMENT

Ferrum Phos.—In the first or initial stage of *la grippe,* for the febrile symptoms, fever, heat, pain, etc., frequent doses.

Kali Mur.—Secondary symptoms, sore throat, white coated tongue, rheumatic pains.

Kali Sulph.—Evening aggravations.—In alternation with *Ferrum Phos.*, to promote perspiration.

Natr. Sulph.—Chief remedy to control the excess of intercellular fluids, especially when there are bilious symptoms present. Dark brown coated tongue, bitter taste or vomiting of bitter, bilious fluids.

Natr. Mur.—Sneezing, with watery discharges from eyes or nostrils—note color of tongue.

Kali Phos.—If severe nervous symptoms are present.

CLINICAL CASES

Natr. Sulph. the remedy pre-eminent:

During the epidemic of la grippe last winter, I was in an excellent position to verify the much-lauded biochemic remedies in its treatment. I am at liberty to state that I frankly believe that influenza, which has been of such dread to physicians in general, has at last met that remedial agent which will render it as susceptible to treatment as any slight catarrhal trouble. The sequelæ are usually not the result of the disease itself, but, in the majority of cases, come from mismanagement of it in the primary stage. As to remedies, I have found that *Natr. Sulph.* will serve the greater number of cases, and have received wonderful results from its use, both at the beginning and when followed by sequelæ.
(Chas. S. Vaught, M. D.)

Natr. Sulph. after other treatment failed:

Mr. R., æt. 26, bookkeeper; went to his employment in the morning feeling perfectly well; about 10 o'clock he began to experience a very tired, weary feeling, and suddenly became very weak. There was considerable sneezing and much lachrymation, with a thin watery discharge from the nares. He was compelled to go home, and then sent for me. The temperature

for the following two days was 103 to 104, with little or no further variation. He complained of great soreness of the muscles, severe backache and bone pains, and of pain in throat up to ear when swallowing. I prescribed the usual remedies, but did not get any perceptible results from their administration. The discharge had now changed from a profuse watery to a profuse greenish mucus, with much accumulation of mucus in the throat and mouth. I then prescribed *Natr. Sulph.*, to be given every hour, about five grains at a dose. The result was striking. In a few hours he felt so much better that it was with difficulty he was kept in the house. The following morning he went to work, and has not been troubled any more with influenza.
(Henry LaDerne, M. D.)

Kali Mur. in rheumatic pains and white-coated tongue:

Carrie M., about 16 years of age, of anemic temperament, was taken sick with la grippe. The symptoms were characterized by profuse discharges from the nares, with some lachrymation. Pains of a rheumatic nature, involving the muscles of the limbs and joints; chilly, with high, continuous temperature; tongue coated white; great depression; felt as though she had been sick for months. *Kali Mur.*, every two hours, cured in three days.
(Dr. Chas. F. Wright.)

LARYNGITIS

(See Aphonia, Hoarseness and Tonsilitis.)

CLINICAL CASES

Severe Membranous Laryngitis:

A little boy, age 5, had been suffering for a day or so from what the parents supposed to be a cold. However, he was given the usual home remedies without relief, and his general symptoms progressed to an alarming condition within a few hours. Consequently, I was called to render medical aid. His physical symptoms were as follows:

Temperature, 102; pulse, accelerated, full, and hard; flushed face, restless, hoarse croupy cough, with respiration labored and difficult. The expiration was noisy and accompanied by a high-pitched stridulous cough. Inspiration was accompanied by a loud crowing noise; some difficulty in swallowing; no soreness or swelling of the lymphatic glands of the neck. However, the child kept putting his hands to his throat as if trying to remove some obstruction. No false membrane appeared on the tonsils or fauces. The parts presented a catarrhal condition, red and tumified.

Diagnosis: Membranous laryngitis, commonly called "membranous croup," and is regarded by many present-day authorities to be identical with diphtheria.

Treatment: Patient kept in a warm, well ventilated room with a temperature of 75 to 80 F. Calomel trit. 1/4 grain every two hours until free bowel movements were produced. *Ferrum Phos.* and *Kali Mur.* were given alternately every one-half to one hour for about twelve hours, or throughout the night. When I called next morning I met the mother of the sick child at the door. She said, "Our boy is very much worse this morning, and we are afraid he is going to choke to death." I made a hurried physical examination and found that his condition had materially changed. Instead of the rapid hard pulse of yesterday, I found a weak and almost imperceptible beat at the wrist; lips and nails livid; great prostration; increased dyspnoea, extremities cold; face pale.

Treatment changed as follows: Spirits of turpentine, spirits of camphor, menthol, and carbolic acid, AA-1 drachm, added to one gallon boiling water. The child was to inhale this hot vapor every one-half to one hour. This caused an increased moisture in the mucous membrane of the larynx, and its stimulating and sedative action, together with the other remedies given, caused the croupous membrane to disintegrate and

be cast off in large casts and slugs and expectorated. *Kali Phos.* for the prostration, and *Kali Sulph.* to stimulate the oxygen carriers of the blood, were given alternately every half to one hour. This treatment was continued for eight hours, when a very noticeable change for the better evidenced itself. However, the croupous membrane was not being cast off as rapidly as I desired, so a few doses of *Kali Mur.* and *Calc. Phos.* were given every two hours until the false membrane loosened, and a large cast, three inches long- was expectorated. The grave symptoms disappeared and the child was soon breathing natural and easy. In ten days he was up and about, enjoying his former good health.
(Dr. Dennis D. Casto.)

Ferrum Phos. in acute Laryngitis with exudative Tonsilitis:

CASE I.—Mr. P., æt. 50; a veteran of the late war. A severe case of acute laryngitis complicated with exudative tonsilitis; voice husky and hoarse; cough irritating and painful, stridulous, nearly croupy, dry; much pain in the larynx and trachea, with much tension across the upper part of the chest; no pain in tonsils, though much swollen, dark red, studded with deep depressions, partly filled with exudative material, more like ulcerations than diphtheria. Never saw so bad a looking throat without pain, but he declared there was not a bit. Pulse 100; temperature 102½ degrees. *Ferrum Phos.*, a large powder, probably fifteen grains, dissolved in half glass of water, a teaspoonful every hour, was given. In twenty-four hours the fever was gone, and much relief was experienced. In two days the tonsils were clean, but looked quite honey-combed, with a loose, painless cough, much less in frequency. In four days from the beginning of the treatment he was nearly well and had resumed his business.

CASE II.—Mrs. D., "fair, fat and forty"; laryngitis; voice sank to a whisper; cough frequent, rasping, dry and painful; pain down the larynx and trachea; aching of head, back and limbs; temperature 100 degrees; chilly; pulse 100. Received the same treatment, with much relief, and voice returned in twenty-four hours; was about well in three days.

LEUCORRHEA

(See Exudations.)

ETIOLOGY

A discharge from one mucous membrane is the same as from another, although the active causes may be different. In this case the discharge may depend upon simple debility, or some affection of the womb of a more or less inflammatory nature. It is frequently seen in delicate, relaxed constitutions, accompanied with falling of the womb, irregular menstruation, etc.

The discharge varies in color and consistency, according to the stage of the disorder; changing from a white, bland, non-irritating discharge to a yellow, yellowish-green, creamy-yellow, dark yellow or yellowish-brown. At times it is non-irritating, but at other times it may cause smarting and soreness of any part it happens to touch. Frequently there is nothing to indicate leucorrhea except a white, flour-like deposit, but at times it is copious and comes in gushes. The above does not describe those discharges which arise from cancer or other malignant disease of the womb; these are usually foul and very offensive.

BIOCHEMIC TREATMENT

Calc. Phos.—Leucorrhea, with *discharge of albuminous mucus;* looks like white of egg before it is cooked. Leucorrhea after menses, when albuminous; weakness in sexual organs, as a constitutional tonic; also a valuable intercurrent remedy in all cases of leucorrhea.

Kali Mur.—In leucorrhea, when the *discharge is a milky-white, non-irritating mucus.*

Kali Phos.—*Scalding, acrid leucorrhea;* when of nervous origin, in alternation with *Natr. Mur.*

Natr. Mur.—*Discharge watery, irritating, smarting, and scalding;* associated with dull, heavy headache and itching of the vulva. After the use of nitrate of silver, to eradicate the effect of the drug.

Kali Sulph.—Discharge of yellow, greenish, slimy or watery secretions.

Natr. Phos.—Leucorrhea, discharge creamy or honey-colored, watery, with acid conditions.

NOTE:. In all cases of leucorrhea, injections of hot water, in which a small quantity of the remedy has been dissolved, should be used with the internal treatment. The cause should also be discovered, if possible, and rectified.

CLINICAL CASES

Kali Mur. effected a permanent cure:

M. M., a young lady, æt. 17, consulted me on account of an obstinate acrid leucorrhea. I tried the whole series of remedies indicated for such cases. All were without effect, so that I could not but wonder at the patience and perseverance of the patient, whom I saw once a week. *Kali Mur.* effected a quick and permanent cure.
(Dr. S. From Schuessler.)

Calc. Phos. in Leucorrhea:

Minnie S., æt. 17, was troubled with an acrid, albuminous, tenacious leucorrhea, which was usually worse after the menstrual periods. The menses were irregular, appearing every twenty-fourth day, sometimes a few days earlier or later; pains in small of back; bearing-down pains in uterus; dull, no ambition; face pale, sallow; general anemia. The symptoms were rather well marked, and *Calc. Phos.* was prescribed every four hours; an antiseptic douche was to be taken every two or three days. The case began to show some improvement after

first prescription, and in a short time the discharge had disappeared completely. *Ferrum Phos.* was also given later for the anemic condition.
(C. R. Vogel, M. D.)

LIVER, AFFECTIONS OF

The articles on Constipation, Diarrhea, Gall-Stone, Hemorrhoids, Malaria or Chills and Fever, give the entire pathology of liver affections.

BIOCHEMIC TREATMENT

Ferrum Phos.—Inflammation of the liver, in the first stage, for the congestion, heat, fever, and pain.

Kali Mur.—Sluggish action of the liver, with white or grayish-white coated tongue and light-colored stools. *Pain in region of liver and under right shoulder-blade. Constipation, with light-colored stools,* denoting a lack of bile. Jaundice, if caused by a chill, resulting in a catarrh of the duodenum, with other symptoms characteristic of this remedy.

Natr. Sulph.—Jaundice arising from vexation, with bilious-green evacuations, *greenish-brown coated tongue, sallow skin, yellow eyeballs. Natr. Sulph.* is indicated by those symptoms of the liver arising from an excess of bile. Bilious attacks, if from excessive study or mental work, alternate with *Kali Phos.* Congestion of the liver, with soreness and sharp, sticking pains; also *Ferrum Phos.*

Kali Phos.—Affections of the liver, with depression of the nervous system. *Bilious attacks from excessive mental work or worry;* also *Natr. Sulph.*

Natr. Phos.—For *sclerosis of the liver and the* hepatic form of diabetes; note coating of tongue.

Natr. Mur.—*Jaundice* arising *from gastric catarrh;* drowsiness and watery secretions; note also the coating of the tongue.

Kali Sulph.—As an alternate remedy, when symptoms indicating this remedy arise.

Calc. Sulph.—Abscess of the liver, with pain, weakness or nausea, to control pus-formation.

CLINICAL CASES

Kali Phos. in Biliousness:

Mr. D., æt. 42; bilious, yellow complexion; large, rather protruding eyeballs; nasty taste in the mouth; under considerable mental strain. I prescribed *Natr. Sulph.*, without effect. I then diagnosed biliousness caused from mental worry, and gave him *Kali Phos.* In two weeks he reported himself greatly benefited.

(J. B. Chapman.)

Kali Mur. in Jaundice:

Last summer my second daughter returned from a visit to New Jersey with an immense wart on her hand. In a few days she was taken quite ill with fever, which I took to be of a bilious nature; gave *Natr. Sulph.* She became deeply jaundiced and grew worse while taking this remedy. I then changed to *Kali Mur.*, and she began to improve immediately and was well in a few days. After she had taken a few doses of the *Kali Mur.* the jaundice began to abate and the wart fell off.

(E. H. H.)

LOCK JAW

(See Spasms, Convulsions, etc.)

LUMBAGO

(See Pain, Rheumatism.)

BIOCHEMIC TREATMENT

Ferrum Phos.—Chief remedy for the pain and inflammatory condition. Alternate with the other remedies indicated.

Calc. Phos.—Backache, in the lumbar region, in the morning on awakening (*Natr. Phos.*).

Natr. Mur.—*Lumbago, relieved by lying on something hard.* Pain, as if bruised, from prolonged stooping. Back weak, worse in the morning.

MARASMUS

ETIOLOGY

This trouble manifests itself in children by an inability to properly assimilate food, causing atrophy and weakness, delayed dentition, and non-development. It is generally due to a deficiency in Calcarea Phos., which prevents the utilization of albumen by the system, although an acid condition from a lack of Natrum Phos., as well as other symptoms from deficiency of Natrum Mur. and Natrum Sulph. may be present from time to time as the disease progresses.

BIOCHEMIC TREATMENT

Calc. Phos.—*Marasmus of children who are bottle-fed.* Abdomen swollen; liver large. Colic after eating. Stools contain undigested food.

Natr. Sulph.—*Inherited sycotic constitution;* bloated abdomen, with much rumbling of wind; *stools watery, yellow, gushing, worse on commencing to move in the morning.*

Silicea.—*Body wasted* while *the head is exceedingly large.* Child perspires easily, is nervous and irritable; face emaciated, decrepit-looking. Aversion to the mother's milk; vomited if taken. *Stools offensive and watery.* Great prostration upon any change of weather.

Kali Phos.—*Atrophy,* whether it be muscular or otherwise, if *accompanied with foul-smelling stools,* etc., needs this remedy.

Natr. Phos.—As a constitutional remedy, if acid, symptoms are present, intercurrently with the chief salt.

Natr. Mur.—Atrophy from improper distribution of the Natr. Mur. molecules in the system, noticeable by *earthy complexion,* constipation, *emaciation of neck in children,* and other characteristic symptoms.

CLINICAL CASES

One case, a child of one year, suffering from marasmus in a very far advanced degree. I gave *Calc. Phos.* alternately with *Kali Phos.,* and after four weeks the child was gaining in flesh rapidly, and was finally cured two months later.
(Dr. Chas. Mildenberger, Brooklyn, N. Y.)

Patient, boy, one year, fed on condensed milk, head large, fontenelles wide open, sweating about head and body, cries all night, sore on being handled, abdomen soft and flabby, legs bowed, can't sit up straight, no teeth, vomits up food, diarrhea green. Changed the food and gave *Calc. Phos.* 3x with most satisfactory results.
(Dr. R. L. Emery, Rockport, Mass.)

MEASLES

ETIOLOGY

Of all acute infections, measles appears to be the most eminently contagious, very few persons being immune. This fact seems to have been generally accepted, and it is commonly assumed that inasmuch as children will almost certainly have the disease some time, they might as well take it now as any other time. Admitting that all children must sooner or later sicken with it, it should nevertheless be endeavored to defer that time until the age at which the mortality is at a minimum has been attained. Infants fortunately exhibit a relative immunity, so that our anxiety concerning them is relatively small. Of the total mortality, four-fifths occurs in children less than five years of age.

Experience shows that, despite the most careful isolation, a case of measles having occurred in a household will almost certainly communicate the disease to all other residents therein. This communicability is due to the early stage of the disorder at which it is possible to communicate the contagium. Numerous examples have been reported to prove conclusively that it may be communicated even before the initial symptoms have been manifested, *i. e.,* when the person about to be taken with it is apparently in the best of health. Isolation then, to be of value, should be practiced at the moment suspicion is first aroused. Time to make suspicion a certainty should not be permitted to elapse.

In measles, the deficiency in potassium chloride is very great, and the fibrinous, albuminous material in the blood is diffused through the system by a rapid circulation, and reaches the surface of the skin at all parts—engorges the pores and glands, and produces a rose-red rash.

Scarlet fever, diphtheria, etc., are produced by exactly the same cause, *i. e.,* fibrin and other organic material on its way out of the system.

BIOCHEMIC TREATMENT

Ferrum Phos.—In all stages of measles, for the inflammatory conditions, fever, redness of eyes, painful congestion of the chest, etc. Especially suited to the first stage of measles.

Kali Mur.—Second stage of measles, hoarse cough, glandular swelling, etc. The tongue is coated white or grayish-white. *After-effects of measles;* deafness; swellings in the throat; diarrhea, loose, light-colored stools. If *Ferrum Phos.* and *Kali Mur.* are given faithfully, and ordinary care is taken, there will seldom arise any after-effects.

Kali Sulph.—In measles or other eruptive diseases, when the rash is suddenly suppressed, the skin is harsh and dry, *Kali Sulph.*, frequent doses, will assist the returning of the rash by promoting perspiration; warm covering should also be applied.

CLINICAL CASES

Ferrum Phos. for the Coryza and Bronchial Catarrh of Measles:

Dr. Kock, of Munich, reports: In thirty-five cases of measles which came under my treatment, coryza and bronchial catarrh were very slight in the premonitory stage. Conjunctivitis and intolerance of light along with it were the more prominent symptoms. Within a few days, the rash appeared, lasting five or six days, and then disappeared. But either during the blush of the rash or the fading of it, painful swelling of one or both glands below the ear set in. The children became feverish and were crying and moaning both day and night. The remedy which I now chose was *Ferrum Phos.*, and, according to the violence of the fever, I ordered a spoonful of the solution every hour or two. I gave it at the premonitory stage, and when I saw that it proved very satisfactory, I looked for no other remedy. For the glandular swelling, external redness and painfulness, I used the same medicine, and my cases ended very satisfactorily.
(From Schuessler.)

MECHANICAL INJURIES

(See Bones, Diseases of.)

ETIOLOGY

In cases of broken or injured bones Calc. Phos. is needed to furnish bone material and Ferrum Phos. to carry sufficient oxygen to the part affected, increasing the rate of speed of blood through the vascular system. An increase of speed will, as has been shown, create heat or inflammation.

An injury to muscular tissue—the flesh—is, of course, repaired only by the blood. Salves, liniments, ointments, oils (inorganic or otherwise), do not possess any building power, and in this capacity they are inert. Nature uses the vital processes and the constituents of blood to build up all the tissues of the human organism.

When the injury to flesh first occurs, Ferrum Phos. is the cell-salt called for, because an extra supply of oxygen is needed at the part affected, oxygen being the creative power that uses the building material.

If in the process of rebuilding a deficiency is caused and other salts are needed, that fact will be made known by the special symptoms that appear from time to time.

BIOCHEMIC TREATMENT

Ferrum Phos.—Is the first remedy in recent injuries of the soft tissues, to supply material for reconstruction. "Nature, in her effort to supply an extra amount of phosphate of iron to the injured part, is obliged to furnish an excessive quantity of blood; this necessitates an engorgement of the blood-vessels, giving rise to inflammation, pain and fever. *Ferrum Phos.* added to the quantity already in the blood allows the deposit of extra material without the engorgement of the blood-vessels. It should also be applied locally." (Chapman.) *Cuts, falls, bruises, fresh wounds and sprains* require this remedy in the first stage; it relieves the congestion and pain, and greatly assists in repair.

Kali Mur.—In the second stage of injuries, when swelling has set in.

Silicea.—Neglected cases, when suppuration threatens, or when discharging thick yellow pus; to be followed with *Calc. Sulph.*

Calc. Sulph.—Neglected cases of injuries, when the process of suppuration continues too long; discharge of thick yellow pus, sometimes streaked with blood.

Calc. Fluor.—Bruises of the bones, shins, etc. (See Bones, Diseases of.)

Calc. Phos.—Injuries to bones. (See Bones, Diseases of.)

Natr. Sulph.—Mental trouble arising from injuries to the head. (See Brain.)

CLINICAL CASES

Ferrum Phos. in injuries of Soft Tissues:

Ferrum Phos. is a most useful remedy in the mechanical injuries of the soft tissues. It keeps down inflammation, relieves pain and supplies material necessary for rebuilding of the tissues. It should be given internally, and applied as a dressing. The cure is rapid, and if attended to at once, swelling and suppuration rarely ensues.
(J. B. Chapman.)

Natr. Sulph.—the first dose cured Epileptic Fits resulting from a fall:

Young man, hurled from the truck in a fire department. He struck his head. Following this for five or six months he had fits. He was very irritable; wanted to die. His fits drove him to distraction. Never knew when they were coming on. They were epileptiform in character. Had constant pain in his head; much photophobia. *Natr. Sulph.* was given, and the first dose cured him. He has never had any pain about the head since; has had no more mental trouble, and no more fits.
(Prof. J. T. Kent, *Medical Advance.*)

Calc. Fluor. in Suppuration following injuries:

In September, last autumn, I was in the Highlands. The dairy-maid of a farmer there spoke to me, saying she had hurt her thumb while sharpening a scythe. The case proved to be this: The whole thumb of the left hand was swollen, and of a bluish-red color, and very painful when touched; much inflamed, and there was a small wound at the extensor side, at the joint above the nail. On pressure there was a whitish-yellow discharge, mixed with white shreds. Both phalanges were easily displaced, and a peculiar noise was heard, which I had observed before in similar cases. This fact made me decide on giving *Calc. Fluor.* The medical man in the village, whom the farmer had consulted, said amputation was the only thing that could be done for the case. She took *Calc. Fluor.*, and some time after, the farmer had occasion to see me, when he informed me that the servant's thumb was quite well. (From Schuessler.)

MENINGITIS

(See Brain.)

Meningitis is an inflammation of the membranes of the brain, due to a lack of phosphate of iron and potassium chloride, causing a rapid circulation and surplus of fibrinous matter at the part affected.

BIOCHEMIC TREATMENT

Ferrum Phos.—In the first stage of meningitis, for the fever, rapid pulse, delirium, etc.

Kali Mur.—The second remedy, when effusion takes place, after or in alternation with *Ferrum Phos.*

Natr. Sulph.—*Violent pains at base of brain,* heavy, crushing pain (also *Kali Phos.* and *Ferrum Phos.*). Dr. Kent says: "In the spinal meningitis of today, if all the remedies in the materia medica were taken away from me, and I were to have but one with which to treat the disease, I would take *Natr. Sulph.,* because it will modify the attack and save life in the majority of cases. It cuts short the disease surprisingly, when it is the truly indicated remedy. The violent determination of blood to the head that we find in this disease, clinically, is readily relieved."

Calc. Phos.—First and chief remedy in hydrocephaloid conditions, open fontanels, flat, depressed, etc. As a preventive in families predisposed to this disease.

CLINICAL CASES

Ferrum Phos. in Meningitis following a fall:

In the case of a little boy, 7 years of age, who had concussion of the brain from a fall, meningitis set in, with its characteristic symptoms, and the first medical man's prognosis was adverse. *Ferrum Phos.* was prescribed. On the third night, however, there was a change, the pulse being in the morning 100, having been 125 on the day before, fell to 49 per minute. *Kali Phos.*, a dose every quarter of an hour, raised it steadily, though slowly, up to 57, where it remained for two days. After that it rose, and the case mended very satisfactorily, the now threatening symptoms, stupor, dilated, immovable pupils, etc., disappearing. A perfect recovery resulted at end of a fortnight. The remedies given were *Ferrum Phos., Kali Phos.,* a few doses *Calc. Phos.*

Ferrum Phos., Kali Phos.:

Mr. D. suffered from meningitis, and a prognosis of the attending physician was designated as at least doubtful, and nothing was prescribed. The case was especially severe, since in his family there was a hereditary brain disease, and his nearest male relatives had died of it. At the time I was called the patient had been nearly two days in a frightful delirium that had increased almost to madness. Consciousness had disappeared; temperature over 104 degrees. I ordered *Ferrum Phos.* and *Kali Phos.* After a week I found the patient free from fever, still somewhat weak, but subjectively fully recovered. To hasten the convalescence I gave

Calc. Phos., and eight days later the patient was able to be out and at his calling.
(Dr. Quesse.)

Kali Phos. in Spinal Meningitis:

I wish to report the splendid action of *Kali Phos.* in controlling extreme nervousness in a case of spinal meningitis. The case, a boy of five years, had been sick about a week with the disease, when he suddenly developed most distressing nervous symptoms. Night and day he kept up constant movement of both the upper and lower limbs, accompanied with a frightened expression of countenance and a pitiful moaning cry. I prescribed *Kali Phos.* To my great surprise and relief, the symptoms noted entirely disappeared in a short time.
(Dr. J. B. Chapman, Seattle, Wash.)

MENORRHAGIA

(See Menstruation.)

ETIOLOGY

This disease is generally caused: *First,* By a thickening of the blood with fibrin, from a lack of potassium chloride to keep it properly diffused. *Second,* A lack of calcium fluoride in the muscular tissue of the *os uteri.*

The fibrinous particles in the blood tend to irritate and break down the blood-vessels, and the mouth of the womb having lost its power of contraction through a lack of calcium fluoride molecules, the creators of elastic fibre, an excessive menstrual flow is the result.

BIOCHEMIC TREATMENT

Calc. Fluor.—Is the chief remedy to tone up the contractile power of the uterus. Menorrhagia, with excessive bearing-down pains, generally associated with displacement of the uterus.

Ferrum Phos.—To be taken between the menstrual periods, to prevent the blood engorging the womb. Discharges of bright-red blood, coagulating quickly.

Calc. Phos.—Intercurrently in all cases to tone up the general system. (See Menstruation.)

CLINICAL CASES

Ferrum Phos. for Anemia of Menorrhagia:

E. S. Bailey, M. D., reports a case of menorrhagia cured by *Ferrum Phos.* The case presented a history of profuse menstruation; the flow was depleting; no pain or local tenderness—in fact, no tangible symptoms, the condition of anemia representing the cause in this case.
(*Clinique.*)

Ferrum Phos. to prevent Menorrhagia:

Mrs. A., æt. 34; profuse menstruation of bright-red blood every three, sometimes every two weeks, lasting from five to six days. Small, thin, anemic; face pale; during the menstrual period just the reverse—face livid, ofttimes of a fiery red, with much heat and burning. Blood coagulates as soon as expelled from uterus, clotting in the vagina. Vomits everything she eats; debility. The case presented a perfect case for *Ferrum Phos.*, a dose every two hours during the period, and night and morning for a week, were given. This treatment was continued for about three months, when the flow became more normal, her complexion better, and she began to feel stronger and much improved in every way.
(C. R. Vogel, M. D.)

Calc. Fluor. in Menorrhagia:

A lady called to see me just after a severe hemorrhage from the womb—in fact, every time she menstruated she almost flooded to death. Upon examination I found the uterus hard and so large that it completely filled the vagina. This had doubtless been coming on for six years, since the birth of her child, as she complained of an increasing weight in that region all the time. I at once began to give her *Calc. Fluor.*, a dose every four hours. This reduced the induration in four to six weeks to its natural size; and five years have passed and no return of the trouble.

(A. P. Davis, M. D.)

MENSTRUATION

BIOCHEMIC TREATMENT

Ferrum Phos.—Painful menstruation with flushed face, quick pulse and discharge of bright-red blood, coagulating readily. Vomiting of undigested food at the menstrual period. These symptoms are due to excessive congestion of the uterus. *Ferrum Phos.* regulates this condition. If the pains are recurrent, the remedy should be given before the period, as a preventive.

Kali Phos.—An important remedy in the treatment of irregularities of menstruation, especially in weak, irritable, lachrymose, sensitive women. Menses too late and too scanty, or too profuse; discharge deep-red or blackish-red, not coagulating, sometimes with strong odor (not always). Pain at the monthly flow in pale, sensitive women. Retained or delayed menstruation, with depression of spirits and general nervous debility.

Kali Mur.—Menses are too late or suppressed from taking cold; tongue has a white or grayish-white coating. Menses too early, too frequent; discharge is very dark, clotted, black, like tar. Menses too long or too early (also *Kali Phos.*).

Natr. Mur.—Thin, watery, pale discharge (alternately or intercurrently, *Kali Phos.*). Menstruation of young girls with anemic conditions, drowsiness, gloominess and dull, heavy headache in the morning.

Magnes. Phos.—For menstrual colic, chief remedy. Painful menstruation or pain before the flow begins. Pains of a constrictive nature, heat relieves. When the flow is scant and associated with great pain, a dose of *Magnes. Phos.* will frequently produce a copious discharge.

Calc. Phos.—Menstrual colic when *Magnes. Phos.* fails. Menstruation irregular in young girls or anemic subjects, as an intercurrent remedy, to tone up the general system. Menstruation during lactation. Too early menstruation in young girls. Throbbing in the genitals, with voluptuous feelings.

Calc. Fluor.—Excessive menstruation, with bearing-down pains. Flooding, to tone up the contractile power of the uterus (also *Kali Phos.*)

Kali Sulph.—Menstruation too late and too scanty, with a feeling of fullness and weight in abdomen; note also the yellow coating of the tongue.

Natr. Phos.—Menses sour-smelling or acrid; note also the creamy coating of the tongue and acid condition of the stomach. Discharge corrosive and causes soreness wherever it touches.

Silicea.—Strong-smelling menses, associated with constipation. Icy-cold sensations during menstruation. Metrorrhagia from working in cold water. Nymphomania.

CLINICAL CASES

Choosing Biochemic Remedies in Dysmenorrhea:

Ferrum Phos., *Kali Phos.*, *Magnes. Phos.* and *Kali Mur.* will handle most cases of dysmenorrhea. *Magnes. Phos.*, given *in hot water* by mouth or hypodermically will relieve the agonizing pains of menstruation in many cases, as quickly as a dose of *morphine sulph.* Miss S., age 20, was subject to these unwelcome monthly visitations. The first time I was called I found the patient screaming with intense, griping uterine pains. *Magnes. Phos.*, one teaspoonful in a glass one-half full of *hot water,* teaspoonful doses each five or ten minutes, brought quick relief. The same remedy taken a few days before the menstrual flow was expected served to control

the pains until such time as the os uteri could be dilated. When the flow is black, like tar, use *Ferrum Phos.* and *Kali Mur.* If accompanied with severe nervous symptoms, *Kali Phos.* Don't resort to narcotics. The relief from them is only temporary and they are harmful to the system.
(Dr. J. B. Chapman.)

Kali Phos. in irregular Menstruation:

Miss H., age 16, high school pupil. Menstruates very irregularly, once in three or four months. No menses for several months past. Nervous and sensitive. Slightly jaundiced. Dark streaks under eyes. Skin dry and rather inclined to be scaly. Poor appetite. Is losing flesh. Gave *Kali Phos.*, a dose three times a day. Two months later the young lady's mother reported that Miss H. was menstruating regularly and was much improved in general health.
(Dr. L. C. Smith.)

Ferrum Phos., Magnes. Phos. and Kali Phos. in Dysmenorrhea:

A lady, 34, two children, youngest eight years old, had been in poor health for about four years, had become very weak and all sorts of trouble during monthly periods—was either too free or vice versa, but always cramps, pains, etc. Combination of *Ferrum Phos., Magnes. Phos.* and *Kali Phos.*, gave five tablets in a wine glass of hot water every hour at the approach of the periods. As improvement set in extended the time to two to four hours—nothing could have done better and no further trouble with dysmenorrhea.
(Dr. L. J. Dorsey.)

MENTAL CONDITIONS

(See Articles on Brain, Delirium and Kali Phos.)

BIOCHEMIC TREATMENT

Kali Phos.—Is the great brain remedy, for the functional disturbance. Depressed spirits, irritability, impatience. Sleeplessness or loss of memory. *Brain-fag from overwork,* study, etc. Inability of thought. Sensitiveness, shyness, restlessness. timidity, dullness, loss of energy, dread of noise. Faint feelings, homesickness, hallucinations, morbid thoughts, longs for the past, melancholy, crossness, lassitude, nervous exhaustion. *Mental illusions, false impressions and fancies.* Always better under cheerful excitement, but desires to be alone. Sighing and depression; looks on the dark side of everything. Sighing and moaning in sleep. Night terrors of children. Excessive blushing from emotional sensitiveness. Easily startled, whining disposition. Crossness and irritability of children; ill-temper arising from nervous disturbances. Fear, fretfulness, crying or screaming in children. Tearful moods. Insanity, loss of correct reasoning power; *chief remedy.* Mania in its various stages and degrees (also *Ferrum Phos.*). Delirium tremens.

Calc. Phos.—Peevish, fretful children. Poor memory; incapacity for concentrated thought; mind wanders from one subject to another; weak minds in those practicing, or who have practiced self-abuse (*Kali Phos.*). Dull, stupid depression of spirits; anxious about the future. Desires solitude. After grief, disappointment, pain, etc.

Ferrum Phos.—Consequence of anger. Violent mania or maniacal moods from hyperemia of the brain.

Natr. Mur.—Sadness, with palpitation of the heart. Worries about the future. Fits of "blues"; consolation aggravates. Low spirits, *spells of sadness,* when *accompanied with constipation* from dryness of the mucous membranes of the bowels. Tearful moods. Delirium tremens.

Magnes. Phos.—Illusions of the senses; *optical illusions.* Indisposed to mental efforts and inability for clear thought. Also *Kali Phos.,* chief remedy.

Natr. Sulph.—Suicidal tendency, due to bilious derangements.

CLINICAL CASES

Kali Phos. in religious Melancholy:

The following is a case of a lady, æt. 44: "I saw," writes Dr. A., of Arnsberg, on the 7th of February, "a lady suffering from mental derangement. Religious melancholy was at the root, although, before this occurrence, she had not inclined to religious excitement. She now declared she was lost forever—lamented, cried, wrung her hands and tore her clothes or pieces of paper which were laid about to prevent her tearing her garments. She did not know those around her, and was unable to sleep. Her eyes had an unconscious stare, and frequently it required two persons to hold her down. Only by holding her nose, and by force, a little food or medicine could be put down her throat. I prescribed *Kali Phos.,* as her condition, though one of excitement, was originally one of depression, to which *Kali Phos. is suited.* Dr. Schuessler says, in his book: 'A functional disturbance of the molecules of this salt causes in the brain mental depression, showing itself in irritability, terror, weeping, nervousness, etc., as well as softening of the brain.' She took *Kali Phos.,* with excellent results. A former experience gained by this remedy led me to select it.

"On that occasion it was in the case of an old man, æt. 80. He suffered from mental derangement, which showed itself in the form of intense hypochondriasis and melancholia. He was tired of life, but had a fear of death. For weeks he had been treated, to no purpose, with many remedies apparently called for, as nux vomica, aurum, bromide of potassium, in large doses. But he was rapidly cured by the continuous use of *Kali Phos.* Even after eight hours from the commencement of the treatment, a certain feeling of calmness was experienced, and that night he had a quiet sleep. I had, therefore, no reason to regret the treatment I selected, as the improvement continued steadily, so that on the 25th of February I discontinued my professional visits.

"I have seen my previous patient frequently, busily engaged in her home with her usual cheerfulness, and she speaks quite calmly of her past illness."
(From Schuessler.)

Kali Phos. in Hypochondriasis:

Patient, æt. 80, suffering from deep hypochondriasis, melancholia, tediousness of life, fear of death, mistrust, downhearted and morose. After the failure of other remedies, he was entirely restored by *Kali Phos.*

Mrs. N., wife of a minister, 50 years of age. Was consulted by the husband who came to consult me regarding the steps to be taken to commit the wife to the asylum, as she had become insane at times. It was the change of life, and I advised to wait a while and treat her, which we did. I gave her four tablets of *Kali Phos.* dissolved in hot water every two hours when awake. Within less than a month she was perfectly recovered, and the asylum was not necessary. Many cases of mental disorders, especially if connected with female trouble, responds nicely and quickly to *Kali Phos.*
(W. E. Daniels, M. D.)

E. S. Age 58, suffered from a severe attack of Neurasthenia, which lasted for several months, finally he partially recovered, with slight attacks every few weeks. But he has never been normal at any time. Examination revealed that he had a systolic pressure of 108 and a diastolic of 65, very nervous, gloomy, possessed with a morbid fear, suspicious of his friends, severe Insomnia, morbid and wanted to be alone. Difficult to get conversation, slow of speech, cold extremities, almost complete anorexia, impotemtoa erigendi, a well defined psychoneurosis and a general depression of all the function. There is no organic heart or lung trouble; blood examination, reds 3,500,000, whites 10,000. Greatly increased eosinophils which is characteristic of such cases. A combination of *Kali Phos., Calc. Phos.* with *Natrum Mur.,* each five grains, brought about surprising results in a few weeks. This was followed every three hours during the day, with an added capsule of Sodium Amytal twice daily. The patient is now perfectly well and feels better than he has for years. The addition of

tablespoonful of Manola three times daily, was of assistance in the way of a general tonic.
(H. H. R.)

A physician who had been doing a large practice for several years was inclined to be nervous, probably from overwork and suddenly he became very dizzy, a drunk-like feeling which made walking very difficult, was compelled to hold to chairs and bed. He had a slight loss of strength and a fear of a complete breakdown. He visited several physicians in St. Louis and had numerous X-rays, including his teeth, etc. He had about decided to quit his large practice, except probably a little office work as he had received no benefit from any treatment. Being a good friend of mine I prevailed upon him to take my little tablets, in which he had no confidence at all. He finally consented to take five celloids of *Kali Phos.* 3x every two hours for 30 days. At the end of that time his nervousness and dizziness had disappeared and he again took up his large practice, which he is still doing now two years later, without any recurrence of symptoms. He was advised to continue for some time with this treatment which I think he failed to do. I think this was a "Life Saver" for the doctor, but yet he cannot conceive of the idea of the little sweet tablets doing him so much good.
(Dr. B. J. Cline.)

Miss E., age 18, a young school teacher, had an unfortunate love affair. She became despondent and neglected her school work. She grew worse until she was seized by suicidal melancholia that caused her to beat her head against the walls of the school house, in her attempt to beat out her brains. I advised that she should place a substitute in her school while she took a short vacation. I prescribed *Kali Phos.* 2x, three grains every hour, during the first day (not at night unless she was unable to sleep), then every two hours. I gave the 2x trituration dry. In two weeks she returned to her school work, thoroughly cured.

(NOTE: I have frequently prescribed *Kali Phos.* 2x for Normal School students whose mental faculties seemed to "flunk" at examination time; and for lawyers and business men who were suffering from brain-fag, and always with the most satisfactory results.)
(Dr. A. E. Wentz.)

Mr. H. C., age 38 years, married, family of three children, oldest 12 years, has always enjoyed good health, owns his own home, is or was manager of a large retail clothing store, had saved some money which he invested in a certain stock." The depression" came, the clothing house went into the hands of a receiver. Mr. H. C. lost his position, his stocks were wiped out. He became despondent, lost interest in everything, did not care for his home or family, was formerly very fond of them. Instead of sleeping, he would worry the night through. *Kali Phos.* 3x one week, same 6x one week, and the 12x third week braced Mr. C. up. Says he feels fine and is looking for a "job."
(J. B. Kersey, M. D.)

Kali Phos. saved her from the Insane Asylum:

Miss M., the daughter of the late Dr. M., has been suffering since her eighteenth year from occasional attacks of aberration of the mind. But as years passed on, these attacks of insanity became worse and more frequent, until it was deemed advisable by her brother to make arrangements with the doctor of the lunatic asylum in the district to have her moved there. As a last recourse, a friend called to see if the new remedies could be of any service in such a hopeless case. Having assured him that *Kali Phos.* would do her good, they gave it very steadily, four doses daily for weeks. This was four years ago. The result was most satisfactory. After taking it, she never had another attack, and is completely cured; able to superintend home duties, receive callers and make calls, which she had not been able to do for years, on account of feeling so nervous and shy during the intervals of the attack. Several cases of a similar nature have been treated with equal success—two of these puerperal mania.
(M. D. W. From Schuessler.)

Kali Phos. in homicidal Mania:

Mr. J., æt. 36; married, cigar drummer by occupation. Living at home with wife and one child, a bright boy of about four years. Had been a great drinker of whiskey, and shortly before placing case in my hands had entirely quit the use of whiskey. Knowing the close sympathy existing between the brain and digestive organs, soon found the following facts to be present: He complained of distress at stomach and in bowels, with more or less bloating of abdomen at times; eructations per mouth, and fetid gases per rectum, with restlessness at night—almost a pronounced insomnia, with that tired feeling, enfeebled, and less than normal; liver torpid; bowels obstinately costive; fetid breath; coated tongue; depressed spirits and flatulence. Hyperemia more or less present every day, of front and apex of head, with feeling of weight when so bothered. The predominant feature of the case was his great fear of doing bodily harm to his little boy, claiming that he feared he would kill him—and the weapon a knife. Claimed that a knife in his own hands, or on seeing a butcher with one, vividly called to mind at once his weakness and fearful desire. After some little reasoning on my part, he placed his case in my hands for treatment. I requested him to sleep apart from wife and child which had been his habit. He, in a few days, informed me that a friend of his, then out of work, was sleeping with him, and also journeyed with him in day-time, whilst attending to his calling. Knowing that a fit of indigestion would be severe in his case—being plethoric—admonished him about regular eating, and but to eat three meals a day, avoiding excessive use of meat foods. As to treatment, I placed him on essence of pepsin, to supply a needed adjunct to digest food and lessen disturbance from same, also administered *Kali Phos.,* one tablet every third hour, allowing same to dissolve in mouth, and to be kept there for a few minutes before swallowing. After two weeks' continuous use of this, and a mild sedative at times at night to overcome the restlessness and insomnia, found decided benefit. I continued the same plan of treatment, save the substitution of papoid et sodæ bicarb. tablets, desiring the added good of the small doses of soda and mint. This treatment I kept up a period of some twelve weeks and discharged him well. This has been some months now and have often seen him since, and in good condition, and no more homicidal tendencies. (O. D. Whittier, M. D.)

METRITIS

BIOCHEMIC TREATMENT

Ferrum Phos.—In the first or inflammatory stage to remove the fever, pain and congestion. Also hot applications over region of womb.

Kali Mur.—Second stage, when the congestion has become chronic or exudation has taken place, causing hypertrophy of the uterus. If of stony hardness, *Calc. Fluor.*

METRORRHAGIA

(See Menstruation.)

CLINICAL CASES

Silicea in Metrorrhagia:

Metrorrhagia of six weeks' standing, in the case of a fat and robust woman of brown complexion. This person, who was a washer-woman at Grenille, and whom I saw only three or four times at my office, attributes her sickness to her constantly standing in cold water. *Silicea* arrested the hemorrhage almost immediately and effected such an improvement in one week that I scarcely knew her again the second week. She did not take any other medicine.

(A. Teste.)

MILK FEVER

(See Labor and Pregnancy.)

MISCARRIAGE

(See Labor and Pregnancy.)

MORNING SICKNESS

(See Vomiting, Labor and Pregnancy.)

BIOCHEMIC TREATMENT

Ferrum Phos.—Morning sickness with vomiting of undigested food.

Natr. Sulph.—Morning sickness, with vomiting of bilious fluids; bitter taste in the mouth.

Kali Mur.—Morning sickness, in pregnancy, with vomiting of white phlegm—white-coated tongue.

Natr. Mur.—*Morning sickness, with vomiting of frothy, watery phlegm;* profuse constant water-brash, like limpid mucus. Great hunger, as if stomach were empty, but no appetite.

Natr. Phos.—Morning sickness, with vomiting of acid, sour masses.

MOUTH, DISEASES OF

BIOCHEMIC TREATMENT

Ferrum Phos.—Inflammation of any part of the mouth in the initiatory stage. Gums are sore, red and inflamed.

Kali Mur.—*White ulcers in the mouths of little children or nursing mothers.* Aphthae, with much saliva (*Natr. Mur.*). Canker of the mouth. Diseases of the mouth, when there is a white-coated tongue. Gum-boils, before matter forms. Gums puffed and swollen; thick, whitish secretions from the mouth.

Natr. Phos.—An excellent remedy for *ulcerations* of the mouth, when the characteristic *creamy, yellow discharge* is present. Canker sores, when due to an acid condition of the stomach.

Calc. Phos.—Pale appearance of the gums, a sign of anemia—a course of this remedy is necessary; follow with

Ferrum Phos. Painful gums during dentition; inflamed (*Ferrum Phos.*).

Kali Phos.—Gangrenous conditions of the mouth. Scurvy. Canker of the mouth; mortification of the cheek, with ashy-gray ulcers; alternate *Kali Mur.* Fetid breath. Bleeding gums. Gums with a bright-red edge.

Natr. Mur.—Salivation. Any disease of the mouth in which there is an *excessive flow of saliva.* Watery blisters around the mouth.

Kali Sulph.—Dryness and peeling of the mucous membrane of the lower lip.

Calc. Fluor.—Hard swellings on the jaw, associated with gum-boil. Indurations.

CLINICAL CASES

Kali Phos. in Stomatitis:

At a meeting of medical men at Schaffhausen, Professor Dr. Rapp said: "In my opinion, the greatest merits of Dr. Schuessler's method lie in the introduction of *Kali Phos.* and *Magnes. Phos.* In ordinary stomatitis, with swelling of the gums, deposit on the teeth and foul breath, *Kali Phos.* has given very satisfactory proofs of its value."

MUMPS

(See Glandular Affections.)

ETIOLOGY

In the condition called mumps, a lack of the molecules of potassium chloride allows the fibrin to become a disturbing element; and on its way out, instead of passing through the lungs or nasal passages, it accumulates in the parotid gland, causing inflammation and swelling.

BIOCHEMIC TREATMENT

Ferrum Phos.—For the febrile symptoms, in the first stage of the disease.

Kali Mur.—*Principal remedy for the exudation* or glandular swelling. Alternated with *Ferrum Phos.*, it will, in most cases, prove sufficient.

Natr. Mur.—*Mumps, with excessive secretion of saliva,* or with swelling of the testicles, alternate or intercurrent remedy.

CLINICAL CASES

Ferrum Phos. and Kali Mur. in Mumps:

I have treated, during the past year, at least a dozen cases of mumps, and I have never had such satisfactory results with other remedies. One case had violent fever, even to delirium, great deal of swelling, pain, etc. The fever was entirely reduced within five or six hours, and the swelling and all the other symptoms were entirely relieved within three or four days by the alternate use of *Ferrum Phos.* and *Kali Mur.* Two cases in one family, with similar conditions, were in a like manner treated with the same results.
(S. Powell Burdick, M. D.)

NERVES

(See Neurasthenia, Neuritis, Neuralgia.)

ETIOLOGY

The nervous system of the human body is the most highly complex, the most delicately balanced, the most finely adjusted mechanism known. And the problem of a healthy nervous system is the most compelling of all health problems, as the condition of the entire body is largely dependent upon it.

The grey matter of the brain cells, as well as the cells of the motor and sensory nerves throughout the body, contains the inorganic cell-salt Potassium Phosphate combined with albumen and oxygen. The cells of the white fibers found in the sheath or neurilemma surrounding the motor and sensory nerves contain the inorganic cell-salt Magnesia Phosphate, which has united with albumen and oxygen. Other substances enter into the composition of the nerve cells, but the basic elements are those mentioned above.

When too severe a strain is put upon the nervous system in any way, overwork, worry, extreme mental or physical shock, and similar departures from the normal demand, cell metabolism is increased, and a greater amount of the inorganic cell salts, Magnesia Phos. or Kali Phos., as the case may be, is required. Frequently, the supply of these salts available in the blood is not sufficient. Thereupon the various forms of nervous disorders, neurasthenia, neuritis, neuralgia, paralysis, etc., result. To overcome these disorders, and restore the nervous system once more to normal, it is necessary to furnish the organism a fresh supply of the lacking inorganic cell-salts, which will unite with organic matter to form the new nerve cells so imperatively required.

There are two other potassium salts in the body besides Kali Phos., namely, Kali Mur. and Kali Sulph. When from continuous strain on the mental processes the lack of Kali Phos. becomes very great or is maintained for a long period, the grey-matter cells must draw upon one of these other potassium salts to supply the deficiency. In this way a deficiency is caused in the potassium salts drawn upon, so that disease may result in some other part of the body.

Modern life, especially in cities, is exceedingly wearing on the nerves. The noises, the excitement, the hurry, the competition, the lack of regular hours and sufficient sleep are enough in themselves to cause a nervous strain. And when hard study, worry, anxiety and similar mental exertions accompany them, the tax on the nerve-cells is apt to become too great to bear. It is for this reason that the number of people suffering from nervous disorders has so greatly increased in the last few decades.

It is for this reason, too, that the patient, suffering from nervous disorders, should have complete rest and quiet, should be free from worry and harassing mental exercise, should have plenty of sleep and fresh air, and, if possible, a complete change of scene. In a word, he should be removed from the environment that has caused too great a strain on his nervous resources. Then by supplying the deficient cell-salts in the form of the indicated Biochemic Remedies at regular and frequent intervals, the nervous system will be able to build itself up again to normal condition.

It will be found advisable to continue the use of Kali Phos. for a considerable time after a cure has been effected, in order that a relapse may be averted. In fact, to a person laboring under constant mental strain, the consistent daily use of this remedy will be of great value in keeping the nervous system in good order.

NEURALGIA

(See Pain.)

ETIOLOGY

Neuralgia is caused most frequently by an impoverishment of the nerves themselves or undue pressure of surrounding tissues. The phosphates of magnesia and potassium enter largely into the formation of nerve fibers; therefore, when these elements are deficient or disturbed, the brain at once receives the warning. A deficiency in other phosphates or sodium chloride often causes nerve pain, also; and it may be caused by albuminous or fibrinous particles clogging in the tissue of the neurilemma, or nerve sheath, and thus preventing free circulation. It matters not in what part the pains are situated, the treatment will be the same.

The symptoms consist of sharp, shooting, darting or intense pains along the course of the nerves. Heat generally relieves, if the pains are not deepseated.

BIOCHEMIC TREATMENT

Kali Phos.—This remedy is indicated where the pain is of a continuous character. Symptoms: Neuralgic pains in neurasthenic subjects. Neuralgia, with irritability, crossness, etc.; pains are ameliorated by gentle motion. Pain is worse when rising from a sitting position or from overexertion. Neuralgic pains and neuritis with depression and failure of strength; sensitiveness to light and noise. Neuralgic headaches, with sleeplessness, nervousness, etc. Pains, with humming in the ears. Threatening paralysis, with feeling of lameness and numbness. (Alternate *Calc. Phos.* for its systemic effect.)

Magnes. Phos.—The chief indication for this remedy is the spasmodic character of the pain. Symptoms: All neuralgic pains and neuritis, when heat gives relief and cold aggravates. Neuralgic pains very sharp, darting and intense. Intercostal neuralgia of a drawing, constrictive nature. Excruciating, spasmodic, crampy pains. Pain in the ends of nerve fibers. Periodical pains, very acute in their character, shooting along the course of the nerves. Neuralgia of the face, better in warm room, worse in open air.

Ferrum Phos.—Alternate with *Kali Phos.* for the following symptoms: Neuralgia due to neuritis. Neuralgia, when caused by congestion. (Cold applications relieve by reducing the congestion.) Neuralgia from chill or cold, with severe throbbing pain, pain in one side of the head, in the temples or over the eye. Follow with *Calc. Phos.*, if this does not give relief. Neuralgic pains, when accompanied by flushed face, burning heat, fever, etc. Tic douloureux.

Calc. Phos.—Neuralgic pains, especially in anemic or undernourished persons, and when the pains do not yield to the indicated remedy. Intercurrently in chronic cases. Neuralgia recurring periodically, coming on at night, deep-seated, as if on the bone. Pains, with sensation of crawling coldness and numbness. Pains worse at night in bad weather. Neuralgia of the anus, pain long-continued after stool.

Natr. Mur.—Severe neuralgic pains, recurring at intervals, with flow of saliva or tears. Darting, shooting pains along the nerve fibers, with flow of tears. The pains of *Natr. Mur.* are quite similar to those of *Magnes. Phos.*, but are easily distinguishable by the excess of saliva or involuntary flow of tears. Irritation of the fifth pair of nerves, also facial nerve, with intense pain and lachrymation. Neuralgia, with constipation from dryness of the bowels, and accompanied with the usual excessive secretions from other membranes.

Kali Mur.—Alternate with the indicated chief remedy where the disease is accompanied by stomach trouble, usually manifested by white or grayish-white coated tongue.

CLINICAL CASES

Magnes. Phos. in Neuralgia:

Neuralgia of face cured by Biochemic Remedies. Male patient, 50 years, suffered with neuralgia of severe type. He was entirely relieved by *Magnes. Phos.* given every twenty minutes. In two hours pain had ceased, but face was very sensitive to touch. Six months have elapsed with no return. (Dr. S. W. Jones, Wilbur, Washington.)

Magnes. Phos.—two doses cured her Neuralgia:

Miss Margaret S. suffered from neuralgia, true nerve fibre pain, darting through her head along the nerves. She had suffered intermittently for three days. Two doses of *Magnes. Phos.* cured her completely.
(M. D. W. From Schuessler.)

Magnes. Phos. regulated the Catamenia; cured the Neuralgia:

Lady, æt. 42, with a hectic appearance, the catamenia scanty, often omitting. For two years, boring over the right eye, after a few minutes spreading over the whole right side to the lower jaw, driving her out of bed. Liver torpid; little appetite. *Magnes. Phos.* overcame all complaints in four days. This remedy regulated the catamenia and all subsequent attacks.

(A. Plate, M. D.)

Post-Influenzal Neuralgia (Supraorbital):

A case of post-influenzal neuralgia (supraorbital).—After the patient seemed to be getting fairly over the fever, and, as I thought, would not need another visit, I was called to him in a hurry to relieve a pain over the eye. I knew the value of *Magnes. Phos.* in neuralgia, but at the time I was out of it, having just sent an order to Luyties Pharmacal Company for a supply. I gave him morphine hypodermically, but with no relief; I used all the remedies of which I had ever heard or read of in the next three days. The man suffered terribly. He was running subnormal temperature, the room had to be darkened—so dark that one had to grope his way to where he was. On the least admission of light he would be wild with pain. The patient was becoming awfully weak and had to be raised to take his medicine. It began to look bad for him.

Toward night of the third day his father announced his intention to call a surgeon as he thought this was a true sinusitis. I asked him to wait for one more mail, because I had some medicine coming in which I had great faith. I received the medicine at 8 p. m. and drove back at once to give him the test, because I had agreed to call a surgeon as soon as it was plain that the medicine would not relieve him.

As soon as I could obtain it, I prescribed five celloids of *Magnes. Phos.* every thirty minutes until he was easier, then five every hour until he was perfectly easy. I left. They told me next day that after the fourth dose of the medicine he was resting and sleeping so well that they would not awaken him to give more medicine, and that he slept soundly and awoke next morning free from pain.

I kept him on the *Magnes. Phos.*, however, for two or three days longer, and he has never felt the pain since. This was a case in which the action of medicine was perfectly marvelous. (Dr. I. M. Howard, Cross Plains, Texas.)

Kali Phos. in Neuralgia from decayed teeth:

Kali Phos. cured a case of neuralgia of the right side of the face from decayed teeth, relieved by cold applications. *Magnes. Phos.*, given at first, did not relieve, probably because there was no relief from warmth.
(W. P. Wesselhoeft, M. D.)

Magnes. Phos. in Neuralgia of Head:

A severe case of neuralgia in the head. The lady had come sixty miles to attend a musical entertainment and was compelled to go to bed on account of the pain. After suffering for several hours I was called, and relieved her completely in an hour with *Magnes. Phos.*, a dose every ten minutes.

Calc. Phos. in Neuralgia of Sacrum:

Ada D., a healthy, robust child, æt. 8. Her only symptom was a severe pain at the lower part of the sacrum, coming on after stool and lasting the entire day until she goes to bed, when it ceases. The pain is so severe as to prevent her walking or even standing. *Calc. Phos.* gave immediate relief.
(R. T. Cooper, M. D.)

Magñes. Phos. in right facial Neuralgia:

Dr. H. C. Allen reports a case of right facial neuralgia, with sharp, quick, spasmodic, lightning-like pains, sensitive to touch, relieved by heat and pressure, accompanied by prostration and night-sweats, cured by *Magnes. Phos.*, after several other remedies had failed to give permanent relief. Also another case cured by the same remedy, where the pains were intermittent, darting, lightning-like, suddenly appearing and disappearing, relieved by heat and pressure; at the same time an annoying constipation disappeared.

Magnes. Phos. in facial Neuralgia:

Miss S., æt. 24; dark complexion; nervous temperament; clerk. She had been under treatment for facial neuralgia for two weeks previous, the principal remedy being *Morphia*, without relief. On being called to the case, I found the patient much prostrated, the right side of the face and supraorbital region somewhat swollen, pains very severe, of a crampy, shooting, darting nature. There was also much tenderness over the affected side. The pains were of an intermittent character, and seemed to affect different parts of the head and face on different days. *Magnes. Phos.* cured the case in twelve hours.

Magnes. Phos. in Neuralgia from exposure:

Miss B., æt. 22; dark complexion; nervous temperament; slight build; had neuralgia from exposure to a strong north wind, and was under the treatment for three days before I was called, and had taken *Bromide of potash* and *Chloral hydrate*, with no relief. I found her in bed, almost frantic with pain, flushed face, eyes injected, with a high degree of photophobia; pain was left-sided and involved the supramaxillary portion of the trigeminus. In character the pain was lancinating, crampy, darting and shooting, frequently extorting cries. *Magnes. Phos.* was given and resulted in a speedy recovery.

Magnes. Phos. in facial Neuralgia:

Miss S., æt. 20; brunette; tall and slender; nervo-bilious temperament; occupation, stenographer. She was taken suddenly with acute pain in right side of face, the pain involving the supra and infraorbital region, paroxysmal, of a darting, tearing character. *Magnes. Phos.* cured promptly.

Calc. Phos. cured; Electricity failed:

Chas. M., æt. 47. Has for a week or two a severe tearing, gnawing pain in region of right scapula, extending into the right upper arm, and down the forearm into the thumb, with numbness, particularly of the thumb, but without loss of motion or use of arm. The pain comes in paroxysms, and is only relieved by hard rubbing and pounding of the flesh; troublesome as well day-times as nights. Has taken several remedies, and had electricity each day for a week or more, without benefit. After taking *Calc. Phos.* for a few days the pain and numbness were much relieved, and being continued, the trouble was cured in about three or four weeks. Any return of it would be at once relieved by this remedy.

A similar case in a young lady, æt. 20, was cured by the same remedy, though she had almost complete paralysis of the hand.

(C. T. M.)

Magnes. Phos. in Faceache:

A lady of healthy appearance had suffered several weeks with faceache, radiating over one-half of the face, lasting five or six hours. Warm wadding relieves. Worse when body gets cold. *Magnes. Phos.*, every three hours, removed the pain in three days.

Magnes. Phos. in Neuralgia:

Lady, æt. 30, had suffered several weeks with pains in face and teeth, right side, changing locality. Appears every two or three hours, and rushes about like lightning. *Magnes. Phos.*, a dose every three hours, relieved in two days.

NEURASTHENIA

ETIOLOGY

Neurasthenia is a condition of general breakdown in the nervous system, due primarily to a lack of the cell-salt Kali Phos. following severe mental of physical strains or shocks.

This results in an exhaustion of the nerve-cells in the brain and spinal cord so that the mental processes become weakened and easily fatigued and the senses deadened.

Usually neurasthenia is a condition resulting from long and continuous abuse of the nervous system, and the cure is, therefore, generally a long process. For when a disease has taken months and sometimes years to manifest itself, one cannot expect it to be cured over night. But it is important that proper treatment should always be given in cases of nerve weakness and that the condition should not be looked upon as one that will naturally disappear in time of its own accord. For by neglecting this trouble, and continuing the abuses that have brought it on, melancholia, nervous breakdown or prostration will surely result.

A neurasthenic condition may be brought on by a steady indulgence of the following: too much and too long continued mental exercise in the form of study, concentration or any other form of mental exertion; worry, harassing thoughts, grief, or other exhausting emotions; over indulgence in stimulants; too little sleep; irregularity of meal hours when combined with long working hours; uncongenial surroundings and occupations that induce a gloomy frame of mind.

Complete rest and quiet is essential to the patient suffering from neurasthenia. He should avoid worry, noise, and excitement; should rest his mind as well as his body; should lead a simple, healthy life. If it is possible for him to travel, a change of scene and environment is greatly beneficial, preferably to some quiet country spot where he can get plenty of fresh air, mild exercise, wholesome food and sleep. The indicated Biochemic Remedies should be taken regularly, Kali Phos. predominating.

BIOCHEMIC TREATMENT

Kali Phos. is indicated in: Depressed spirits, irritability, impatience. Sleeplessness or loss of memory. Brain-fag from overwork, study, etc. Inability of thought. Sensitiveness, restlessness, dullness, loss of energy, dread of noise. Faint feelings, hallucination, morbid thoughts, melancholy, nervous exhaustion. Sighing and moaning in sleep. Night terrors of children. Easily startled; whining disposition. Crossness and irritability of children; ill temper arising from nervous disturbances. Fear, fretfulness, crying or screaming in children. Insanity, loss of correct reasoning power.

Calc. Phos.—Alternate with *Kali Phos.* for children and anemic subjects, for its constitutional properties.

Ferrum Phos.—Alternate with *Kali Phos.* where there is fever, flushed face, hectic appearance, to increase the hemoglobin content of the blood.

Magnes. Phos.—Alternate with *Kali Phos.* where the neurasthenia is accompanied by pains, convulsions, neuralgia, etc. This cell-salt is found in the white fibers of the nerves and muscles and, if deficient, will cause the fibers to contract, producing cramps, convulsions, etc.

Natr. Mur.—Alternate with *Kali Phos.* in cases where neurasthenia is accompanied by constipation owing to dryness of the mucous membranes of the bowels. Also in tearful, lachrymose subjects. *Natrum. Mur.* is found in combination with water, especially in the mucous membranes, and this cell-salt regulates the proper degree of moisture in the tissues.

Natr. Sulph.—Alternate with *Kali Phos.* for bilious conditions. This salt works with bile and keeps it in a normal consistency.

CLINICAL CASES

Nervous Breakdown:

Mr. H., a young married man, 26 years of age. Nervous temperament, hard mental worker. School teacher; had been teaching five years. Some reverses in way of dissatisfaction among directors and trouble in church work confined him to his room. Photophobia marked, would scream when touched, had much pain in all parts of body; weak digestion, illusion, delusions, hallucinations, slow mental activity.

He had services of local physician and nerve specialist. Both gave grave prognosis. I was called—gave him *Kali Phos.,* five grains every two hours. Second day, some improvement. At the end of the first week, he was able to go away to a sanitarium for change of environment, rest, etc. After two weeks he was able to leave the sanitarium, return home and in a little while resume his school duties. He took *Kali Phos.* for three months. He is still teaching. However, occasionally, he sends for a little *Kali Phos.,* as he uses a great deal of brain energy.

I have a number of other cases where *Kali Phos.* has done as much as above.
(Dr. H. O. Young.)

Kali Phos. in Nervous Exhaustion:

Mrs. G. M., age 36, married fifteen years. One child which died in thirty-six hours, cause unknown; history otherwise negative. Always nervous, had abdominal operation ten years ago: appendix, one tube, and ovary removed; somewhat better since then. Menstruation irregular, misses occasionally, is taking on weight, no nausea. Present complaint: always tired, weak, occasional attacks of vertigo, very nervous, always thirsty and hungry, forgets where she is or where she is going; must concentrate and think for a few minutes before she can remember; cannot sleep until about 2 a. m., and is rested when she awakes; has tired aching in legs most of the time.

Examination. Lungs and heart normal. Urinalysis, no albumen or sugar, sp. gr. 1025. Uterus normal size and position, cervix normal. Wassermann was returned negative.

Treatment. *Kali Phos.,* two tablets four times daily. Reported January 13, feeling quite well, no flighty nervous spells, feels much stronger, is sleeping well. A urinalysis and examination of the reflexes at this time was negative. Patient has been to office since above date, but with other little troubles. February 16, last call. The first troubles have not returned. She is at the climacteric and is getting through with very slight difficulty. She comes in on the slightest symptom.
(Dr. G. R. Reay.)

Kali Phos. in Neurasthenia:

Miss G. F., age 27. Employed as a typesetter in job printing office. Neurasthenia: Became despondent, wanted to be alone, broke into tears while talking, lost all interest in life, had lost several pounds, and could not eat or sleep. I prescribed outdoor walks with pleasant company, and *Kali Phos.,* five grains every two hours. After three weeks she experienced a marvelous change, was cheerful, could eat and sleep well and was gaining flesh. She returned to her work and has had no further trouble in past two months. Still taking *Kali Phos.* every four hours. I could enumerate a number of cases so treated with brilliant results. I am satisfied it will pay any physician to investigate and use the Biochemic Remedies. They are very pleasant and effective.
(Dr. J. W. Kannel.)

The Five Phosphates in Neurasthenia:

Give the five phosphates, *Calc., Ferrum, Kali, Magnes.,* and *Natrum.* *Kali Phos.* and *Magnes. Phos.* will take care of the nerves. *Calc. Phos.* and *Natr. Phos.* will aid digestion and *Ferrum Phos.* will oxygenize the blood. These remedies will need to be given over a long period of time, and must be accompanied with dietary and hygienic measures.
(Dr. J. B. Chapman, Seattle, Wash.)

Kali Phos. in Neurasthenia:

Married lady, aged 28, nervous temperament, made greatly worse by a succession of deaths in her family, also some considerable financial trouble. The functional nervous derangement was so intense that her friends though her hopelessly insane, and were seriously considering placing her in an asylum. I diagnosed the case as one of aggravated neurasthenia and at once placed her on *Kali Phos.*, five celloids every hour for twenty-four hours, then every two hours, and was gratified to find her rapidly recover her normal mental and physical equilibrium. Two years since, she has remained in excellent health.

(Dr. B. A. Sanders.)

NEPHRALGIA

(See Kidneys, Diseases of.)

NEPHRITIS

(See Kidneys, Diseases of.)

NEURITIS

ETIOLOGY

Neuritis, or "inflammation of the nerves," is caused by a deficiency of one or more of the cell-salts *Kali Phos., Magnesia Phos.* or *Ferrum Phos.* This deficiency may be the result of exposure to cold or dampness, injury, excessive use of stimulants, etc. Neuritis is a rather rare disease: neuralgia often existing to a severe degree, without inflammation of the nerve substance itself.

The chief remedies are Potassium and Magnesium Phosphate, the former indicated in deep-seated, continuous pains, the latter in spasmodic, cramp-like pains Other cell-salts may, and usually are, also indicated, and should be given according to the symptoms present.

For further treatment, see *"Neuralgia."*

NIPPLES, SORENESS OF

BIOCHEMIC TREATMENT

Ferrum Phos.—Principal remedy, especially if there are cracks which bleed. Give internal and apply locally each time after the child nurses. *Calc. Fluor.* will be found useful in obstinate cases.

OPHTHALMIA

(See Eyes, Diseases of.)

BIOCHEMIC TREATMENT

Ferrum Phos.—The remedy for all inflammatory symptoms.

Natr. Phos.—Infantile ophthalmia, *purulent discharge from the eyes of new-born children;* discharge from eyes, creamy.

Kali Sulph.—Discharge purulent, greenish in character.

Calc. Sulph.—Ophthalmia, with quick, purulent discharges, sometimes mixed with blood.

ORCHITIS

BIOCHEMIC TREATMENT

Kali Mur.—Inflammation and swelling of the testicle, *chief remedy, if caused from suppressed gonorrhea.*

Ferrum Phos.—For the inflammatory conditions, fever, heat, pain, etc.

Calc. Phos.—As an intercurrent remedy, or when the disease has reached the chronic stage.

CLINICAL CASES

Calc. Fluor. in Orchitis:

A little more than a year ago I received an injury which resulted in orchitis of a stony hardness. I used about all of the remedies I knew of besides some recommended by notable medical writers. None of them did any apparent good. Finally I consulted one of my brother practitioners who advised the use of ichthyol one part, vaseline two parts; mix, 1 oz. to 2. This mixture reblistered the scrotum.

I reduced the ointment twice by adding one ounce of Lanoline each time, but the use of it always caused the blistering of the scrotum. Now I thought was a good time to test the Biochemic Remedies. I had a bottle of 1,000 1-grain tablets of *Calc. Fluor.*, which had not been opened, made by Luyties.

I commenced the use of these by taking five or six every two hours when possible, and putting a two-dram vial of them in my vest pocket to use when on the road.

At the end of six weeks the testicle was reduced to normal size and condition. I took in all about five hundred tablets, or a little more.
(Dr. Z. T. Riggs, Biloxi, Miss.)

OTALGIA

(See Ear, Diseases of.)

OTITIS

(See Ear, Diseases of.)

BIOCHEMIC TREATMENT

Ferrum Phos.—With painful and inflamed soft parts.

Calc. Sulph.—Otitis media; discharge of matter from the middle ear, sometimes mixed with blood. Deafness, with middle ear suppuration, swelling of the glands, etc.

Silicea.—External ear inflamed; swelling of the external meatus. *Suppurative otitis, when discharge is thin, ichorous, offensive* and *attended with destruction of bone.*

OTORRHEA

(See Ear, Diseases of.)

CLINICAL CASES

Calc. Sulph., Ferr. Phos. and Silicea in Otorrhea:

I herewith report a very interesting case of otorrhea, with enlarged glands almost to the point of suppuration. I treated the case with *Calc. Sulph., Ferrum Phos.* and *Silicea.* I arrested further development, thus preventing suppuration, and brought the case to a happy termination in 12 days.

I consider this a very grave case, and comparing it with former cases, treated by other methods, I realize more satisfactory results in half the time.
(Dr. A. B. Couch, Houston, Texas.)

Rapid cure in Otorrhea:

Patient came from Dallas, had left ear discharging pus for two weeks, also large swelling in front of ear. Had not lain down for two weeks at night, owing to pain. *Kali Mur.* and *Magnes. Phos.* relieved him in a week, then followed with *Silicea,* which brought about a rapid cure.
(Dr. F. V. Bryant.)

Silicea in Otorrhea:

In May a lady came to me with chronic ear trouble in one ear which was discharging pus, and said she had been under a doctor's care over a year. She said she had washes to keep the ear clean, but was not any better; if anything, the discharge was worse.

I gave her *Silicea,* to take three times a day. I gave her quite an amount, and told her to return when the medicine was gone. I did not see her any more until about September 1st, and asked her why she did not come back when her medicine ran out. She said that the ear quit discharging before the medicine was gone, and that she was well.
(Dr. J. S. Leachman.)

OZENA

(See Catarrh.)

PALPITATION

(See Heart, Affections of.)

PAIN

(See Neuralgia and Headache.)

BIOCHEMIC TREATMENT

Ferrum Phos.—Pain from inflammatory causes in any part of the body. Neuralgia, backache, pains in the back and loins and over kidneys. All *Ferrum Phos.* pains are ameliorated by cold, applied directly to the seat of disease; but if the pains are deep-seated, heat will be necessary, applied to the surface as a counter-irritant.

Magnes. Phos.—*Pains* of a *sharp, shooting, darting, spasmodic* or constrictive nature, relieved by heat and aggravated by cold. Pains vivid, boring, intermittent and neuralgic.

Kali Mur.—Useful after, or in alternation with, *Ferrum Phcs.*, if swelling exists. Movement causes pain. Tongue coated white.

Kali Phos.—Laming pains; the parts affected feel powerless; gentle movement relieves pain and stiffness, but too much exertion aggravates. Neuralgic pains in anemic, irritable persons. Pains are worse when beginning motion, but gentle exercise relieves. Pains are better under cheerful excitement.

Calc. Phos.—Pains associated with feeling of numbness, coldness, or with a creeping sensation, worse at night or in bad weather. *Pains resulting from exhausting diseases.* Lumbago, alternate with *Ferrum Phos.*

Natr. Mur.—Pains, when accompanied with excessive secretion of saliva or flow of tears; the tongue also is covered with bubbles of frothy saliva. *Dull, heavy pains in the head, with flow of tears.* Neuralgic pains, resembling those of *Magnes. Phos.*, but with a flow of tears. Pains are generally worse in the morning.

Kali Sulph.—*Pains of a shifting characte, flitting from one place to another,* require this salt. Pains are generally worse in the evening, in a warm room or heated atmosphere; better in cool, open air.

Natr. Phos.—Pains, especially rheumatic, if the tongue has a yellow, creamy coating. *Pain after taking food, with acid conditions.*

Calc. Fluor.—Backache simulating spinal irritation. Pains in the lower part of the back, indicating confined bowels, hemorrhoids or fali of the uterus.

PALSY

(See Paralysis.)

PARALYSIS

ETIOLOGY

A great diminution, or total loss of the power of motion in one or more of the voluntary muscles. This condition is known by many different names; such as: Paralysis agitans, ascending paralysis—beginning in the legs and ascending to other parts of body; diphtheritic, hemiplegic, paraplegic, reflex, writer's paralysis, etc. A deficiency of the inorganic salts that furnish organic matter to make and keep up the supply of nerve and muscle fluid sufficient to keep them in order, or working condition, is the first cause of paralysis.

It sometimes occurs that the condition is aggravated by an accumulation of organic waste matter, albuminous and fibrinous, in the connective tissue and interstices surrounding nerve plexuses or muscular fibres, causing an engorgement and thus preventing free circulation, which cuts off the vital supply.

BIOCHEMIC TREATMENT

Kali Phos.—*This is the first remedy* to be considered in all cases of paralysis, whether creeping or sudden in its onset. Paralysis of vocal cords, causing loss of voice. Locomotor paralysis, creeping paralysis, with atrophic conditions, vital powers are reduced and stools have a putrid odor. Facial paralysis, partial paralysis, hemiplegia, facial or infantile paralysis requires *Kali Phos., the chief remedy.*

Magnes. Phos.—Paralysis of the white nerve fibres. Palsy, involuntary shaking and trembling of the hands or of the head (*Calc. Phos.*). "*Muscular paralysis* caused by a disturbed or diseased condition of the efferent nerve fibres which convey the motor stimulus to the muscles." (Walker.) Alternate with *Kali Phos.*

Calc. Phos.—Coldness, numbness, creeping sensations in the lower limbs. Creeping paralysis; intercurrently with the chief remedy.

Silicea.—Paralysis from tabes dorsalis. Paralytic weakness of the joints. (*Natr. Phos.*)

CLINICAL CASES

Kali Phos. and Mag. Phos. in Paralysis:

Was called to see Mrs. R., age 36. Paralysis of left side. Had been treated about one month by another M. D. I found her in bed, unable to walk. I put her on *Kali Phos.*, every four hours in alternation with *Magnes. Phos.* every four hours. Her improvement was soon noted, and after two months' treatment she was walking the streets with almost complete use of the paralyzed parts. No other remedies were used. Have had other similar cases with same results.

(Dr. W. J. Grimes, East Liverpool, Ohio.)

Biochemic Remedies in Paralysis:

My brother, who is 61 years old, suffered a stroke of paralysis on May 8, 1924. His condition was so grave that no hope for his recovery seemed possible as he could not move hand nor foot and could not speak. He was as helpless as a baby. I began at once to give him the following Biochemic Remedies. *Kali Phos., Calc. Phos.* and *Magnes. Phos.*, five tablets of each together at 8 a. m., 12 noon, at 4 p. m., and 8 p. m., and five of *Silicea* on retiring.

I had him out of bed in 30 days, able to help himself. He is now walking and talking and his eye sight came back and his general health is better than for years.

(H. L., M. D.)

Calc. Phos. in Paralysis of hands and feet:

A. G., in order to kill herself, took poison, which left her paralyzed hands and feet. I gave her six doses of *Calc. Phos.*, and four weeks later she wrote me that she could go around the room by taking hold of furniture. She received six more doses, which completed her recovery.

Kali Phos. in facial Paralysis:

Henry K., æt. 24, was brought to the office by his father for treatment. Right side of face, from the ramus of jaw to above the tempero-parietal suture, paralyzed. Entire loss of sense of touch in the cheek, which he said felt numb, causing impediment in speech. Mouth was drawn to left side. Walked with a shuffling gait, which led me to anticipate a general paralysis or a tendency toward locomotor ataxia. Suspected onanism, which was denied. His hands would occasionally shake involuntarily, "as if he had the palsy," his father explained. Hands and feet cold.

Concluded that his trouble was due either to his working in water at his occupation, or else to sexual excesses, or both. Prescribed *Kali Phos.* and *Calc. Phos.*, in alternation, every three hours for two weeks, discontinued for one month, and then continued giving the *Kali Phos.* alone. Improvement

has been gradual, till now, after nearly three months, the facial paralysis is hardly perceptible, has considerable feeling in affected side, walks more regular, stepping somewhat naturally—and improvement in general. I might add that at a subsequent visit he admitted masturbating, and after the proper advice he promised to try to quit, and I think this, too, has aided some in his present improvement.
(C. R. Vogel, M. D.)

PARTURITION

(See Labor and Pregnancy.)

PELLAGRA

ETIOLOGY

Pellagra has been recognized for over 250 years, the name being given to it by Frapolli of Milan in 1771. In the United States the first case was not adequately reported until 1902 by Sherwell.

The first large series of cases which called general attention to the malady was reported by Searcy in 1907, the patients being in an insane asylum in Mt. Vernon, Ala. Since that time hundreds of other cases have been recorded.

The cause of pellagra is disputed, some claiming that it is transmitted by the bite of an insect, while others believe that it is due to corn which has been impaired in its nutritional value, or contains a fungus which is productive of the symptoms. In any event, whatever may be the cause, it produces in the sufferer a lack of certain cell-salts, which fact is evidenced by characteristic symptoms. It is only after the exciting cause of the trouble has been removed and the lacking cell-salts restored, that a return to health can be expected. It is noteworthy, also, that care as to corn used as food prevents the disease.

Symptoms. Pellagra is a non-contagious and non-hereditary disease, characterized by great variety in its manifestations. In the first stages its symptoms are a drowsiness and increasing physical and mental fatigue and depression. The alimentary symptoms include a coated tongue with stomatitis, nausea, vomiting and diarrhea.

There is also an erythematous appearance of the forearms and hands on the extensor surfaces, and of the face.

The trouble usually develops in the spring months, and if mild, the symptoms gradually disappear, recurring again and again yearly, or if severe, there may be no period of immunity.

An acute type of pellagra which pursues a very rapid course is rarely met with, death usually occurring after a period of about two to six weeks. It has its onset in a sharp attack of headache, vomiting and diarrhea, the diarrhea frequently resembling dysentery. Blood may occur, not only in the stools, but even from the lips and tongue.

The more severe symptoms of pellagra appearing in those who have the well-developed type consist of obstinate diarrhea, the tongue being denuded of epithelium and sometimes ulcerated. An erythema appears on the back of the hands and other parts exposed to the weather. The erythema at first disappears on pressure. Later on it is not affected by pressure. Finally it disappears. After several repetitions of this the skin atrophies, appearing as a thin, parchment-like membrane. In the wet type of the disease ulcerations may extend as deeply as the tendons of the hand. Even these deep lesions may heal.

In the second stage of the disease nervous manifestations take place. The languor of the first stage changes into a more or less profound melancholia and sometimes there are suicidal tendencies, especially by drowning. In other instances delusions of persecution are met with and finally stupor and coma develop.

In the alimentary canal, an intractable diarrhea may develop, often as early as the erythema, which is often dysenteric in character.

In the last stages of the disease there is a typhoid like condition present, as well as the stupor or coma before described.

Prognosis. Much depends on the severity of the symptoms and whether the patient's condition of life can be changed as to habits, food and climate. Even the administration of the lacking cell-salts cannot bring about a permanent improvement, unless the original source of the disease is removed.

BIOCHEMIC TREATMENT

Kali Phos.—Should be given for the nervous manifestations of this trouble. Headache, mental depression, and melancholia, even with suicidal tendencies.

Natr. Sulph.—Diarrhea, simple or resembling dysentery, with blood in the stools. Nausea and vomiting.

Calc. Sulph.—Skin yellow, with suppuration threatened, or where suppuration has already occurred. Dry parchment-like appearance of the skin.

Ferrum Phos.—When there is fever, especially with vomiting of blood.

Hydrotherapy should also be employed, in the form of warm or cold baths, or douches—particularly for the relief of the nervous symptoms. The diet should include fresh vegetables and fruit in the early stages.

In chronic cases, a milk diet should be instituted, with the addition of eggs as soon as possible, then cereals, and later fresh meats and vegetables. It is best to prohibit corn and maize.

A mouth wash of an antiseptic solution such as boric acid or sodium bicarbonate, one teaspoonful to eight ounces of water, will be found very helpful for the stomatitis. Ice will also relieve the vomiting.

CLINICAL CASES

Ferrum Phos., Natr. Sulph. and Calc. Phos. in Pellagra:

On November 22, I was called to see a lady 23 years old who had previously been treated by five different physicians for pellagra. I found her extremely emaciated, mouth sore, copious diarrhea, mind wandering, and unable to turn herself in bed.

Her case appeared practically hopeless, and I so informed the family. However, I put her on *Ferrum Phos.* and *Natr. Sulph.,* five grains each every two hours, alternately, with an occasional dose of *Calc. Sulph.,* five grains.

On January 14 I discharged her, cured. Three months from the beginning of treatment she resumed her work in a textile mill; and at his writing, a year later, there has been no return of the malady.

I have treated five other cases of pellagra of less gravity on the same lines with the same gratifying results. I did not restrict the diet in any of the cases, but ordered them fed with wholesome, nourishing food.

(Dr. J. A. Mourfield, Lenoir City, Tenn.)

Biochemic Remedies in Pellagra:

In June I was called to see my first pellagra patient, a woman, 45 years old. She had been suffering with the disease for several weeks, was so weak she had to be lifted on a sheet, could not retain any kind of food on her stomach, vomited large quantities of bile, for which condition I gave her five grains *Natr. Sulph.* every two hours. She also showed an evening temperature of 101 to 102 degrees, also vomited some red blood. For this condition I gave her *Ferrum Phos.* in alternation with the *Natr. Sulph.* On every seventh day

I gave my patient *Calc. Sulph.* To overcome the yellow condition of the skin, and the threatening suppuration, the *Calc. Sulph.* was given every hour during the day and night, then proceeded as before. In addition to the above treatment, I had the patient bathed all over the body in alcohol followed by pure olive oil. In eight weeks the patient was dismissed, cured.
(Dr. A. E. Johnson, Minneola, Florida.)

PERITONITIS

ETIOLOGY

This trouble is an inflammation of the serous sack or peritoneum which lines the abdominal cavity, and covers in its reflections the organs which this cavity contains.

It originates in a lack of *Kali Mur.*, which causes an excess of fibrin in the serous membrane of the peritoneum, and thus provides a breeding place for micro-organisms. Cold and abdominal strains frequently play a part in this, as they make severe demands upon the mucous and serous membranes and tend to break up the union between *Kali Mur.* and fibrin.

Peritonitis itself is due to germ invasion, most frequently from the extension of infection from appendicitis, or from disease of the Fallopian tubes. The *bacilli coli communis* is, perhaps, the most frequent producer of peritonitis under these circumstances, but the *streptococcus, pneumococcus, staphylococcus,* and others may also be present. In the acute peritonitis occurring after labor, the so-called septic peritonitis, the streptococcus is the chief factor.

Peritonitis usually is very sudden in its onset, the first symptom being a chill, followed by fever running as high as 102-104°, with a tense, wiry pulse. Accompanying this is an intense, cutting pain in the abdomen, which is extremely sensitive to the slightest touch. The thighs are kept flexed, to relieve abdominal pressure. Frequently there is anorexia, with nausea and vomiting, especially after eating. Constipation is usual. The face has a typical pinched and anxious look.

In treating peritonitis, the basal cause must be first considered. This is a deficiency in Kali Mur., which by the consequent excess of fibrin in the serous membranes, has provided a bacterial breeding place. Kali Mur., therefore, with Ferrum Phos. for the fever, is the indicated remedy.

At the same time the patient should be given absolute rest in bed, on a liquid diet, milk, peptonized or otherwise, and light broths.

Hot, light compresses should be applied to the abdomen; if there is gas present, the compresses should be sprinkled with turpentine and sweet oil, equal parts. The ice-bag should be employed in circumscribed inflammation. The lower bowel may be cleared with a laxative enema, but purgatives should never be given.

BIOCHEMIC TREATMENT

Ferrum Phos.—Principal remedy in this disease, for the inflammatory conditions; fever, heat, pain, etc. Give copious injections of hot water in which a quantity of *Ferrum Phos.* has been dissolved.

Kali Mur.—Second stage of peritonitis, swelling of the abdomen, white coated tongue. Alternate with the chief remedy, *Ferrum Phos.*

CLINICAL CASES

Ferrum Phos. for Peritonitis caused by eating berries:

Was called late one night to see a child, æt. 8; had eaten a large quantity of berries the day before. Found the patient partially delirious; pulse 130; temperature 103½; bowels hard, hot and swollen. I diagnosed peritonitis, caused by the berries and stoppage of the bowels. The parent had given two doses of a cathartic medicine, but without effect. I ordered a copious injection of hot water, in which was dissolved about twenty grains of *Ferrum Phos.* A large movement of the bowels occurred, after which I followed with Ferr. Phos. internally. Nothing could have acted better, as the patient was all right in the morning. Some think me radical on the subject of water, but if I am, I have cause to be proud. Its proper use will greatly facilitate the action of the salts. An injection will relieve the bowels instantly, without fear of causing diarrhea; copious drinks of *hot* water will relieve pain, inflammation, spasms, etc.

(J. B. Chapman, M. D.)

Ferrum Phos. in Peritonitis following acute inflammation of bowels:

After every other remedy had failed *Ferrum Phos.* was resorted to, in a case of acute inflammation of the bowels. The effect was a brilliant one. The fever abated; the pains decreased rapidly. This medicine was continued until the fever had quite subsided, and profuse perspiration commenced. At this stage *Kali Mur.* was given, which caused the absorption of the rather profuse effusion.

Ferrum Phos. in chronic Peritonitis:

Mrs. E., æt. 38; suffered for many years from chronic peritonitis and ovaritis. She would have subacute attacks, which would last for several months, confining her to her bed or room. Hardly would she be well of one attack before another would be induced by a cold or some slight overexertion. Was nervous and much depressed. One evening was seized with severe pain in the uterine and left ovarian regions, extending over the whole abdomen, which was very sensitive to the slightest touch. Pulse 120; temperature 104. *Ferrum Phos.* was given in water every fifteen minutes, for two hours, when the pains were somewhat less. The remedy was then given every hour for several days, until the pain and sensitiveness had gone. The patient was kept under treatment for two weeks longer, when she was obliged to go away. She gradually grew stronger and better, and now two years have passed and she has never

had the slightest sign of the trouble, which she had had for so many years, and is well and strong.
(G. H. Martin, M. D.)

PERTUSSIS

(See Whooping-Cough.)

PHTHISIS PULMONALIS

(See Consumption.)

CLINICAL CASES

Silicea in an exceptional case:

Mr. T., æt. 30; of sanguine, bilious temperament; rather dark complexion; five feet ten inches high; weight, in health, 166 pounds; family consumptive, two sisters and a brother have already died, leaving a brother still enjoying tolerable health. Had several hemoptyses in the summer while in the hay-field, and had constantly declined from that time. Saw him in April following; he having passed through the hands of several physicians, and at that time was so low that his physician said he could not live six weeks; and such was my opinion on seeing him. There was a large cavity in the right lung, at the second intercostal space, at about three inches to the right of the sternum; there were heavy rales in the left bronchi, with decided indications of breaking down of the parenchymatous structure and cavernous lesions there; also the sputa was very heavy and largely purulent; there was the odor of the cadaver already present, musty and offensive enough from septicemic influences; he had no appetite and sat up hardly longer than to have his bed made; skin had a cold, clammy feeling, and he was drenched with night-sweats. Case was marked with absence of vital warmth; indeed, so forbidding was the case that I refused his brother when he asked me to visit him again in a week; he lived forty miles away.

He was given a dose of *Silicea* every other night, and ordered to report by mail in a week. He had been very much harassed with his night-sweats and cough, which was worse from motion. The first mail brought me the intelligence that the medicine acted like a charm, and he wanted more of the same kind. I sent so that he got a dose of *Silicea* twice a week, and so treated him till June, when he paid me a visit. Left lung appeared to be cleared up, night-sweats no longer troubled him, appetite was good, he was steadily gaining in flesh and strength. Nevertheless, in the right lung there yet remained traces of the cavity, which now was much smaller and secreting only a small amount of muco-purulent matter. He was furnished additional medicine and went home, and by the middle of June was on his mowing machine. Patient was alive four years after and enjoying fine health. No man could be more surprised than myself at these results. Were we all deceived? Three physicians of the leading school of medicine agreed about the diagnosis, and I do not think there is left a possible ground for doubt. The case is exceptional, we agree, but is it not full of suggestions?

(G. N. B., in Brigham's "Phthisis.")

A typical case:

Case of a lady who had been bedridden for nine months. Mrs. McH. was considered by the doctors as beyond medical treatment. The doctor's diagnosis ran thus: Both lungs diseased, especially the right lung. The heart is greatly dilated, especially the right cavity. The lung disease produced by neglected cold. When her case was brought under treatment by biochemic measures, four years ago, she was also suffering from dropsy. At the stage she came under the new treatment, it took sometimes an hour and more before she could find the right position to rest in. She would often rather spend the night on a sofa than venture to go through the fatigue of going to bed. Her cough and expectoration were very bad; breath extremely short, and palpitation constant. She did not know what it was to have a good night, and rarely slept. By pa-

tiently adhering to the Biochemic remedies she has improved greatly, her lungs appear to be healed up, and her dilation of heart almost removed. She now lives in comparatively good health, so that she was able to nurse her husband during a severe illness, where night watching was necessary. To reassure all concerned, a diagnosis was made. Dr. H., a specialist, concurred in the statement that her right lung, of which a large portion is gone, is now fairly healed up, and dilation of heart has almost entirely disappeared.
(From Schuessler.)

PILES

(See Hemorrhoids.)

PLEURISY

(See Pneumonia.)

BIOCHEMIC TREATMENT

Ferrum Phos.—For the febrile conditions, *first stage,* dependent upon this disease, such as fever, pain, stitch in side, short cough, etc., short oppressed breathing. Hot applications to the surface.

Kali Mur.—*Second stage,* when there is plastic exudation, white or grayish-white coated tongue, etc.

Calc. Sulph.—Third stage, when pus has formed in the cavity.

CLINICAL CASES

Ferrum Phos. relieved Pleurisy entirely, second day:

Boy, æt. 5, with right-sided pleuritic stitch; worse when coughing and on deep inspiration. Rheumatic pains in right shoulder-jont. General heat of the body; very little thirst. *Ferrum Phos.* every two hours relieved entirely on the second day. I noticed an unnatural excitement about the child the day after having taken *Ferrum Phos.* He desired to get out of bed and wished to run around, but was too weak and fell over; very talkative and hilarious.

A similar excitement I noticed in a lad, æt. 7, to whom I had given *Kali Mur.* during a gastric fever, with great benefit. (W. P. Wesselhoeft, M. D.)

Ferrum Phos. in acute Pleurisy:

Miss G. R., æt. 20. Was called about midnight to see this young lady, who was said to be suffering with a pain in her side. I found her to be suffering with the symptoms common to an acute attack of pleurisy: high fever and severe pain in the left side of the chest. Called next morning: found the fever somewhat less, but pain not relieved. Called at 4 p. m.: about the same, pain still severe; gave *Ferrum Phos.* in solution. Called at 9 p. m.: the fever had abated, and the pain was much less. Called the next morning: no fever and pain nearly gone. She continued to improve, and after a few days was up and about, as usual.
(C. T. M.)

PNEUMONIA

ETIOLOGY

LIKE all other diseases of the respiratory organs, pneumonia is always preceded by a weakening of the mucous membrane of the air passages. This is ordinarily due to the effect of cold and electrical changes in the atmosphere, which cause a deficiency in the cell-salts Kali Mur. and Ferrum Phos. The deficiency in Kali Mur. sets free a quantity of fibrin, which seeks an outlet from the system through the mucous membrane of the lungs. Thus the mucous membrane is weakened, and a breeding place provided for the pneumococcus of Fraenkel, which is the exciting cause of pneumonia.

At the same time, the deficiency in Ferrum Phos. deprives the blood of a certain amount of its oxygen carrying ability, and it is obliged to circulate much faster in order to supply the tissues with the requisite quantity of oxygen, thus creating the condition commonly known as fever.

As the pneumonia continues, there is a hyperemia of the intervesicular tissues of the affected lobe or lobes of the lung. Soon there is an exudation intó the air vesicles and smaller bronchi of white cells, red cells, and plasma containing fibrin.

This soon forms a solid exudate, so that the affected portion of the lung becomes impervious to air, and absolutely useless for breathing. This puts a still greater strain upon the circulation, on account of the smaller amount of lung surface available for supplying oxygen to the blood, and the fever ordinarily becomes higher. This is known as the stage of red hepatization, since the exudate is colored red from the red blood cells, and the consistency of the organ to touch and on section resembles that of fresh liver, hence it is said to be hepatized or liver-like.

Shortly after the stage of red hepatization has been reached, that of gray hepatization begins, in which the exudate loses its color. Then resolution sets in, during which the exudate is gotten rid of by absorption and expectoration.

During the entire course of the disease, which lasts ordinarily nine days and ends by crisis, the patient suffers from a greater or less degree of toxemia, due to the poisons created by the invading micro-organisms and from the changes produced in the tissues of other organs than the lungs by the growth of the pneumococcus or by its toxins.

BIOCHEMIC TREATMENT

The Biochemic treatment of pneumonia should always be begun as promptly as possible. Realizing that the basic cause is an excess of fibrin in the mucous membrane of the lungs, thus furnishing a breeding place for the pneumococcus. it is evident that this breeding place can only be destroyed supplying the Kali Mur. which is lacking, to unite with the fibrin in the lungs. When this is done, the lung membrane will be restored to normal, and the pneumococcus will disappear.

For the fever, inflammation and congestion, Ferrum Phos. should be given. Thus a fresh and increased supply of oxygen is furnished, and the strain on the heart and circulation lessened.

A frothy sputum indicates Natrum Mur. also. During the stage of consolidation, when the skin is very dry, Kali Sulph. should be given until the moisture at the surface is well established. A few doses given in hot water rarely fails to start perspiration.

The bowels, also, should be carefully looked after. An overloaded colon or rectum will seriously depress the heart's action. An enema of warm water should be given daily.

Ferrum Phos.—*In the first stage of inflammation of the lungs,* for the pain, fever, congestion, short breathing, etc., also *Kali Sulph.* to establish free perspiration. Cough in pneumonia, without expectoration, or expectoration of blood or rust-colored sputa. Short, acute, hacking cough. Hot applications to the chest are very beneficial to relieve the congestion. Frequent doses of the remedy should be given.

Kali Mur.—*Second stage, when there is fibrinous exudation into the lungs;* cough, with white expectoration (alternate with *Ferrum Phos.,* for the febrile symptoms); note color of tongue.

Kali Sulph.—If free perspiration is not established by the use of *Ferrum Phos.,* alternate with *Kali Sulph.* Pneumonia, with wheezing and *expectoration of loose, rattling, yellow phlegm* or watery, yellow mucus; sometimes mucus slips back and is swallowed.

Natr. Mur.—Inflammation of the lungs, with *loose, rattling phlegm, clear and frothy;* tongue has frothy bubbles of saliva on the edges. Short, dry, hacking cough, when *Ferrum Phos.*

fails to relieve. Tickling cough with characteristic tongue. Distressing cough, with flow of tears and heavy, beating headache.

Calc. Sulph.—Inflammation of the lungs with expectoration of pus and matter.

CLINICAL CASES

Acute Lobar Pneumonia.

Mrs. H., age 71, married and the mother of several grown children, had been ailing for several years with a chronic bronchitis. However, she enjoyed apparently moderately good health, until the night of January 19, 1924, when she was seized about midnight with an intense chill which lasted almost an hour. As the chill terminated there was rapid rise of temperature to 104 F., accompanied by a deep stabbing pain located under the right nipple, and aggravated by coughing on deep inspiration. Pulse, rapid and compressible; respiration, 40 to 50; flushed face, headache, nausea and vomiting; dull pains in the back and limbs with great prostration; circumscribed red spot on the right cheek; slight dullness on percussion over the lower lobe of the right lung, with an increased vocal resonance; diminished respiratory movements on the right side; crepitant rales, muttering delirium.

Diagnosis: Acute lobar pneumonia.

Treatment: Patient placed in a large, well ventilated room with a temperature of 70 to 75. *Ferrum Phos.* and *Kali Sulph.* were given every half hour. The former for the fever, pain, and local congestion. The latter for the dry, hot skin, until a mild moisture on the surface was established. However, it only required a few doses of the *Kali Sulph.* in hot water to produce this effect, when *Kali Phos.* for the prostration was substituted, and given alternately with the *Ferrum Phos.* every one to two hours. The chest was incased in a flannel jacket which served to protect the surface from sudden changes of temperature; and applications of camphorated oil were frequently made over the diseased lung. The diet was given in a liquid form, and consisted largely of milk, coffee, meat broths, custards, and soups.

The above treatment was given for the first three or four days when the character of the expectoration changed to a white albuminous matter. *Kali Mur.* was given alternately every two hours to control the fibrinous exudation. This treatment continued till the seventh day of the disease, when the stage of gray hepatization was reached, and the sputa changed to a thick yellow. Very tenacious; prostration very marked. *Kali Phos.* alternated every three hours with a triturate of nitrate strychnine, 1/40 grain. *Kali Sulph.* took the place of *Kali Mur.* and continued alternately with the *Kali Phos.* and strychnine until the crisis, which occurred on the tenth day. *Calc. Phos.* was given over a period of two weeks for its tonic effect on the general system, at the expiration of which time the diseased lung had entirely cleared up, and her recovery was complete.

The case got along remarkably well considering her previous physical condition and her extreme age. As there were no complications or sequelae I attribute her speedy recovery to the use of the "Biochemic Remedies."
(Dr. Dennis D. Casto.)

Ferrum Phos. cured:

Case of pneumonia of left upper lobe, with well-marked crepitation and profuse expectoration of frothy, pink mucus, yellow watery diarrhea, green vomiting. *Ferrum Phos.* every two hours produced immediate improvement, although we considered her moribund (she had tuberculosis); the diarrhea and vomiting were unaffected.
(W. C. Goodno, M. D.)

Lobar Pneumonia:

Mrs. S., lobar pneumonia. Upper lobe left lung. Temperature 104, pulse 120, respiration 40. Treatment. *Ferrum Phos.* and *Kali Mur.* in alternation. The crisis occurred on

the fifth day. Temperature 99 2/5. Sixth day, chill. Temperature 103, lower lobe of right lung involved. Treatment persisted in fifteenth day, crisis again. I left patient on *Kali Sulph.* in alternation with *Kali Phos.* Cured. This case I considered desperate from the beginning to the end, and did not think she would get well, but I persisted in the remedies and she recovered, to the surprise of all concerned. Sputum bloody at first when each lobe was attacked.
(Dr. G. A. Budd, Frankfort, Kentucky.)

Ferrum Phos. and Kali Sulph. in lobular Pneumonia:

Dr. A. L. Fisher quickly relieved a child of lobular pneumonia, with high temperature, with *Ferrum Phos., Kali Sulph.,* given on account of thick, yellowish expectoration, speedily cured the case.

Ferrum Phos. and Kali Mur. in Pneumonia from exposure:

Archibald Herbert, suffering from chronic bronchitis, had an attack of pneumonia. An iron moulder by trade, he was exposed to great heat; he had lain down on a form in a state of perspiration, took a severe chill, and inflammation in the right lung was the result. His case was a bad one, complicated by bronchial affection; fever high; cough distressing; a pain, deep-seated, in the right side; expectoration tenacious, rusty-colored. *Ferrum Phos.,* in alternation with *Kali Mur.,* a dose every half hour, was taken for twenty-four hours, then every hour. For his prostration and sleeplessness, a few doses of *Kali Phos.* were taken now and then. The improvement every way was very marked in two days. As the color of the sputa changed to yellow, he took *Kali Sulph.* instead of *Kali Mur.;* and as this condition was remedied, *Natr. Mur.* and *Calc. Phos.* completed the cure in a little more than ten days. He returned to work free from inflammation and bronchitis.
(From Schuessler.)

Ferrum Phos. and Kali Mur.; marked improvement in twenty-four hours:

A case presented itself with the following conditions: Extensive extravasation, with solidification, great pain, hard and

exhaustive cough, with characteristic expectoration, little or no sleep. After being treated for about ten days with the ordinary remedies, without improvement, and as the case was assuming graver proportions than any I have had for years, I placed him upon *Ferrum Phos.* and *Kali Mur.*, in alternation. In twenty-four hours a marked and amazing improvement resulted, which continued to the termination of the disease, with rapid convalescence. The case was a grave one, for the reason that he had been laid up three months with a fractured arm, and was in a very reduced condition when the pneumonia appeared.
(S. Powell Burdick, M. D.)

Broncho-Pneumonia of infant rapidly relieved:

M. R. Broncho-pneumonia. Age 3 years, temperature 103, respiration 30, pulse 120. Both lungs full of crepitant rales with much mucus. *Ferrum Phos.* alternated with *Kali Mur.* cured the case in four days.
(Dr. G. A. Budd, Frankfort, Kentucky.)

Ferrum Phos. brought relief in a few hours:

The worst case of pneumonia that I ever saw recover—the pain and rapid respiration producing a veritable agony—was relieved beautifully in a few hours with *Ferrum Phos.*, after the best selected remedies had failed for days to make any change for the better. In this case we had complete hepatization of the left lung and of the lower lobe of the right lung, with a strong tendency to hepatization of both lungs, a rapid pulse, small and weak, with a temperature of 103 to 104 degrees. The fever left and the pulse steadied and became better in a few days. Suppuration ensued, however, for the remedy was not administered early enough, or, I have no doubt, it would have arrested it before suppuration ensued. The duration of this case was eleven weeks. He was about 28 years old, and of rather robust constitution. The amount of muco-purulent sputa expectorated was simply enormous. He has made a good recovery, and seems to be in excellent health.

Ferrum Phos. and Kali Mur. in Bronchial Pneumonia:

Was called in night to see baby P., 3 years old. Had been sick several days, under treatment by another M. D. Found him cyanotic, blue lips and finger nails. Breathing almost nil with some external applications. I placed him on *Kali Mur. and Ferrum Phos.* Next morning I found him greatly improved. Continued same treatment until well.
(Dr. W. J. Grimes, East Liverpool, Ohio.)

PREGNANCY

(See Labor and Pregnancy.)

PROSOPALGIA

(See Neuralgia.)

PRURITUS

Calc. Fluor.—Pruritus ani—from piles; to be used externally as a lotion, and in enema.

PUERPERAL FEVER

(See Labor and Pregnancy.)

BIOCHEMIC TREATMENT

Ferrum Phos.—First stage for the fever, chills, headache, quick full pulse, tenderness over the region of womb, and other febrile disturbances.

Kali Mur.—Chief remedy in this disease. Suppression of the milk and lochia, white-coated tongue, distention of the abdomen.

Kali Phos.—When the disease has progressed so far that the mind is affected; delirium, anxiety, nervousness, listlessness, foul odor from the vaginal discharges. Tongue coated brown or like stale liquid mustard, foul breath; putrid symptoms.

Natr. Mur.—In the lower stages—low, stupid conditions; low muttering; tongue parched and black, intercurrent with the main remedies.

Calc. Phos.—Intercurrently through the course of the disease or steadily when convalescence begins. There should also be given frequent vaginal injections of hot water containing *Kali Phos.*

CLINICAL CASES

Ferrum Phos. in a case of Puerperal Fever:

A case of puerperal fever. Chill, followed by fever. Suppression of the lochia, milk and urine. Hilarious delirium; profuse critical diaphoresis without thirst or much coated tongue; bowels confined, and extensive tympanites over abdominal parieties. *Ferrum Phos.*, a dose every hour. In ten hours all uremiform symptoms had subsided; patient cheerful and comfortable. Lochia and milk secretions returned, and urine voided freely. A good recovery followed.
(F. A. Rockwith, M. D.)

PULSE

(See Heart, Affections of.)

RACHITIS [Rickets]

ETIOLOGY

This disease is an inflammation of the spine, caused by an abnormal cell-growth of the bone tissue. There is a great deficiency of the phosphate of lime: and the albuminous substances not containing enough lime to create proper bone tissue, a spongy structure is the result; hence, abnormal conditions prevail, producing symptoms called rickets, or disease of the spine and other bony substances. Calc. Phos., Kali Phos. and Magnes. Phos. are all frequently needed in this disease.

BIOCHEMIC TREATMENT

Calc. Phos.—This is pre-eminently the *leading remedy in* the treatment of a majority of *children's complaints due to poor assimilation,* causing conditions unfavorable to the deposit of the phosphate of lime. Delicate, emaciated children, with sallow, earthy complexion, open fontanels, *retarded dentition,* etc. Curvature of the spine; bones of skull soft and thin; inability to hold the head up, due to a deficiency of lime phosphate. *Calc. Phos.* should not be confused with lime-water, so frequently used. Lime-water is beneficial only from its tonic action, while *Calc. Phos.* (a combination of phosphoric acid and lime) is in the identical form as that used by nature in the formation of the organism.

Diarrheas of rachitic children are met by this remedy "There are a number of well-authenticated cases on record wherein the fetus was treated through the maternal ingestion of *Calc. Phos.,* and was born healthy, whereas all previous children by the same mother had been born rachitic." (Dr. Chapman.)

Natr. Phos.—*Natr. Phos.* is a very useful remedy in *rachitic children, when caused from non-assimilation of food;* usually accompanied with acid symptoms.

Silicea.—In those cases when there is *profuse sweat about the head* and offensive diarrhea, intercurrently with *Calc. Phos.,* the chief remedy.

Kali Phos.—Wasting of the body, when putrid-smelling stools occur (intercurrently).

CLINICAL CASES

Calc. Phos. and Kali Phos. in Rickets:

Lizzie Macquillen was brought to the dispensary on October 15th; 4 years of age; to all appearances an imbecile; her head large, broad and flat, but the rest of the body undeveloped, like that of an infant, denoting her case to be that of a class of rickets; also curvature of the long bones, etc.; the face pale and triangular; no teeth; the neck too weak to keep the head steady; constant movement of the eyes, showing no intelligence. The mother stated the little girl seemed to be well enough until four or five months old, when she took fits till the end of the twelfth month. Since then she had scarcely grown any bigger; never had the power of holding anything in her tiny hands; and if food was held to her, did not know it was for eating; had to be fed; never attempted to use her legs; could only sit when resting her elbows on the flat cross-bar of her chair, fixing her mouth on the knuckles of her hands. In bed she could not turn herself over. She had frequently been under medical treatment, but without benefit. The mother persisted in the statement that she had lost her first and second set of teeth. The case seemed a very hopeless one. Having great doubts of doing much good, prescribed *Calc. Phos.* in alternation with *Kali Phos.*, a dose every hour, and told the mother to come back in six weeks, as I could give her an additional remedy then. She called back at the appointed time, quite proud of her little thing. The change was marvelous, scarcely any rocking of the head, and as I turned over the leaves of the entry-book, the little creature looked up wistfully, bent over and stretched out her hand to take hold of them. The mother expressed her gratitude for the change in her child, saying the last week or two many neighbors had called to see little Lizzie and her father was now happy to dandle her on his knees. The remedies, *Calc. Phos.* daily, alternate doses of *Kali Phos.* and *Kali Mur.*, day about, were continued another six weeks. The improvement has continued steadily, she nibbles crusts out of her own hands; the

intelligence developing apace, she begins to say some words, can now stand holding by her chair, which she pushes before her and moves through the room. To crown all, she has cut two front teeth.
(J. B. C.)

Calc. Phos. during Gestation, to prevent Rickets:

Dr. Knuppel, of Magdeburg, reports cases in which children had formerly been born rachitic, but through the maternal ingestion of *Calc. Phos.* during last months of pregnancy, all subsequent children were born perfectly healthy.

Calc. Fluor. relieved the distress:

Child, æt. 2 years, with right thigh swollen to three times its natural size from hip-joint to knee, stony hard, having existed for six weeks; yielded promptly to *Calc. Fluor.* In this case even touching the limb was followed by the greatest distress, even prolonged crying.
(J. W. Ward, M. D.)

RETINITIS

(See Eye, Diseases of.)

RHEUMATISM

ETIOLOGY

It is now quite generally conceded that rheumatism, especially articular rheumatism, arises from an acid condition of the blood. A lack of a proper amount of the alkaline salt sodium phosphate in the blood, by producing a deficiency of alkali in the synovial fluids, allows the acids to predominate and cause deposits of urates in the tissues adjacent to the articulations. This lack of sodium phosphate may be due to an unusual demand being made upon it by the system as a substitute for a deficiency in calcium phosphate. A lack of potassium chloride, which controls fibrin, causes a collection of fibrinous matter, which will give rise to swellings and pain—hence inflammatory rheumatism. A deficiency in the salts that furnish muscular and nervous fluids will cause nerve and muscular pains and stiffness of the limbs also called rheumatism.

BIOCHEMIC TREATMENT

Ferrum Phos.—This is the *principal remedy in the initiatory stage* of rheumatism and rheumatic fever, for the febrile symptoms. If given frequently at the onset, it is often the only required remedy. Arthritis, acute articular rheumatism, which is very painful and when movement increases the pain. Acute inflammatory rheumatism of any part. Soreness and stiffness all over the body. Lumbago; stiff neck from cold. All rheumatic pains aggravated by motion.

Kali Mur.—Second stage of rheumatic fever, after *Ferrum Phos., when exudation has taken place and swelling results.* Rheumatic, gouty pains, if worse from movement and accompanied with a white-furred coating on the tongue. Arthritis, for the swelling of the joints (alternate with *Ferrum Phos.*). Tenalgia crepitans. *Chronic rheumatism,* with swelling, white-furred tongue, and when movement causes pain.

Natr. Phos.—*Acute and chronic rheumatism of the joints,* with profuse, sour-smelling perspiration. Arthritis, when acid conditions are present; creamy, yellow coating on the tongue and tonsils. Acute and chronic gout; chronic rheumatism. "Drs. Schuessler, Walker and others have lately begun to realize the importance of *Natr. Phos.* in the treatment of rheumatism, especially articular rheumatism. It has long been suspected that one of the principal causes of the excessive pains in the joints was due to an acid diathesis; this, then, will account for the salutary action of *Natr. Phos.* in this disease. I am, therefore, led to believe that it would be expedient to exhibit it as an intercurrent remedy in all cases of a rheumatic nature." (Dr. Chapman.)

Magnes. Phos.—Acute, sharp, *spasmodic pains in articular rheumatism.* Excruciating violent pains in rheumatic fever; intercurrentlv with the chief remedy.

Kali Sulph.—Rheumatic *pains* which are of a *wandering, shifting* nature; worse in heated room or in the evening; feels better in cool, open air. Chronic or acute rheumatism of the joints, when shifting from one place to another. Arthritis. Rheumatic headaches, with evening aggravation, or worse in a warm atmosphere. Pains in the back, neck or limbs, with the above symptoms.

Kali Phos.—Acute or chronic *rheumatism, with stiffness of the parts;* pains worse on beginning to move, but relieved by gentle motion. Rheumatic pains which are worse in the morning or when rising from a sitting position; gentle motion relieves, but continued exertion or fatigue tends to increase the pains.

Calc. Phos.—Rheumatism which is worse at night and in bad weather, alternate with *Ferrum Phos.* Rheumatic pains aggravated by heat or cold, worse with change of weather. Rheumatism of the joints, with cold, numb sensations. Stiffness of neck from cold and dampness, alternate with *Ferrum Phos.* Severe pain in the nape of neck, worse at night. Lumbago (also *Ferrum Phos.*). *Rheumatic gout,* worse at night and in bad weather. Dropsical swelling of the knee or hip-joints.

Natr. Sulph.—Gout; in the acute stage this remedy should be alternated with *Ferrum Phos.* It is the *chief remedy in chronic gout;* patient should abstain from wines and liquors and rich foods. Rheumatic pains associated with bilious conditions, and which are worse in wet weather.

Natr. Mur.—Chronic rheumatism of the joints, with cracking of the joints and corresponding watery symptoms. Rheumatic fevers, after *Kali Mur.*, and with characteristic symptoms.

Calc. Fluor.—*Enlargement of joints from gout;* in alternation with *Natr. Sulph.*

Calc. Sulph.—Articular suppurations (also *Silicea*); the discharge must govern the selection of the remedy.

CLINICAL CASES

Kali Sulph. in Rheumatic Fever:

Dr. Schlegelman reports the following case: L., of Regensburg, a strong, healthy man, æt. 26, had taken a cold during a state of perspiration and contracted acute rheumatism of the joints. (Rheumatic fever.) At first, the right shoulder was attacked; the patient had violent pains and high fever. Remedies which seemed decidedly indicated here, had no other effect, except that the pain on the next morning had changed its seat and had appeared in the left knee. I gave *Kali Sulph.* The result was very favorable. The wandering pains ceased changing their location, and the pain confined itself to the right shoulder again, but was far less violent than before. Under the continued use of this medicine, the fever and pains gradually disappeared; sleep and appetite returned, and no other joints were implicated. Eight days after giving the first dose of *Kali Sulph.*, the patient was dismissed as convalescent. No relapse occurred.
(From Schuessler.)

Kali Mur. in Rheumatism of Joints:

Dr. Brisken was called to a case on the eighth day after seizure. All the joints were swollen, and the patient had not been able to stay in bed a single night. In the morning he received *Kali Mur.*, with such good results that during the next night he was able to stay in bed, and in twelve days was completely cured.
(From Schuessler.)

Ferr. Phos. and Kali Mur. in acute Rheumatism:

A gentleman, æt. 70, had acute rheumatism in the shoulder and elbow-joints. He had been cupped, which made it worse.

His joints were wrapped in pine-wool, with no effect. He had not been in bed the last two nights, as on lying down the pains were worse. On the third day he came under Dr. Brisken's treatment. After giving him *Ferrum Phos.,* the fever ceased in a few days, after which *Kali Mur.* was given. In a short time complete recovery resulted.
(From Schuessler.)

Ferrum Phos. in Rheumatic Fever:

Dr. Brisken mentions three cases of rheumatic fever. One case was that of a bookbinder, middle-aged, whom Dr. Brisken had treated three years previously for this malady. On that occasion his recovery took from eight to ten weeks. The patient was again attacked in the joints of the hands and knees, when he received *Ferrum Phos.* every hour; and as the fever had abated, *Kali Mur.* was given the same way. On the fifth day he was able to return to his work.
(From Schuessler.)

Ferrum Phos. and Kali Mur. in Rheumatism of Joints:

Edward B., æt. 12, had been complaining a few days, when pains began in all the principal joints, but mostly in wrists and elbows, attended with redness and swelling, with some fever; there was most pain on moving, and he had to sit quiet to be in any comfort. Gave him *Ferrum Phos.,* dissolved in one glass and *Kali Mur.,* dissolved in another, to be taken alternately every two hours while fever lasted, then continue *Kali Mur.* alone. These remedies soon relieved him, and he was out in a few days. A second attack the next year was cured by the same remedies in a short time.
(C. T. M.)

Kali Sulph. in Rheumatism from getting wet:

Robert D., æt. 34. This patient lives on the bank of the lake, and goes frequently into the water, and often gets wet fishing and shooting. Has had pains about him for a year or two, at times. They are sometimes in one joint, and then in another, seem to shift about, and are becoming very trouble-

some, hindering him from work, and he desires a remedy, if possible. I gave him *Kali Sulph.*, several powders, one to be dissolved in water, a dose four times each day. This remedy, after a few weeks, completely cured his trouble, and he has not complained now for a year or more.
(C. T. M.)

Magnes Phos. in lightning-like pains:

J. D., a man æt. 69, had been complaining for several weeks of pains in the limbs, which settled in the right leg, from the hip down to the ankle, but were worse at joints, being of a shifting nature—intermittent—sometimes shooting and darting, like lightning, causing the patient to change his position frequently. Warmth gives him relief. He is unable to leave his bed; is almost in despair, thinking he is dying. *Magnes. Phos.*, a dose every three hours. The improvement on taking this remedy was marked and rapid, but whenever he stopped with the medicine he felt worse again. By continuing steadily with *Magnes. Phos.*, a complete cure was effected.
(From Schuessler.)

Ferrum Phos. and Kali Mur. in Rheumatic Fever:

I was called to attend a girl, æt. 12; she had had, some time ago, an attack of rheumatic fever. I found the little patient, who had been taken ill the previous day, in bed. The joints of both knees were swollen, somewhat red and very painful. The joints of the vertebræ at the nape of the neck were implicated, and every movement out of the constrained position of the neck and back was very painful. Her friends expected that salicylic acid would be applied, which they had already seen used, but I gave her *Ferrum Phos.* and *Kali Mur.*, alternately, every three hours. Next day, to the astonishment of the friends, the fever and pains were less, and knees were quite free from pain. Now I ordered *Kali Mur.* to be given alone for the swelling, and the next morning on my return I found all the symptoms worse. I repeated the *Ferrum Phos.* again, and there was a rapid improvement. But in the same degree as the pains were leaving and the swelling decreasing, spasmodic pains in the abdomen set in. There was also an occasional vomiting of bilious matter. As soon as these latter symptoms come on, I ordered the little patient some *Magnes. Phos.,* dissolved in water, in frequent sips, which removed all these symptoms in twenty-four hours. *Ferrum Phos.* and *Kali Mur.* were continued, in less frequent doses. Six days after my first visit the patient was able to leave her bed, and was quite well.

(Dr. Schlegel.)

Calc. Phos. and Natr. Sulph. in Rheumatic Gout:

Miss A. W., æt. 10½, was taken with a chill on January 1st. The next day I found her with a very high fever, pulse 120; severe pains in back and limbs; nausea and vomiting; joints, small and large, greatly inflamed; hands, feet and limbs edematous. Could not bear to be touched or moved. Great sensitiveness in every part of the body and limbs. Pains became very much worse at night, increasing to such an extent that her screams could be heard by the neighbors on each side of the house. Constant crying for cold water; vomiting of food and drink almost as soon as swallowed. Tongue coated yellow, with horrible bitter metallic taste. Great prostration. Hereditary, gouty-rheumatic and dropsical diathesis. Has had for some time back a ravenous appetite, especially for sweet things, which was freely indulged. TREATMENT: After wasting much time of the first week with various remedies, with no improvement, I determined to adhere to the system of Schuessler. For the fever, vomiting of food and drink, and the inflammation, I gave *Ferrum Phos.,* pains aggravated at night, *Calc. Phos.,* for rheumatic gout, edema, dropsy, yellow-coated tongue with bitter taste, *Natr. Sulph.,* about ten grains in half a goblet of water, a teaspoonful every other hour, in alternation with the first two, which were given dry and at the same time. From the commencement of this treatment, decided improvement began, and by the fourteenth day of her sickness she was able to sit up. Previous to her sickness she

had become so stout that she could not stoop to button her shoes, and her cloak could scarcely be buttoned around her. It was so uncomfortable buttoned, she would go with it opened almost all the time. After her recovery, she was able to stoop, and her cloak lapped several inches.
(E. H. Holbrook, M. D.)

Ferrum Phos. in Rheumatism during Catamenia:

From the reports of a Medical Congress at Dortmund, by Dr. Stens, Jr. I should like to report on a case of rheumatism which was cured by *Ferrum Phos.* in a very short time, after having tried several of the most reputed remedies which seemed indicated. A lady of about 42 years of age (catamenia normal, though scanty), had been treated by me for the last few years. She suffered from digestive derangement, and sometimes from violent attacks of megrim. This lady awoke one morning with an acute pain in the right upper arm and region of right shoulder, being of a tearing nature; she had walked the previous evening through a damp meadow, getting her feet wet. The pains were worse if she moved her arm quickly; not as bad on moving it very gently; she was, therefore, careful to use gentle motion. The parts affected were painful on being touched. Several nights perspiration had been excessive, and afterwards made its appearance every morning between 2 and 6 o'clock, when the pains were always worse. The patient complained of a pain in the right hand—powerlessness—which prevented her from lifting anything heavy. She often felt rather exhausted, and had to lay down. I gave her no less than five remedies, which seemed to suggest themselves, but without success. From the lady's anemic condition and partly Dr. Schuessler's recommendation, made me think of iron. I prescribed his own preparation of *Ferrum Phos.*, to be taken night and morning. The result was that after taking the medicine for six days, the pains, with their accompanying symptoms, did not return, even though soon after this wet weather set in, when she had generally felt her pains to be worse.

Ferrum Phos. in Rheumatism:

Miss H. came to me with a sore throat and expressed the hope that it would not terminate in an attack of inflammatory rheumatism as it had on a former occasion, but it did. The patient's joints became inflamed and swollen and so painful that it was necessary to turn her with a sheet. For a time the fever ran high, but this was finally controlled by *Ferrum Phos.* and the swelling reduced by *Kali Mur.* Nervousness was overcome by *Kali Phos.* and the attendant stomach derangements by *Natr. Phos.* At one time the patient complained of severe pain in the leg, but seemed unable to describe the character of the pain. Various remedies were given for nearly a week without relief. One morning she said it seemed to want to draw her leg up. I then gave her *Magnes. Phos.* with the result that the pain disappeared in a few hours and the patient made a satisfactory recovery.
(Dr. J. B. Chapman, Seattle, Wash.)

Ferrum Phos. in inflammatory Rheumatism:

Reuter, a shoemaker, æt. 40, was taken ill, after catching cold, as he stated. There was fever and violent pains in the right shoulder. The first visit I paid was on the third day after he had been taken ill, November 21st. Temperature high, pulse full and quick, thirst and loss of appetite. The right shoulder was very red, and sensitive to the touch. He was not able to lie in bed, as the pressure of the pillows was unbearable. He was lying on the sofa, supported with cushions, so that the shoulder should be free from pressure. I gave my patient *Ferrum Phos.*, 15 grains, dissolved in a half glassful of water, and a teaspoonful of the solution given every hour. Improvement was felt, even after a few hours. During the night the patient was able to sleep, and on the following day the fever abated. On the 25th of November the patient was able to move the arm pretty freely. November the 28th, he tried to work, but feeling the weight of his hammer too much, he rested a few days longer, when he felt himself quite well.
(Dr. L. Sulzer.)

RHINITIS

(See Colds.)

SCALDS

(See Burns and Scalds.)

SCARLET FEVER

ETIOLOGY

Scarlet fever, or scarlatina, as it is frequently termed by the laity, is an acute infectious disease, to which children are particularly prone, though it occasionally occurs in adults who have not had the disease in childhood. Scarlet fever, as a rule, never attacks the same person twice.

The basic cause of this trouble is a deficiency in the cell-salt Kali Mur., which results in an excess of fibrin. This fibrin, trying to find an outlet from the system through the mucous membrane of the mouth and throat, produces a condition which provides a breeding place for the micro-organism that is responsible for scarlet fever. This micro-organism has not as yet been satisfactorily identified, but is practically always associated with a variety of the streptococcus, which produces many of the pathological conditions found in the disease.

The onset of scarlet fever may be either slow or sudden, the rapidity of onset frequently measuring the severity of the attack. The first symptom may be an attack of severe vomiting after eating. The temperature will run from 101-103 degrees, the eyes are bright and shining, the skin is hot and dry, while the child feels tired and listless. The mouth and throat are dry and red. Sometimes there is a complaint of sore throat. In from twelve to twenty-four hours after these symptoms appear, the typical scarlet fever rash begins to manifest itself, beginning, as a rule, on the neck and upper part of the chest. In other cases the onset is more deliberate, consisting of indisposition, slight chill followed by moderate fever, and accompanied by vomiting.

The scarlet fever rash is punctated, that is, it appears darker about the hair follicles in the skin, while the rest of the skin surface is literally "as red as a lobster." It appears rapidly, the whole body and extremities being frequently involved in four or five hours.

The eruption usually lasts from three to seven days, and then gradually subsides. Desquamation, in which the skin comes away in large flakes, begins about the twelfth day, but sometimes not until the twentieth day. A week to three weeks are required for desquamation, but this period may be shortened by anointing the child frequently during the illness with some oily substance.

The extent and severity of the rash may vary greatly in different cases. It may be so mild as to make diagnosis difficult, or so severe that the patient is speedily overcome by toxemia. Occasionally only parts of the body will be covered by the rash, and it may only last for a day or two.

The temperature in scarlet fever varies with the severity of the attack. It may go as high as 105 degrees within twelve hours, but generally falls to about 103 degres in a day or two, and disappears as the rash fades away.

Outside of the possibility of profound infection from the disease itself, the chief danger in scarlet fever is the renal irritation or inflammation which so frequently accompanies it. Slight albuminuria is an almost constant symptom, and this is always liable to develop into acute nephritis, especially if the child is exposed to cold air during the period of desquamation, when the skin is particularly sensitive, and congestion of the kidneys is easily brought about.

Extension of the septic inflammation from the throat through the Eustachian tube of the middle ear is another frequent complication in scarlet fever. Permanent deafness frequently is the result.

BIOCHEMIC TREATMENT

In treating scarlet fever biochemically the urgent need is to destroy the breeding place of the micro-organism which is causing the trouble. Kali Mur. will accomplish this, as it unites with the excess of fibrin which is irritating the mucous membrane of the respiratory passage, thus enabling the mucous membrane to return to a normal condition, and depriving the micro-organism of its breeding place. Ferrum Phos. is also needed for the fever, and other cell-salts, as the symptoms calling for them appear.

Ferrum Phos.—For the fever, quick pulse, etc., *in the initiatory stage;* in alternation with *Kali Mur.*

Kali Mur.—This remedy alone may suffice in simple cases. Alternate with *Ferrum Phos.*, for the inflammatory conditions. Give as a preventive during epidemics.

Kali Sulph.—Peeling of the skin; it assists desquamation and development of the rash. *Sudden suppression of the rash.* High temperature.

Kali Phos.—*Putrid conditions of the throat in scarlet fever,* symptoms of exhaustion, stupor, etc.

Natr. Mur.—Scarlet fever, when *vomiting of watery fluids, drowsiness and twitching* occur; note also tongue symptoms. NOTE: For the "after-effects of scarlet fever, such as induration of glands, abscesses, boils, etc., see under the separate heads. But if the remedies are given faithfully from the commencement, there will be no "after-effects."

Natr. Sulph.—Frequently an important remedy to control the excessive engorgement of blood to the head. Also when bilious symptoms are present.

CLINICAL CASES

Kali Mur. in Scarlet Fever and as a Prophylactic:

Two boys admitted to the Institution from Portsmouth, O., with clear certificates of health, were placed in separate cottages. Both came down with scarlet fever in eight days and nine days, slept in a crowded dormitory with 18 other boys each, went to the main dining room for breakfast, reporting to my clinic at 7 o'clock a. m., covered with rash, and having bad throats. Gave all boys along the line *Kali Mur.* and had no more cases.

Three boys were circumcised and put in one of my rooms together, two of them in one bed. During the night one vomited freely and had a fully developed case of scarlet fever. The other two boys were given *Kali Mur.* and neither took scarlet fever. Dr. Wm. Galloway of Xenia heard my lecture on scarlet fever, and some time later had a woman confined and the same day one of her children in a family of six came down with scarlet fever. He came out to me and I told him to use *Kali Mur.* three times a day for two weeks, and gave him the remedy. No other members of the family took the disease.

Dr. Anderson of Alpha, Ohio (near Xenia) had a similar experience in a family of five, scarlet fever appeared in one of the children three days before confinement of the mother. Dr. Galloway was called in consultation and brought Dr. Anderson out to see me. I gave him a supply of *Kali Mur.* and no more cases were had in the family.

Dr. Whittaker of New Burlington was called to the public schools of that village to see a sick teacher, found her with scarlet fever and all the school badly exposed. He came to Xenia and I gave him a pound bottle of *Kali Mur.* tablets and he used it freely, and did not have another case. I could give you a number of other experiences I have had here and without a failure. I would add that I had early in my experience here an epidemic of scarlet fever that lasted over two years and that in institutions it is very difficult to root out. (Dr. W. C. Hewitt, Resident Physician, Ohio Soldiers' and Sailors' Orphans' Home.)

Kali Mur. in Scarlatina; no results from other remedies:

A. S., the child of a post official visiting here, was taken ill with an attack of very slight scarlatina. The rash had disappeared after scarcely twenty-four hours. The throat symptoms, at first threatening to be severe, disappeared in three or four days. On the seventh day almost complete retention of urine set in, as in twenty-four hours only a very small quantity was passed, although the child drank a good deal. The urine contained some albumen; the feet were swollen; the abdomen very much distended. As the child was all this time in high fever and at night delirious, I advised the parents, on my visit on the morning of the eighth day, to consult a second physician. Dr. Gerster, who was called in to consult with me, agreed completely to my diagnosis. When I told him that I had not had any results from any of the medicines prescribed, we agreed to give *Kali Mur.*, every two hours a small powder. In the evening the little one was already better. She had passed a tolerable quantity of urine free from albumen; the pulse steadier; the skin moist. The following night the little girl slept quietly for several hours. In the morning, almost free from fever, and could be considered convalescent. We continued the use of *Kali Mur.*, and in a few days after she was able to return home perfectly well.
(From Schuessler.)

Kali Mur. in Scarlatina—curative and preventive:

Dr. Holbrook reports a case of scarlatina treated with *Kali Mur.* alone, making a good recovery; and, given to the rest of the children in the home, prevented their having it, though with the sick one nearly constantly.

Natr. Sulph. in Scarlatina:

Several cases of scarlatina this winter did not do well under the usual remedies, but were speedily relieved and cured by

Natr. Sulph. The rash, instead of being smooth, was rough and pimply, and in some cases rising of mucus in the throat. (E. H. H.)

SCIATICA

(See Rheumatism.)

BIOCHEMIC TREATMENT

Kali Phos.—The *chief remedy* in this disease. "Affection of the sciatic nerve, which extends down the back of the thigh to the knee; dragging pain, torpor, stiffness, great restlessness and pain; nervous exhaustion; lack of motor stimulus; moving gently for a little time gives relief." (Dr. Walker.)

Magnes. Phos.—For *spasmodic excruciating pains,* give in hot water, frequent doses, intercurrently with the chief remedy.

Natr. Sulph.—When symptoms of gout exist, this remedy should be alternated with *Kali Phos.*

Ferrum Phos.—Should there be febrile symptoms present, which is frequently the case, *Ferrum Phos.* should be alternated with the indicated remedy.

Calc. Phos.—A useful intercurrent remedy in this disease also when *Magnes. Phos.* fails to bring relief.

CLINICAL CASES

Kali Phos., Ferrum Phos. and Kali Mür. in Sciatica:

Man, aged 36. When I was called he was in bed. He had a severe pain in left limb from hip to ankle. I put him on *Kali Phos.* every three hours, *Ferrum Phos.* and *Kali Mür.*, of each three doses a day, and *Magnes. Phos.* to be taken when the pain was severe. In three days he was out of bed and on the tenth day he was at work and has had no symptoms of it since.

(Dr. H. Whisler, Tingley, Iowa.)

Kali Phos. in Sciatica:

Mr. B. has been suffering for seven months with sciatica in left leg; the pain was very severe and fast undermining his health; he had been treated by a very skillful physician all this time, and almost every known remedy was tried, until the physician himself gave up the case and said that he could do nothing more. I was called, found patient suffering with a dull, tensive pain, extending the whole length of the sciatic nerve of the left leg; worse on slightest motion. Prepared a small quantity of *Kali Phos.,* in half glass of water, and gave a teaspoonful every ten minutes for an hour, when the pain was much better; patient then slept until morning. Next night the pain returned; gave same remedy, but with no result. The next night gave *Kali Phos.,* and very soon the pain was relieved; continued *Kali Phos.,* every two hours a small dose for a week, and then four times a day for a month; once during that time had a slight attack, which was soon stopped by putting a small quantity in half a glass of water, and giving a teaspoonful every ten minutes for a while. A year has passed and there has been no return of the trouble.

(G. H. Martin, M. D.)

Ferrum Phos. and Natr. Sulph. in Sciatica:

A lady who had to be brought home from camp-meeting, I found suffering from an intense pain down the sciatic nerve. There was some fever and extreme soreness to the touch or movement. She would cry out with pain from the slightest movement. Tongue was coated greenish-yellow. Gave *Ferrum Phos.* and *Natr. Sulph.* in water, alternately. The next day she could move without much pain, and was able to shift herself from one side of the bed to the other. The third day she was able to sit up and was soon convalescent.

(E. H. H.)

Magnes. Phos. cured his Sciatica:

A man who had been washing sheep had sciatica, and could not lie down. All the sleep he got was in a chair, and hot

applications to the right sciatic nerve alone relieved. *Magnes. Phos.* cured him without much trouble.
(H. P. Holmes.)

Magnes. Phos. in Sciatica:

I was called to see a woman about 50 years old, who had been suffering with sciatica for some time. In spite of drastic treatment, she did not improve. A few doses of *Magnes. Phos.* eased the pain, and within a week she was entirely free from it. She had been under treatment for three weeks previous to my visit.
(Dr. J. S. S. Chesshir.)

SECRETIONS

(See Exudations.)

SKIN, AFFECTIONS OF THE

(For Pathology see Exudation.)

BIOCHEMIC TREATMENT

Ferrum Phos.—In the *initiatory stage of skin disease,* for the inflammation, fever, pain, congestion, etc.

Kali Mur.—Second stage of inflammations of the skin, after *Ferrum Phos. Eruptions of the skin, with thick, white contents,* or when connected with stomach derangements, white-coated tongue, etc. Pimples and pustules, with the above conditions. *Eruptions* on the face, *with deranged uterine functions.* Bunions, *warts,* sycosis, shingles, etc. Erythema, for the swelling. *Lupus, the principal remedy.* Eczema, crusta lactea of little children, flour-like scales and characteristic tongue. Eczema arising from vaccination with impure lymph or from deranged uterine functions. Vesicular eczema, with thick, white secretions. Local applications of the remedy are also very useful.

Kali Sulph.—Eruptions and eczema, with *discharges of watery, yellow and effete matter.* Sudden suppression of eruptions or eczema from a chill or any other cause. Dryness of the skin during the course of any disease (alternate with *Ferrum Phos.,* to promote perspiration). Diseased condition of the nails, interrupted growth. Desquamation or peeling of the skin secretions are sticky. Dandruff, with yellowish or white scales, requires this remedy internally and also as a wash. In selecting a remedy for skin diseases, note also color of the tongue.

Natr. Mur.—*Eruptions* on the skin, *with clear, watery contents;* small vesicles or blisters, with the above secretions. *Eczema,* white scales, with watery secretions, *from eating too much salt.* Soreness of skin in children (chafing), with watery secretions; internal and external. Dandruff (if *Kali Sulph.* does not cure). Pemphigus, rupia, sycosis, etc., if the watery symptoms correspond. Bites and stings of insects; externally as soon as possible—it will stop the pain. Herpes zoster, herpetic eruptions, occurring through the course of any disease, with corresponding watery symptoms.

Natr. Phos.—Eczema and other skin diseases, *with creamy, honey-colored, golden-yellow* scabs or *discharges.* Skin diseases, with symptoms of acidity; creamy, yellow coating on the root of the tongue. Crusta lactea, with above conditions. Soreness and chafing of children, with acid conditions. Rose-rash, hives, itching all over the body, like insect bites, sore patches on the skin, etc., if accompanied with symptoms of acidity or creamy, yellow discharges.

Kali Phos.—Eczema and *eruptions* of the skin, if *accompanied with malignant* or putrid *conditions,* nervous irritation or oversensitiveness. Malignant pustules; greasy scabs, with offensive smell; secretions on the skin, causing soreness and itching; chafed skin; bloody watery secretions. Scurvy, with malignant conditions. *Itching of the skin, with crawling sensations.* Chilblains, for the tingling and itchy pain; alternate with *Kali Mur.* Exhausting perspirations, with heavy odor, or during meals, with weakness at pit of stomach.

Calc. Phos.—Eruptions (especially of the face) containing albuminous fluid; yellow-white scabs. *Eczema, generally associated with anemia.* Eruptions on the skin, with itching (intercurrently). Freckles are lessened by this remedy. Lupus in scrofulous subjects, intercurrently with *Kali Mur.* Troublesome *itching of the skin,* often *in aged persons* (*alternate with Kali Phos.*). Excessive or too frequent perspiration, especially about the head. Acne in young people during puberty or in anemic persons.

Calc. Sulph.—Skin affections, with *discharge of thick, yellow matter* or yellowish scabs, after *Kali Mur.* Suppuration of skin after inflammation. Pimples, if matter forms on the heads. Scald-head of children, with yellow, mattery crusts or scabs. Suppurating chilblains, after *Kali Mur.*

Calc. Fluor.—Chaps and cracks on the skin; fissures in palms of hands; use also externally with vaseline, after thoroughly cleansing the hands with soap and water. *Suppurations, with hard, callous edges;* horny skin, intensely sore; crack or fissure at the anus; also locally.

Silicea.—Little blind boils on the skin. Diseases of the skin, when there is pus, or blood and pus secretions. Perspiration of the feet, excessive or with offensive odor, or when suppressed by a chill. Perspiration of the head in children.

Natr. Sulph.—Eczema; eruptions of *vesicles contain yellowish, watery secretions.* Moist skin affections, with yellowish scabs or scales, associated with bilious conditions. Chafing of the skin; edematous inflammations, with bilious symptoms.

CLINICAL CASES

Natr. Mur. in Lichen:

Dr. S. writes: "Mrs. S., æt. 24, of Regensburg, who had been suffering for several years from lichen (skin affection), had used various well-known medicines, which had done her no good. I tried various remedies, and at last cured her. A few months ago she came again, and the lichen was worse than ever. My former remedy had no effect. I gave her *Calc. Sulph.,* night and morning, in five-grain doses, and in a fortnight the cure was complete."

Natr. Mur. in Pemphigus:

The following is a most striking case, showing what has been done with one remedy—*Natr. Mur.*—in pemphigus, pronounced incurable. The son of a gentleman came under my treatment at the age of 15 with this disease, which he had had since childhood; he was little and stunted in growth. He had never been able to wear ordinary clothes, but wore sandals and a loose garment with a girdle. He had a tutor, as he could never go to school. The whole body, face and feet were covered more or less with the vesicles and incrustations in their various stages. All the highest authorities on skin diseases had been consulted and their medicines tried without any lasting effect. The whole—the symptoms and pathological conditions—pointing so clearly to *Natr. Mur.,* he received this, the only remedy, to take internally and also for outward application. The effects were such that in less than three months he wore his first tailor-made suit, and has since then (now eight years) enjoyed good health, and is quite the strongest and tallest of the family.

Rapid cure of Eczema of long standing:

Mr. C., age 32. Subject to severe eruptive skin disease for ten years. Intolerable itching with yellow discharge. Had tried all kinds of salves and lotions with but little relief. I diagnosed eczema. The Biochemic Remedies which were used were *Ferrum Phos.* and *Natr. Phos.,* ten grains of each, one powder at 9 a. m. and 3 p. m., and *Silicea,* ten grains at noon and 6 p. m. Low protein and starch dietary was used. The treatment lasted from January 16 to February 16, after which the skin was almost cleared of all eruption. Itching but little felt except when over-heated.

(Dr. Ford Wilson, Vancouver, B. C., Canada.)

Kali Mur. in Eczema Capitis:

Eczema in a child; on cheeks, chin, and behind ears; skin swollen and inflamed, and underneath it indurations. Pustules developed early. Cured in one week by *Kali Mur.*, every four hours.

(D. B. Whittier, M. D.)

Calc. Sulph. cured Sycosis:

Dr. H. Goullon reports in the *Pop. Zeit.*, a case of sycosis cured by *Calc. Sulph.* The case presented the yellow purulent conditions calling for this remedy.

Calc. Phos. for Eruptions:

Julia C., æt. 3; eruption all over the face and on the hands, which are kept covered to prevent scratching; has been afflicted eight months and been under the best treatment without benefit. Gave her at first *Kali Mur.*, in solution. This remedy was continued for some time, but without much benefit, if any. Gave her then *Calc. Phos.*, in solution. This remedy produced a change for the better in a week and, it being continued, cured the case in two months. The heat of the following summer seemed to produce a relapse, when the same remedy again cured it, and she remains well.

(C. T. M.)

Kali Sulph. in recurring eruptions of Pimples:

Case of skin disease lasting for five years, consisting of a recurring eruption of fine red pimples, and, when very severe, the pimples run together, the surface presenting a red, swollen appearance. A strong alkaline fluid oozes out copiously; after this exudation the inflammation subsides, and the cuticle comes off in fine scales. Eruption itches and stings intensely, and, although formerly relieved by cold water, the irritation has become relieved lately by heat. He has also used *Acetic acid,* except on the face, which allayed the itching and redness. He has taken in the last year Fowler's solution, but without relief. The attacks are worse in the fall and spring, and the eruption is mostly on the face, arms and chest. Constipation

is present. After using *Kali Sulph.* a few days, commenced having boils and had a great many, after which the skin was better than it had been for years; bowels also better.
(C. H.)

Ferrum Phos. in Erythema:

Lady, blonde, æt. 20; fair skin ordinarily. Consulted the writer for erythema. For two days cheeks were swollen, fiery-red and burnt like fire; no itching, eruption or roughness. One dose *Ferrum Phos.* In thirty minutes the fiery redness was gone, and there was no return, the cure being perfect.
(Boardman.)

Kali Sulph. in Ivy-Poisoning:

Case which had suffered from effects of ivy-poisoning (*Rhus tox.*) for eight months. Was formerly treated by external remedies, but has repeatedly broken out again, with small, hard herpetic vesicles, forming into a thin scab, with itching and some moisture. The eruption appears in the left axilla, about the neck and on the backs of both hands. She has a sensation of faintness at stomach and befogged feeling in head, fearing to lose her reason. Very vivid dreams. Two doses of *Kali Sulph.*, taken in water, morning and evening, for four days; cured the case in four weeks.
(W. P. Wesselhoeft, M. D.)

Kali Sulph. in Alopecia:

Case presenting the following symptoms: Bald spot as large as a silver dollar on left side of the head. Hair falls out easily, when combing, all over the head, also of beard. Came on after gonorrhea a year ago, and has probably taken much potash. After taking *Kali Sulph.*, every third day a dose for three weeks, the hair ceased falling and the bald spot is covered with hair.
(W. P. Wesselhoeft, M. D.)

Silicea for papillary Eruptions:

Th., æt. 15; thick crop of papules on forehead, face and both hands; red looking; itches and burns in day-time only.

The spots on forehead are much worse when he takes off his hat. Not at all annoying in the evening, when warm or at night. The entire eruption vanished in less than a fortnight under *Silicea.*
(R. A. Cooper.)

SLEEPLESSNESS

(See Kali Phos.)

ETIOLOGY

"Sleeplessness, pathologically, is an abnormal condition of the brain-cells, kept vivified or awake by the blood supplied to them, when it should be lessened by the contracting of the vessels supplying the brain; and shows loss of stimulating power of the nervous centres to cause muscular contraction of the vessels and diminished supply of blood to the brain. During sleep the brain is anemic and pale, and should be so. Sleeping draughts, morphia, etc., are dangerous and deadening in effect, and can produce death. *Kali Phos.,* the true remedy, restores normal stimulating power in the grey nervous matter, and consequent contractions of the artery, which diminishes the flow of blood to the brain, and natural healthful sleep results. Sometimes a course of the remedy is needed." (Dr. Walker.)

BIOCHEMIC TREATMENT

Kali Phos.—The *principal remedy for disturbances of sleep, when due to mental overwork, excitement, business troubles, worry or general nervous causes.*

Yawning and stretching. Somnambulism; a steady course of this remedy is needed.

Ferrum Phos.—Alternately with *Kali Phos., in sleeplessness from hyperemic conditions of the brain.* Restless, anxious dreams, drowsy in the afternoon.

Natr. Mur.—Excessive sleep, constant desire to sleep, drowsiness. *Unnatural sleep,* sometimes *with saliva dribbling* *from the mouth,* or constipation. Excessive sleep, if traced to an excess of moisture on the brain. Usual amount of sleep is unrefreshing; feels tired and languid in the morning. Excessive drowsiness and stupor during the course of low fever.

Natr. Sulph.—Drowsiness, when the precursor of jaundice, or bilious symptoms are present. Sleepiness, when the tongue has a grayish or brownish-green coating, bitter taste in the mouth, etc.

CLINICAL CASES

Kali Phos. acted like Morphia:

"Mrs. C. says when she had a severe pain in back of neck and head, and so nervous she could not allow anyone to talk to her, could not lie still nor sleep, one dose of *Kali Phos.* would relieve her in a few minutes, and she would sleep as if she had taken morphia, and would feel sleepy for the entire day and night following the dose." Dr. J. C. Nothingham, who prescribed the *Kali Phos.,* believes the symptoms were due to sexual excesses.
(*Medical Advance.*)

Kali Phos. did him much good:

A gentleman who has suffered from great sleeplessness, depression and occasional tendencies to suicidal mania, writes: "I do not know how to thank you for the medicine you gave me; it has done me so much good. I have taken the *Kali Phos.* very faithfully, and will continue to do so, as it keeps me right."
(From Schuessler.)

Natr. Mur. in Insomnia:

Mrs. W., æt. 60; much sleeplessness, with great nervous irritability and coldness of extremities for three months. She cannot keep them warm in any manner; coldness is subjective, but not objective. *Natr. Mur.* promptly cured the insomnia, "soothed her nerves," and cured the other symptoms.
(J. C. Burnett, M. D.)

Magnes. Phos. overcame the difficulty:

I have treated many cases of that affection with *Magnes. Phos.*, where I suspected the cause to be of nervous origin. Generally a good dose of that medicine in two or three tablespoonfuls of water, teaspoonful doses every four or five minutes, overcomes the difficulty after half a dozen teaspoonfuls have been taken.

(E. A. de Çailhol, M. D.)

Kali Phos. in Sleeplessness:

Frank .H., grocer, became involved heavily in debt, due to speculation; his troubles weighed heavily on his mind and he could not sleep soundly at night; often when sleeping would walk about the room; muttered and talked in his sleep; restless, could not lie still when sleeping or awake; nervous; stretches and yawns a good deal, mostly after meals. Constantly worrying and fretting about his business; peevish and irritable; wants to be by himself. Had been taking chloral and morphia, by the advice of his physician, when he came to me. Recommended a change of scene, daily baths, good nourishing food, and *Kali Phos.*, five-grain tablet every three hours. He went to the Alleghanies, and a letter from him informs me that he is much improved in every way. Continued treatment; one tablet every night on retiring.

(C. R. Vogel, M. D.)

SMALL-POX

(See Exudations.)

ETIOLOGY

Small-pox is an eruptive disease of the skin, the basic cause being a deficiency in the cell-salt *Kali Mur.*, which causes an excess of fibrin in the system. This fibrin attempts to escape through the skin, and thus furnishes a breeding-place for the micro-organism of small-pox.

The disease itself consists of four stages: incubation, eruption, suppuration, dessication.

The period of incubation lasts from 5 to 20 days, severe fever, with nausea and headache, appearing during the last few days. The temperature may even go to 106°.

The eruptive stage begins three or four days after the fever appears, the eruption making its appearance on the face in the form of red points, which increase in size and elevation, and soon spread over the arms, hands and whole body. These red elevations have a peculiar, loose feeling, like shot beneath the skin. With the appearance of the eruption, the temperature lowers, but rises again during the stage of suppuration.

During the suppurative stage, the macules become vesicles, and then pustules, which frequently slough. The amount of scarring resulting from small-pox depends upon how deeply these pustules have invaded the true skin, in any given case. The stage of suppuration generally continues three or four days.

The stage of dessication consists of the drying up of the pustules, which may either leave a cicatrix, or form a scab, the abatement of the fever, and gradual subsidence of the swelling. The disease usually runs its course in from four to five weeks.

Small-pox is highly contagious, and the strictest isolation and quarantine should be observed. To avoid pitting or scarring the patient should be prevented from scratching, and the pustules should be protected from the air by carbolized vaseline.

Kali Mur. is the chief remedy in small-pox, as in this way the excess of fibrin is utilized, and the breeding place of the small-pox organism destroyed. Ferrum Phos. is also indicated for the fever, and various other cell-salts as the symptoms calling for them arise.

BIOCHEMIC TREATMENT

Ferrum Phos.—*The first remedy in small-pox,* for the febrile disturbances, high fever, quick pulse, etc., in alternation with the chief remedy.

Kali Mur.—*Kali Mur.* is the *principal remedy* in this disease, *as it controls the formation of pustules.*

Kali Phos.—Adynamic symptoms indicating blood decomposition. Putrid conditions, stupor, exhaustion, etc.

Kali Sulph.—To assist desquamation and facilitate the formation of new skin.

Natr. Mur.—Low forms, when there exists drowsiness, stupor or salivation. Confluence of pustules.

Calc. Sulph.—When the pustules are ripe and are discharging matter.

CLINICAL CASES

Ferrum Phos. and Kali Mur. in Small-Pox:

I am in receipt of a letter from Dr. M., of Muncie, Indiana, who has had a number of small-pox cases during the epidemic in that city the past few months. He says: "I am exceedingly glad to be able to report favorably the action of the Biochemic remedies in the cases of small-pox in which I have used them this summer. The cases, while rather severe while at their height, resulted more favorably under the tissue remedies than did those treated by my friends, who used various other remedies. *Ferrum Phos.* was prescribed during the initiatory stage, for the febrile disturbances, followed by *Kali Mur.* The pustule formations were not so well marked as in some of the cases treated by others, while when they did suppurate, *Calc. Sulph.* seemed to abort the usual profuse discharge. *Kali Sulph.* aided in the stage of desquamation and also assisted and hastened the new skin. I am well satisfied with the result, and think this dreaded disease can, if taken at once in the first stage, be handled without any difficulty, with a decreased mortality, with *Ferrum Phos., Kali Mur.* and *Kali Sulph.*"
(C. R. Vogel, M. D.)

SORE THROAT

(See Diphtheria, Croup, etc.)

BIOCHEMIC TREATMENT

Ferrum Phos.—Inflammatory conditions of the throat, arising from any cause, need this remedy in frequent doses; also a gargle. Sore throat, with fever, great pain, etc., to reduce the congestion. Ulcerated sore throat; acute stage of laryngitis. *Sore throats of singers and speakers,* "clergyman's sore throat," to reduce the inflammation and strengthen the muscles. (*Calc. Phos.* intercurrently.)

Kali Mur.—*Second stage* of inflammatory conditions of the throat, *when exudation has taken place,* with swelling of the glands or tonsils. Ulcerated throat, with grayish-white patches, tongue covered with a thick, white fur. Diphtheria. Should also be used as a gargle in hot water.

Kali Phos.—Gangrenous and malignant conditions of the throat. Accompanied with foul breath.

Calc. Phos.—"Clergyman's sore throat" (chronic); *constant scraping of the throat, with expectoration of albuminous phlegm.*

Calc. Fluor.—Tickling in the larynx, due to relaxed condition of the uvula. Tickling cough upon lying down.

Natr. Mur.—Inflammation of the throat, when the *tonsils are covered with a transparent frothy mucus.* Sore throat accompanied with watery secretions. Relaxed uvula, when watery symptoms are present (*Calc. fluor.*).

Magnes. Phos.—*Spasms of the throat,* with sensation of choking on attempting to swallow.

Natr. Phos.—Inflammation of the throat or tonsils, when coated with a creamy, golden-yellow mucus. *Raw feeling in the throat in the morning;* covered with a creamy, yellow coating.

Calc. Sulph.—Last stage of ulcerated sore throat and tonsillitis, when suppurating; thick, yellow matter, sometimes streaked with blood.

Natr. Sulph.—Sore throat, with *feeling as of a lump in throat on swallowing.*

SPASMS, CONVULSIONS, ETC.

(See Epilepsy.)

ETIOLOGY

The direct cause of all spasms is a deficiency of the inorganic salt which controls the white fibres of nerves and muscles. Many cases may work to produce this result. Vicious habits, worms, great fear, over-taxing the nervous or muscular system, and thus consuming the cell-salts faster than the digestive and assimilative processes can furnish them. Magnes. Phos. and Calc. Phos. should be used in combination in all cases of spasms.

BIOCHEMIC TREATMENT

Magnes. Phos.—Spasms of every kind or in any part of the body are met by this salt. Convulsions, twitchings, contractions, cramps, fits, etc., give frequent doses in hot water. Lockjaw, rub it into the gums. Spasmodic stammering. Writer's cramp. Spasm of throat on attempting to swallow; twitching of corners of mouth or muscles of face.

Calc. Phos.—Fits and spasms, after *Magnes. Phos.* In teething disorders or spasms and convulsions due to a deficiency of the lime-salts, to prevent recurrence of the spasm; spasms in anemic, pale subjects.

Kali Phos.—Fits, from fright, with pale or livid countenance. Alternate with *Magnes. Phos.* for the spasm.

Kali Mur.—Almost a specific for epilepsy, to prevent the spasms; *Magnes. Phos.* when the spasm is on.

Ferrum Phos.—Convulsions in teething children, for the febrile disturbances.

CLINICAL CASES

Magnes. Phos. in muscular Spasms:

Magnes. Phos. is doing noble work for me in treatment of agonizing pains that accompany muscular spasms, especially of the involuntary muscles. Some physician said within my hearing last year, that when you felt morphine to be an urgent necessity, try *Magnes. Phos.* first—the solution in hot water at frequent intervals, to insure prompt absorption. It has been especially valuable to me in the treatment of intestinal and uterine colics, and should be also valuable in that accompanying the passage of stone. I have no experience with it in the latter. I value it especially as a prophylactic against the tendency of such muscular spasms.
(Dr. A. L. Monroe.)

Calc. Phos.—Thirty convulsions in twenty-four hours—cured:

A very interesting case came under my treatment, which deserves the attention of the profession. I was called to a lady advanced in years. She had been suffering for nearly five weeks from fearful attacks of convulsive spasms. During the last twenty-four hours she had had thirty attacks. The spasms darted through her body like an electric shock, so that she fell to the ground. The attack lasted a few minutes, after which she felt well enough, but rather exhausted. The sufferer did not venture to leave her bed now, afraid of being injured. She had been treated by her first doctor with flor. zinci, Fowler's solution, and friction, without success. When I saw the lady, I thought of trying the Biochemic remedies. Knowing that *Magnes. Phos.* and *Calc. Phos.* are the two prescribed for allaying spasms (cramp), I chose the latter, *Calc. Phos.*, under those circumstances. Next day, to the astonishment of those about her, I found the old lady walking about the room. She met me with a smile, exclaim-

ing: "Ah, doctor, my spasms are cured!" And so it was. She has not had another attack.
(Dr. Fechtmann.)

Magnes. Phos. in convulsive Sobbing:

Dr. F., of Also, Hungary, reports: I was requested to go into the country to see a man who had been suffering the last three days from spasmodic convulsive sobbing. He was lying in bed. Subcutaneous injections of morphia, friction with chloroform and sinapisms (mustard poultices) were all of no use. Although the sobbing was mitigated for two or three hours, it returned with more violence than ever. I gave him a powder of *Magnes. Phos.* in half a tumblerful of water. After the second tablespoonful the sobbing ceased altogether, to the astonishment of all those present.
(From Schuessler.)

Magnes. Phos. in Writer's Cramp:

Miss Carrie W., employed in a large wholesale house addressing envelopes, consulted me regarding what turned out to be a typical case of writer's cramp. After an unusual amount of work, she found that her hand became suddenly very tired, and she was compelled during her subsequent writings to rest her hand frequently. Then she noticed a cramping at the first three fingers, only slight at first, when it became so bad that she could not hold the pen. The cramping extended throughout the hand, and involved the entire right arm to shoulder in a trembling spasm, making it an entire impossibility to use the hand at writing at all, and she was compelled to give up her position. I prescribed *Magnes. Phos.*, every two hours, bathed the arm in hot water twice daily, applying friction with a crash towel. This treatment was given for over two weeks, when she became so much better that she could again resume her position. She used the hand only moderately, and a thick, though light, penholder. To-day, over six months after, has had no return of the spasm. Still gave *Magnes. Phos.*, two doses every day.
(C. R. Vogel, M. D.)

Spasms during Catamenia:

A. R. V. G., a young lady, æt. 18, had visited, along with her mother, in the past summer, a hydropathic establishment. Without being ill, she had used the baths, even during her catamenia. Immediately after this, she took violent spasms or cramps, which set in daily and continued after having returned home. A medical man was consulted, as the disease increased in spite of the different medicines she took. A second doctor was consulted, who quite agreed in the diagnosis, as well as the treatment adopted by his colleague. Injections of morphia, very strong, and repeated several times daily, was the main remedy applied; but the distressing ailment could not be removed; on the contrary, the cramps increased in violence and frequency. The medical men in attendance finally declared that there was no chance of improvement until the patient would take special medical baths in the Spring. The parents were afraid that their daughter would not live to see the Spring, and if she did, that she would not be fit to be removed. They therefore telegraphed, requesting a visit from me. On the 6th of September last, I saw the patient for the first time. I had known her formerly, and was astonished to see, instead of the blooming healthy girl she had been, a pale, emaciated figure, whom I should not have recognized. During my presence she had an attack, her features were distorted, the eyes turned upward, froth came to the mouth, and then a fearful paroxysm of beating and striking with the hands and feet, such as I had never seen before. This was only the commencement. Suddenly the trunk of her body was contorted in an indescribable manner, the back of the head pressed deeply into the pillows, the feet forced against the foot of the bed, her chest and abdomen became arched like a bridge, drawn up almost half a yard. In this unnatural position she was suspended several seconds. Suddenly the whole body jerked upward with a bound, and the poor sufferer was tossed about for some seconds with her spine contracted. During the whole attack, which lasted several minutes, she was quite unconscious;

pinching and slapping had no effect; dashing cold water in the face, or applying burnt feathers to the nostrils, was ineffectual; the pupils were quite insensible to the light. When the spasms came on again with such violence that the bedstead gave way, I ordered *Magnes. Phos.* After taking this remedy, on the 10th of October, the catamenia appeared, but her condition otherwise was in no way changed. The spasms continued with the same violence. Then, remembering Schuessler's injunction to use *Calc. Phos.* where *Magnes. Phos.,* though indicated by symptoms, proves ineffectual, I gave her *Calc. Phos.* on the 16th of October, a full dose every two hours. Immediately the spasms became less frequent. On the sixth day there was an attack, weak and of short duration. From this date she had peace until the 6th of November, the day of the return of the catamenia, which was preceded by a short, slight attack. On the 14th of December I had a call from the young lady, looking well, who wished to consult me for a slight bronchial affection. She told me she was entirely cured of her attacks. and at the beginning of December she had been quite regular without experiencing any inconvenience.

(From Schuessler.)

Magnes. Phos. in Convulsions:

A child has been having convulsions for two or three days and was treated by physicians without any relief when I was called to take charge of the case. A few doses of *Magnes. Phos.* soon checked the convulsions and he was about again in a few days.

(Dr. E. H. Holbrook.)

Natr. Phos. in Convulsions:

A little boy who had indulged too freely in candy, bananas and various other things, had an attack of sour vomiting, followed by convulsions and mild typhoid fever symptoms. *Natr. Phos.* promptly removed the trouble.

(Dr. J. S. S. Chesshir.)

SPERMATORRHEA

ETIOLOGY

The meaning of the word is, to flow. The condition is caused by a weakness of nerves and muscles that control the fine network of blood-vessels (tunica vasculosa) which supplies the secreting substances.

This weakness frequently extends to the prostate gland and the *corpora cavernosa,* thereby weakening erectile tissue, and the spermatic cord. The discharge is not all semen, but is largely a catarrhal discharge or secretion from the fibrous capsule or tunica albuginea.

According to Biochemistry, this condition could not prevail unless a deficiency first occurred in the cell-salts that control the organic matter which builds up the tissue and furnishes the elastic fibre and contractile power to these glands, nerves, muscular tissue, etc.

BIOCHEMIC TREATMENT

Natr. Phos.—Seminal emissions, with acid conditions; semen thin, watery, and stale odor; *emissions, when followed by weakness and trembling.*

Kali Phos.—For the *nervous symptoms* arising *from excessive sexual excitement* or other disorders of the sexual organs.

Calc. Phos.—Seminal emissions; *chief remedy for the general weakness of the system, to tone up the sexual functions* to a normal standard. Tendency to masturbation in the young.

CLINICAL CASES

Calc. Phos. and Kali Phos. cured Spermatorrhea:

Mrs. P. consulted me for a case of spermatorrhea in her son, 18 years old. He was tall, emaciated; complexion, sallow; bashful; did not want to tell me about his condition; hypochondriacal. His mother informed me that he complained very frequently of dizzy spells and headache, always feeling tired; no ambition; aversion to company; saw spots before the eyes; letters blurred in reading; trembled so at table would often drop his knife or fork. Spasmodic cramps of fingers, with jerking. He would have the emissions as often as three or four times a week, usually accompanied by lascivious dreams. I questioned him privately, being almost positive that he was an onanist, and through his tears he admitted that such was the case and that he was willing and anxious to get relief and do anything he could to stop the habit. *Calc. Phos.*, was prescribed for the general weakness of the system, in alternation with *Kali Phos.*, a dose every four hours. A quick sponge-bath of cold water was taken night and morning; avoiding all meats, confining himself to a light diet. Improvement was gradual but certain. The emissions having ceased entirely, feels stronger, is brighter mentally, more active physically, and as he expresses it: "I am a changed man, doctor, in every way, for which I have your medicine and advice to thank."

(C. R. Vogel, M. D.)

SPLEEN, INFLAMMATION OF

BIOCHEMIC TREATMENT

Ferrum Phos.—First stage for all the acute febrile symptoms; pain, inflammation, high temperature, quick pulse, tenderness to pressure.

Kali Mur.—Second stage; tumefaction and enlargement, white-coated tongue, etc.

Calc. Phos.—Intercurrently in all cases. See "*Inflammations.*"

SPINE DISEASES

(See Rachitis and article on Calc. Phos.)

BIOCHEMIC TREATMENT

Calc. Phos.—*Spinal troubles* arising *from a deficiency of the lime-salts;* spinal weakness; spinal curvature; anemia of the spine. Backache and pains in the lumbar region. Rachitis, child not able to hold up its head; open fontanels; emaciated children, peevish and fretful. In spinal curvature, mechanical supports are necessary; give *Calc. Phos.* steadily, one or two doses per day.

Natr. Mur.—Spinal irritation and weakness of back. The general condition of the system and watery symptoms, with corresponding dryness of some of the mucous membranes, must govern the selection of this remedy. In spinal weakness a good method is to briskly rub the spine with a solution of common table salt.

Kali Phos.—*Softening of the spinal cord,* with deadening of the nerve centres. Spinal anemia from exhausting diseases. Laming pains in the spine, worse on beginning to move about, but better from gentle exercise.

Kali Mur.—Wasting of the spinal cord; intercurrently with other indicated remedies.

Natr. Phos.—*Spinal anemia* arising *from an acid condition. Natr. Phos.* is a solvent of lime, and, therefore, promotes the deposit of *Calc. Phos.*

Silicea.—*Spinal irritation, with offensive foot-sweat.* Spinal irritation of children, depending on worms; in alternation with *Natr. Phos.* Sweat about the head in children. Suppurative diseases of the bony structure of the spine.

Calc. Fluor.—Spina ventosa, in alternation with *Magnes. Phos.* Weak back, with dragging, down-bearing pains, associated with constipation.

STOMACH, INFLAMMATION OF

(See Gastric Derangements.)

STOMATITIS

(See Mouth, Diseases of.)

SUN-STROKE

BIOCHEMIC TREATMENT

Natr. Mur.—*Natr. Mur.* is the *principal remedy* in this disease, which arises from a sudden abstraction of moisture from the tissues, causing a dryness of the membranes. *Kali Phos.* will frequently be found necessary, to control the brain symptoms.

CLINICAL CASES

Natr. Mur. in Sun-Stroke:

On a stifling morning last July, I was summoned to see a young man who had been "sun-struck." Patient unconscious; general convulsions; face flushed; breathing deep and labored; pulse rapid, though feeble. Inhalations of *Amyl nitrite* resuscitated him, and I then gave him *Natr. Mur.*, every two hours for about one week. He recovered completely, with none of the usual unpleasant after-effects.

(Frank E. Miller, M. D.)

SQUINTING

BIOCHEMIC TREATMENT

Magnes. Phos.—Spasmodic squinting or twitching of the eyes.

Kali Phos.—Squinting from paralytic conditions; frequently after an attack of diphtheria.

Natr. Phos.—Squinting, if caused by irritation from worms, or acid conditions.

Calc. Phos.—Intercurrently with or after *Magnes. Phos.*, if that remedy fails to act.

SWEATS

BIOCHEMIC TREATMENT

Silicea.—Copious night-sweats with prostration in phthisis. Sweat about the head in children. Offensive sweat of feet and of the armpits. Copious sweats when no disease is apparent.

Natr. Mur.—Weakening and profuse night-sweats, smelling sour; weakening sweats of intermittent fever.

Kali Phos.—Perspiration from debility or weakening diseases.

Calc. Phos.—Excessive sweats in phthisis if *Silicea* fails to relieve. Cold, clammy sweat on the face and body.

SYPHILIS

ETIOLOGY

THIS disease is probably one of the oldest in the world. Brought into Europe from the Far East during the Middle Ages, it at first decimated whole communities, but as it became more common, a certain degree of immunity to it was established, and its virulence somewhat abated. To-day it is found everywhere, with the exception of savage peoples who have had no contact with civilized communities, and its frequency and virulence are not modified materially by geographical conditions or climate.

The basic cause of syphilis is a lack of the cell-salt Kali Mur., which causes an excess of its organic associate, fibrin

This fibrin, in attempting to escape from the system, weakens the skin or mucous membrane at its point of exit.

Thus a breeding place is supplied for the *spirocheta pallida,* as the micro-organism found in all cases of syphilis is termed. This organism usually invades the body during sexual intercourse, although it can also be acquired in many other ways. Obstetricians, nurses and midwives have become infected through a break in the skin of the finger. Children, while nursing, have infected the nipples of the nurse, and *vice versa,* have themselves been infected in the mouth. Knives, forks, spoons, pipes, drinking vessels, and even kissing, have also been known to convey the infection. At any time during the first and second stages of the disease all secretions from its lesions are capable of producing the disease in another person, but never through unbroken skin or mucous membrane.

Sufferers from syphilis pass through three stages, the first stage being characterized by the appearance of the primary lesion, or chancre, which may or may not be visible, according to its position in the body.

The chancre begins as an erosion or papule with a smooth, shiny base, covered with granulations. It soon begins to discharge a thin, watery fluid, and the edges of the chancre become hard and indurated, while the inguinal glands become enlarged. This stage lasts from three to ten days or two weeks, and is followed by the development of the secondary stage.

During the secondary stage fever is common, even rising as high as 104°, and the syphilitic skin symptoms become more pronounced. This may be a roseolus rash, occurring in limited areas, or over the whole body, or a macular syphilide, consisting of reddish-brown macules scattered over the trunk. The eruption may become papular or even pustular during this stage, mucous patches appear at the junction of skin and mucous membrane, while a rapid development of anemia is often observed. The secondary stage lasts from twelve to eighteen months, and is usually followed by an intermediate period, during which the symptoms are modified or almost completely disappear.

Usually, however, in the majority of untreated cases the diseases progresses to the tertiary stage, which embraces more severe skin lesions than the secondary, including tuberculous and ulcerous formations of a subacute or chronic character. There is also a growth of new tissue, with a marked tendency to necrosis, usually found in circumscribed nodes, and known as gummata. They develop in the skin, muscles and internal organs, and may cause serious trouble, especially in the brain.

Cases of syphilis vary greatly in their severity, some progressing rapidly to a fatal result, while in others a chronic condition may be established that will last for years.

In treating syphilis the organism itself may be combatted by the use of salvarsan or neosalvarsan intravenously, or the older plan of treatment by mercury or the iodides. At the same time, however, the basic cause of the trouble must be recognized, and the breeding place of the organism destroyed by replacing the lacking Kali Mur. As is usual in such troubles, there will probably ensue a lack of other cell-salts, and these should also be supplied, as occasion arises.

BIOCHEMIC TREATMENT

Ferrum Phos.—Bubo, for the heat, tenderness, throbbing and other febrile disturbances.

Kali Mur.—Bubo, for the swelling. Soft chancre, with characteristic symptoms. *Chronic stage of syphilis. The principal remedy in this disease;* internally and as a local application.

Natr. Sulph.—*Condylomata of anus, of syphilitic origin;* internally and local application.

Natr. Mur.—*Syphilis, in the chronic stage, when accompanied by serous exudations,* and other watery symptoms.

Kali Phos.—*Phagedenic chancre* or malignant conditions.

Kali Sulph.—Syphilis, with characteristic symptoms.

Calc. Sulph.—Suppurating stage of syphilis, to control the discharge. Bubo, in the suppurative stage (alternate with *Silicea*).

Silicea.—*Bubo, in the suppurative stage* (alternate with *Calc. Sulph.*). Chronic syphilis, with suppurations or indurations. Ulcerated *cutaneous* affections, where *mercury has been given in excess;* nodes in tertiary syphilis.

Calc. Fluor.—Hard and *indurated chancres* or other pathological indications for the use of this remedy.

CLINICAL CASES

Kali Mur. in chancroid ulcers:

Chancroid ulcers, surrounded by congested areola, grayish exudation covering surface. Deep excavations, wider at bottom; painful micturition. *Kali Mur.*, every three hours. Improvement soon set in, the pain on urinating disappeared, and the ulcers rapidly healed.
(F. A. Rockwith.)

TAPE WORMS

(See Worms.)

TEETHING

(See Dentition.)

TESTICLES, DISEASES OF

(See Hydrocele.)

BIOCHEMIC TREATMENT

Ferrum Phos.—First or *inflammatory stage* of all diseases of the testicles, for pain, heat, etc

Kali Mur.—*Second stage* of inflammation of the testicles, with swelling. *Diseases of testicles, if from suppressed gonorrhea.*

Calc. Phos.—Orchitis, hydrocele (after *Natr. Mur.*). Hernia, also mechanical support (alternate with *Calc. Fluor.*).

Calc. Fluor.—*Dropsy of the testicle,* to strengthen the contractile muscles (*Calc. Phos.*). Hernia.

Natr. Mur.—Dropsy of the testicle. See Hydrocele. Spermatic cord and testicles sore and painful. Aching in testicles. Violent itching on scrotum. Loss of hair from pubes.

THROAT

(See Hoarseness, Tonsilitis and Sore Throat.)

CLINICAL CASES

Ferrum Phos. for Bronchial Irritation of public speakers:

Having a large acquaintance among clergymen and public speakers, I have an excellent opportunity of testing the tissue remedies in the throat troubles which annoy that class of people. For the slight bronchial irritation immediately after speaking, *Ferrum Phos.* acts quickly by allaying the inflammation. When the affection has become chronic, and there is much scraping of the throat, with expectoration of albuminous phlegm, a course of *Calc. Phos.* is needed. Should the phlegm be watery or poor in albumen, *Natr. Mur.* is the indicated remedy.

(J. B. Chapman, M. D.)

Kali Phos. in fetid breath:

An actor, Mr. E., consulted me for a severe irritation in the throat that interfered much with speech, and on account of an exceedingly bad breath. This was especially disturbing, as he was obliged to appear in a role, three days later, in which proximity with his fellow actors was necessary. From an examination, I concluded that it resulted from a deficiency

of *Kali Phos.*, and so I ordered this remedy. On the evening of the second day Mr. E. informed me that he was fully recovered of the foul breath; there was not a trace to be perceived. He also stated that he was able to notice an improvement even after the second dose.
(Dr. Quesse.)

THRUSH

(See Mouth, Diseases of.)

TINNITUS AURIUM

(See Ear, Diseases of.)

TONGUE AND TASTE

BIOCHEMIC TREATMENT

Kali Mur.—Coating of the tongue, white or grayish-white, dry; *heavy white fur on tongue.* Inflammation of tongue, for the swelling.

Ferrum Phos.—Inflammation of the tongue, with dark-red swelling; alternate with *Kali Mur. Red tongue,* indicating inflammation of some part of the body.

Kali Phos.—*Coating like stale, brownish, liquid mustard,* excessively dry, especially in the morning, with *bad taste* and *fetid breath.* Inflammation of tongue, with dryness and exhaustion during epidemics of low fever.

Natr. Mur.—*Tongue coated with clear, slimy or watery mucus;* also when small bubbles of frothy saliva cover the sides. Clean, moist tongue and excess of saliva.

Kali Sulph.—*Yellow, slimy coating of tongue;* sometimes with whitish edge. Insipid taste.

Natr. Phos.—*Creamy, golden-yellow, moist coating* at the root of tongue and on the tonsils; sometimes with acid taste.

Natr. Sulph.—*Coating of tongue dirty, brownish-green or grayish-green.* Slimy tongue, much thick tenacious slime in the mouth. Bitter taste, indicating bilious derangement.

Calc. Phos.—Tongue thick, stiff and numb (also *Kali Mur.*).

Calc. Fluor.—Tongue, for induration and hardening after inflammation (also *Silicea*). Cracked appearance of tongue, with or without pain.

Calc. Sulph.—Suppurating stage of inflammation of the tongue.

Magnes. Phos.—"Yellow, slimy coating, especially when there is pain in the bowels, and a sensation of pressure in the stomach." (Dr. A. P. Davis.)

Note: The color of the coating on the tongue usually indicates the remedy to be given; but in cases of chronic catarrh of the stomach, if an acute disease arises, the color of the tongue will not govern the choice of a remedy for the acute disease.

TONSILLITIS

(See Diphtheria.)

ETIOL GY

The same pathological conditions exist in tonsillitis or inflammation of the tonsils as exist in any other inflammatory disease. The same process is observed, *i. e.,* first, inflammation; second, exudation, and, third, suppuration. The exciting cause may be taking cold in the tonsils, the accumulation of food particles in the interstices of the fauces, or irritating effects of stomach disease. Whatever the exciting cause may be, the pathological condition is primarily a disturbance of fibrin. Potassium chloride is the inorganic cell-salt which controls fibrin, therefore when the particles of this salt, for any reason, fall below the standard a portion of fibrin, not having the proper cell-salt to unite with, becomes non-functional and is thrown out of the circulation.

BIOCHEMIC TREATMENT

Ferrum Phos.—in the *first stage,* for the pain, inflammation, fever, etc., frequent doses; also a gargle of the remedy in hot water.

Kali Mur.—The second remedy, for the swelling of the tonsils. White or *gray spots on the tonsils;* also gargle frequently. Chronic or acute tonsillitis, *white-furred coating on the tongue.*

Calc. Sulph.—Last or *suppurative stage* of inflammation of the tonsils.

Calc. Phos.—*Chronic swelling of the tonsils,* sometimes with difficulty of swallowing; intercurrently with other remedies.

Natr. Phos.—Catarrh of the tonsils, with golden-yellow coating at base of tongue, indicating an acid condition of the stomach. Tonsils inflamed, when covered with above coating.

Natr. Mur.—Inflammation of the uvula, with characteristic tongue and watery symptoms.

CLINICAL CASES

Natr. Mur. in Salivation after Merc.:

I have used *Natr. Mur.* repeatedly, and especially in obstinate cases of salivation, with excellent results. One case in particular was cured with remarkable rapidity by this remedy. A young lady, æt. 20, who suffered from severe inflammation of the tonsils, so that she could scarcely swallow milk or water, had received from me a preparation of mercury. The inflammation of the tonsils was reduced very quickly, but another evil set in, namely, violent salivation. The gums were loosened, bleeding easily and standing back from the teeth, and the teeth were slackened. I thought of curing this affection also with *Mercur.*, with which I had often before succeeded in such cases, but by continuing the remedy the evil was only increased. Now, I ascertained from the patient that in the previous summer she had been ill at N., and the doctor had given her a good deal of calomel, which caused fearful and long-continued salivation. She was afraid the evil would again become very tedious, as it had been so bad at N. I now stopped the mercury and ordered *Natr. Mur.*, a dose the size of a bean, every two hours. The success surpassed my most sanguine expectations. In twenty-four hours the swelling of the glands had distinctly diminished, and in three days a complete cure was effected.

(From Schuessler.)

Calc. Phos. in enlarged Tonsils and Deafness:

J. D., æt. 5; a thin, delicate-looking boy; very tall for his age; for two years suffered from partial deafness, which has much increased since he came to Southampton, two months ago. His mother is frightened, fearing he is becoming incurably deaf. At first he would, or rather could, not allow me, from the excessive pain it occasioned, to examine his throat (he was then suffering from exacerbation); but it was evident, from the external swelling and the history, where the true cause of the dyscrasia lay. The tale his mother tells is that he was vaccinated when three years old; that, after much constitutional disturbance, eruption subsided, leaving the tonsils in their present swollen condition. Symptoms are worse after coming in from open air and in damp weather. *Calc. Phos.* had an immediate beneficial effect, so that in three days the throat could be examined. Both tonsils were swollen and red, and formed an almost complete embankment between the mouth and throat. In three weeks hearing was quite restored and swelling subsided.

(R. T. Cooper, M. D.)

Fever in Tonsillitis rapidly dissipated:

Boy seven years old; tonsillitis. Throat swelled until nearly shut and very red. Pulse 140; temperature 106 F. No medicine at hand except *Ferrum Phos.* celloids. This was at 5 p. m. Very reluctantly I gave the *Ferrum Phos.* and advised calling me at 10 p. m. His temperature was decidedly going down. The medicine had been given every fifteen minutes. The child made a fine recovery in three or four days with no other treatment.

(Dr. Z. R. Chamberlain, Perrysburg, Ohio.)

Ferrum Phos. and Kali Mur. in true Quinsy:

Dr. W. had a severe attack of tonsillitis, involving both tonsils, which were very much enlarged, causing difficult and painful deglutition. Temperature 102; pulse 130; patient exceedingly nervous. Gave *Ferrum Phos.* and *Kali Phos.* in alternation, every fifteen minutes. Saw the patient in six hours, and all symptoms were worse; then gave *Kali Mur.*, instead of *Kali Phos.*; continued *Ferrum.* The next morning found that the patient had passed a fair night. Then combined with *Ferrum Phos. and Kali Mur.* In six hours found the patient very much improved; less pain, less swelling; temperature 100; pulse 100; continued the remedies, and in two days the patient was out and suppuration did not take place. This was as truly a case of quinsy, which usually goes on to suppuration and runs a seven days' course, in spite of all we can do, as any case I ever saw. The patient remarked that he could feel the effects of the remedies all through his body, quieting and soothing the nervous irritability immediately after every dose.

(G. H. Martin, M. D.)

Kali Mur. gave quick relief:

One evening a gentleman brought to my office his son, aged 8 or 10 years. As he stood before me, I noticed that he labored terribly in breathing. I found both tonsils inflamed and very much enlarged. He was very feverish, and the tongue

was coated white. I gave him some tablets of *Kali Mur.*, and ordered them to be given every half hour for three hours, and then every hour through the night. The next morning, quite early, I called and, to my astonishment, found him sitting up in bed, quite bright and breathing naturally. His breathing had assumed a more normal form, and the tonsils were considerably diminished in size. The same remedy was continued throughout the next day, and the next morning the little fellow met me in the parlor, comparatively well.
(E. H. H.)

Kali Mur. in Tonsillitis:

Mr. P., brought his little boy to my office to be treated for sore throat. Looking into his throat, I found his tonsils greatly enlarged and very difficult breathing. *Kali Mur.* given every few minutes soon relieved the conditions and he was well in a few days.

Many cases of croup and other throat troubles have been cured with this remedy.
(Dr. E. H. Holbrook, Baltimore, Md.)

Tonsillitis and Sinus Trouble:

Was called for consultation by Mr. Ewing, found him with a temperature of 102½. Headache, backache, was unable to swallow freely.

Diagnosis.—Tonsillitis. *Ferrum Phos.* celloids reduced fever and relieved inflammation of throat. Several days later was called to see him again.

Found him suffering with pain in right supraorbital sinus. Codeine failed to relieve.

Diagnosis.—Catarrhal inflammation of sinus, threatening suppuration. *Calc. Sulph.* in hot water relieved the pain in a few days, and cured the case.
(Dr. H. Clifton Neff, Dunkirk, Ohio.)

Ferrum Phos. and Kali Mur. in Quinsy:

J. W. A groom taking care of horses at fair grounds. History: Many attacks of quinsy. Consulted me about throat and examination revealed tonsils inflamed and badly swollen with engorged veins in pharynx and intense pain and soreness. Ordered *Ferrum Phos.* and *Kali Mur.*, three celloids alternate every two hours.

Thirty-six hours later the inflammation was entirely gone and cure perfect.
(Dr. B. H. Burd.)

TOOTHACHE

(See Neuralgia.)

BIOCHEMIC TREATMENT

Magnes. Phos.—Neuralgic toothache, excruciating pain, when hot liquids give relief and cold aggravates. *Pain very intense and shooting along the nerve.* Pains are relieved by pressure; worse in cold air.

Ferrum Phos.—*Toothache from inflammation of the gums or nerves.* Pains are relieved by cold liquids or in the cool open air; worse from heat. Gums red, sore and inflamed.

Kali Mur.—Toothache, with swelling of the gums or cheeks, to reduce the swelling. (Alternate with *Ferrum Phos.*)

Kali Phos.—Toothache of nervous, pale subjects, or those worn out with great mental strains. Pains are better under pleasant excitement. Toothache, when the gums are inclined to bleed easily or when there is a bright-red line on them.

Calc. Phos.—Toothache, when the tooth is decayed. *Too rapid decay of teeth. Teething disorders* (see Dentition). Toothache which is worse at night.

Kali Sulph.—Toothache, with evening aggravation or worse in a warm room; better in cool open air.

Natr. Mur.—*Toothache, with involuntary flow of tears,* or excessive secretion of saliva characteristic of this remedy.

Calc. Fluor.—*Toothache, with looseness of the teeth;* teeth are sensitive to the touch of food. Deficient enamel. (See Dentition.)

Silicea.—Toothache, when abscess is forming, pain is deep-seated, pulling on the tooth gives relief. *Toothache caused by sudden chill suppressing foot-sweat.* Pains are very violent at night; neither heat nor cold gives relief.

CLINICAL CASES

Silicea in Toothache:

Miss S., a small, pale, nervous little woman, came to me with a severe toothache, involving the molars and bicuspids of the right side of the inferior maxillary, first: then extending to the superior maxillary and to the bones of the face. Pains of a tearing, boring nature all the time; felt worse at night; could not sleep, was compelled to walk the floor, the pains being so severe. Ulceration of the roots of the teeth was the cause of the trouble. Had used hot salt bags locally. Cocaine on the gums, and creosote in one of the teeth, which was hollow from decay. No relief. *Silicea,* five-grain tablet in hot water, brought prompt relief. Consulted her dentist afterwards for treatment, and had the teeth filled.
(C. R. Vogel, M. D.)

TRAUMATIC TETANUS

(See Spasms, Convulsions, etc.)

CLINICAL CASES

Natr. Mur. in Traumatic Tetanus:

On August 19th I was called to see a boy, æt. 2 years, who had thrust his left foot into a large hand corn-sheller while in motion. The terms "compound comminuted fracture," with extensive laceration, will best describe the condition of the foot. I set the bones and brought the torn edges together as best I could with adhesive strips; applied a dressing; gave internally *Ferrum Phos.* every two hours, and left my little patient feeling quite comfortable. On the second day I was hastily called, and found him having convulsions, as many as eight in an hour. So I dissolved three five-grain tablets of *Magnes. Phos.* in hot water, and gave a teaspoonful every fifteen minutes, with the result that after the third dose the child had no more convulsions. Temperature during this time, 103.

On August 26th the parents, thinking the boy was not getting on as well as he ought, called in another physician, who ordered my treatment discontinued, applied a dressing of iodoform, gave nothing internally, ordered the dressing repeated in five days and left. On September 1st, according to orders, the parents attempted to remove the dressing, found it stuck so fast that every attempt to remove it caused profuse bleeding. So they wrapped the child up, put him into the buggy and brought him to my office. When I removed the iodoform dressing the odor was extremely offensive; but the worst was, the child threw himself back into his mother's arms with his head drawn back at right angles with the trunk, his jaws firmly set, the muscles of his neck rigid. A sudden case of opisthotonos with trismus. I again applied the dressing, gave in turn *Magnes. Phos.* and *Calc. Phos.*, but under these and some other means, such as injections of chloral hydrate, the body remained rigid and the jaws firmly set. On the fourth day after I removed the dressing of iodoform, I discovered small air bubbles of saliva coming from between his teeth, which led me to think of *Natr. Mur.*, which greatly relieved the case in twenty-four hours. Allow me to state that we nourished the patient, during the time, by rectal injections of milk and eggs. The yolk of one egg beaten in one-half pint of unskimmed milk, night and morning. At this writing the boy is doing well, able to feed himself, eats anything he wants. The foot is now almost well.

TUBERCULOSIS

(See Consumption of the Lungs.)

ETIOLOGY

Tuberculosis is a disease characterized by the presence in the body of the bacillus tuberculosis. These cause first inflammation and then areas of necrosis. In these areas are found small nodules which appear as gray, or white, or sometimes yellowish bodies called tubercles. From these tubercles the title "tuberculosis" has been given to the malady.

Before the bacillus tuberculosis can obtain any hold upon the system, however, it is necessary that the tissues be in a receptive condition for their propagation and growth. This can only occur when inorganic cell-salts are lacking, and when, consequently, the cells in which they are found are in a debilitated condition, and are not functionating properly.

Tuberculosis may occur in almost any part of the body, the most common locations being the lungs, where it is commonly called "consumption" (see page 175), the various glands, the peritoneum, and the long bones, especially in the vicinity of the hip.

To overcome tuberculosis, and restore the system to health, it is necessary, not only to follow the rules now generally accepted in regard to diet, hygiene, fresh air, and exercise, but also to restore the missing inorganic cell-salts, and thus remove any possible breeding place for the bacillus.

BIOCHEMIC TREATMENT

Ferrum Phos.—For the febrile symptoms of tuberculosis, such as high temperature and flushed face. Hemorrhage from any part of the body, but especially in consumptive cases. Also very useful where the patient is pale and anemic, to increase the percentage of hemoglobin.

Calc. Phos.—In the run-down condition common to practically all sufferers from tuberculosis, *Calc. Phos.* makes new blood cells, overcomes the anemia present, and improves the general condition of the system. Should be given as an intercurrent remedy in all cases of tuberculosis.

Natr. Mur.—In large doses to check hemorrhage, in alternation with *Ferr. Phos.* General weakness and prostration after exertion. Useful in tuberculosis of the lungs, when the expectoration is watery, clear, and frothy, also when there is bloody sputa.

Silicea.—For profuse night-sweats, burning of the soles of the feet, and hectic fever. Constipation. Very offensive foot sweats. Valuable in the later stages of consumption, with profuse easy expectoration of thick, greenish-yellow pus.

Kali Phos.—For the nervous weakness common in tuberculosis. Shortness of breath, putrid sputa. General weakness and prostration. Sleeplessness.

CLINICAL CASES

Tuberculosis of the Bones:

A case of tuberculosis of the bones in a boy ten years of age was entirely cured by the use of *Calc. Phos., Calc. Fluor.* and *Silicea.* For a time I also gave him small doses of fluoric acid to promote deposit of the lime salts. This case had been treated for nearly three years by the old method of bone-scraping.

(Dr. J. B. Chapman, Seattle, Wash.)

Tubercular Sinus:

Mr. G., æt. 45, had a tubercular sinus of the left hip. The discharge was so profuse that it had to be dressed two or three times a day. *Silicea,* in four weeks, stopped the discharge, and healed the sinus. This was five months ago and the cure still holds.

(Dr. J. S. S. Chesshir, Little River, Kans.)

Silicea in Tubercular Abscess:

A young man, age 19. Father and older sister died of tuberculosis. First symptom, a limp favoring right hip. X-ray showed affection of hip joint. He moved to Muncie, Indiana, and I did not see him for six months. He had been in plaster cast for weeks, he told me; and when I saw him again he was on crutches with a tubercular abscess of right hip joint. On removing dressing the discharge was very profuse. Emaciated, night sweats. *Silicea* (no other medicine) was given with little hope and no encouragement to anxious mother. But improvement was noticed in three or four weeks. The boy was faithful with his "tablets" and at the end of seven months laid aside one crutch and at the end of a year both crutches. Favored hip for a while by using a cane, then no cane. Saw him recently: walks without limp; hip is well; no night sweats; gained in weight, etc.

(Dr. I. N. Agenbroad, Dayton, Ohio.)

TUMORS AND CANCER

ETIOLOGY

Tumors vary in their composition, but they all arise, primarily, from a deficiency in Kali Mur., which causes an excess of fibrin in the system. Occasionally this fibrin collects in masses, and a tumor results.

Sometimes these tumors contain only fibrin, and their cure is very difficult, as there are no blood vessels in them, and consequently no method of introducing Kali Mur. into them to unite with the fibrin. In other cases they are filled with fat, still others with water and other liquids. In all cases, however, Kali Mur. is the chief remedy, with such other cell-salts as suppuration and other complications may call for.

The cause of cancer has so far not been discovered, but all present evidence points to the fact that the cancer cannot begin to grow until the vitality of the tissues surrounding it is lowered. It is therefore evident that the logical method of preventing cancer is to maintain the normal vitality of the tissues by watching for any symptoms of lacking cell-salts, and replacing them as soon as possible.

This same rule also holds good after a cancer has become established and the administration of whatever cell-salts the symptoms show to be lacking should be continued even where surgical, electrical, or other forms of treating the active manifestations of the cancer are adopted.

BIOCHEMIC TREATMENT

Kali Sulph.—Epithelial cancer; cancer on the skin, with characteristic *discharge of thin, yellow matter.* Externally and internally.

Calc. Fluor.—Tumors, knots or hardened glands in the breast. *Blood tumors on the heads of infants.* Hard swellings in any part. Ganglion, encysted tumors, from strain of elastic fibres.

Kali Phos.—Cancer, with offensive discharge and discoloration of the tissues. Greatly ameliorates the pain in cancer.

Natr. Mur.—Soft, watery swelling under the tongue. (*Calc. Phos.*).

Ferrum Phos.—For pain in the cancer; alternate with the chief remedies.

Calc. Phos.—Cancer in scrofulous constitutions. Goitre, cysts, house-maid's knee, etc.; also as an intercurrent remedy.

Silicea.—Swelling of glands, lumps, tumors, etc., which threaten to suppurate. Uterine cancer; scirrhous induration of the upper lip and face. Scrofulous tumors of the neck.

Natr. Phos.—"Cancer of the tongue has been greatly benefited by *Natr. Phos.*" (Walker.)

Cancer, using the term to include all malignant growths, is rapidly taking the lead as the principle cause of death in the fourth and fifth decades of life. The apparent increase in incidence of cancer may be due, in part to more accurate diagnosis, but must be to some degree attributed to dietary and other factors of our mode of life.

Although the exact cause of cancer has not yet been determined, certain observations lead to the theory of local irritation being at least one of the factors involved. For this reason it is advisable to remove constant sources of irritation wherever they may be found and in particular those special ones which seem to be concerned with the development of certain common sites of cancer.

The repair of damaged tissues in the uterine cervix has been definitely established as a valuable prophylactic measure against cancer of that organ as has also the removal of sharp roots of teeth and the irritation of the mouth from other sources as a means of prevention of cancer of the mouth.

Scars, moles and other low grade growths on the surface of the body are prone to undergo malignant degeneration and should be removed at the first sign of activity. As such a preponderance of all lumps in the female breast ultimately prove to be malignant, their early removal is an insurance against subsequent dangerous change.

Whatever the background for the changes which result in the growth of cancer, it is certain that the cell metamorphosis is at an early stage entirely a local process and if all the involved tissues be removed at this time, malignant degeneration at that point may be prevented. Therefore the early diagnosis of such change is of the utmost importance and constitutes the greatest factor of safety against the increasing incidence of this great menace to life and health. To stop the progress of a well developed cancer, is with the present knowledge and armamentarium of the medical profession, usually an impossibility and it is therefore largely a problem of time. The only time a cancer is amenable to our treatment is early in its life history and our greatest efforts must be bent toward discovering the incipient malignancy soon enough to attack it while still localized.

The early diagnosis of cancer is dependent on two factors, the education of the public in the early signs of danger that they may present themselves for examination before it is too late and the mental alertness of the medical profession to recognize and to properly evaluate these signs and to act promptly to eradicate the growth while still sufficiently localized to be amenable to cure.

CLINICAL CASES

Calc. Fluor. cured; other medicines failed:

A hard swelling under the chin, about the size of a pigeon's egg, disappeared completely in about four weeks, under the use of *Calc. Fluor.*

(Dr. F. From Schuessler.)

Calc. Phos. in House-Maid's Knee:

Dr. Fuchs, of Regensburg, reports: In August I cured a lady, æt. 40, who had suffered for a considerable time from an effusion in bursa of the knee-cap. Twelve doses of *Calc. Phos.*, two doses per diem, according to Dr. Schuessler, removed this chronic condition of house-maid's knee.

(From Schuessler.)

Calc. Phos. in Nasal Polypi:

Mrs. R. had nasal polypi in both nostrils; large, gray and bleeding easily. *Calc. Phos.*, a powder every morning for a week. The third week reported entirely free. The larger ones came away entirely; the smaller ones were absorbed.

(J. G. Gilchrist.)

Silicea in Multiple Cheloid:

Multiple cheloid, which appeared, after the excision of a tumor, in the scar. It was excised at St. Bartholomew's Hospital, but rapidly returned and increased in size, till the patient, a girl, was put on *Silicea*, night and morning. The gradual disappearance of the growth under this treatment was one of the prettiest things I have ever seen in medicine.

(John H. Clarke.)

TYPHLITIS

(See Peritonitis.)

BIOCHEMIC TREATMENT

Ferr. Phos.—In the initial stage, for the febrile symptoms, fever, inflammation, pain, high temperature, quick pulse, etc.

Kali Mur.—For swelling, hardness, tenderness, etc.; alternate with *Ferr. Phos.* Give copious injections of hot water, in which a quantity of the remedy is dissolved.

Silicea.—Calc. Sulph.—If abscess forms. See under Abscess for characteristic symptoms indicating these salts; also see note under Typhoid Fever on the value of injections.

Natr. Sulph.—"Dull pain in right ileo-cecal region. Shifting flatus; tenderness to pressure and coated tongue." (J. W. Ward, M. D.)

CLINICAL CASES

Ferr. Phos. and Kali Mur. in Typhlitis:

I was called, on the morning of April 14th, to attend to Mr. E. K., a young man, æt. 22, with hereditary tendency to phthisis pulmonalis, who resided in Connecticut, and was sojourning in our city for the benefit of his health, and found him suffering with agonizing pain in the right iliac region. He had been attacked suddenly at 2 o'clock a. m. with this pain, and had vomited several times before I saw him. Upon examination, I found a tumor in the right iliac fossa, so tender to the touch that he could not bear even the weight of the bed-clothing. His bowels had moved twice within a few hours. I learned that he had eaten of a mince-pie at dinner the day before, and had passed a quantity of currant seeds in one of his movements. There could be no doubt as to the diagnosis—typhlitis—and that a currant seed was the casus mali. His temperature was 103 F., and pulse 120. For several inches around the tumor the belly was as hard as a rock, showing a great amount of infiltration. I at once gave him *Ferrum Phos.* and *Kali Mur.*, to be taken every half hour, in alternation, day and night; poultices of flaxseed were kept constantly applied, as hot as could be borne, to alleviate the pain. At the end of thirty-six hours his temperature had fallen to 100 F., and pulse to 90. This treatment was continued without intermission, and the inflammatory symptoms steadily improved, and the size of the tumor gradually lessened. At the end of a week the temperature and pulse became normal, the tumor had entirely disappeared, the belly was soft and a mere trace of the tenderness remained. He took no other medicines. The result in this case is, I think, phenomenal, since in this class of cases the prognosis is always unfavorable; and the credit of the case can be clearly given to the iron and potash, the one removing the inflammation, the other causing the absorption of the infiltration, thus bringing about resolution and aborting perityphlitis and the consequent suppuration. Dr. Burdick, of Oakland, and Dr. Brigham, of San Francisco, were both called in consultation, and both agreed with me as to the disease, and both acquiesced in the treatment. We have no medicine which is the peer of *Ferrum Phos.* as a fever remedy, whether idiopathic or symptomatic; and none better than *Kali Mur.* to cause the absorption of infiltrations. *Calc. Fluor,* rapidly absorbed an indurated and sensitive growth extending from the cecum to the lower border of the liver. (Dr. I. E. Nicholson.)

TYPHOID FEVER

ETIOLOGY

Typhoid fever is a germ disease, the organism responsible being the bacillus of Eberth, or, as it is more frequently termed, the bacillus typhosus. It is necessary, however, in order that the germ can live and propagate in the system, that a suitable breeding place for it shall exist.

If the mucous membrane of the digestive tract is in a normal, healthy condition, the individual is in no danger of contracting typhoid. But if, through a lack of Kali Mur. the mucous membrane has become weakened by the presence of an excess of fibrin, which is trying to find an outlet from the system, a suitable breeding place for the bacillus typhosus is provided, and typhoid fever results.

The method of treatment is obvious. The mucous membrane must be restored to a normal condition, and the bacillus thus deprived of a breeding place. This can be accomplished by supplying the lacking Kali Mur., which will unite with the excess of fibrin that is irritating the intestinal mucous membrane, and relieve the condition. As soon as the mucous membrane is normal again, there is no longer a breeding place for the bacillus typhosus, and the disease disappears.

During the course of an attack of typhoid, other cell-salts than Kali Mur. may be lacking, and have to be supplied.

In the first stage of typhoid, Ferrum Phos. and Kali Phos. are usually indicated, in addition to Kali Mur. If the skin be dry, with a chilly sensation, Kali Sulph. should be given instead of Kali Mur. This treatment, with copious injections of hot water for the bowels and the observation of proper dietary precautions, will frequently break up the condition in two weeks, if taken at the very onset.

When the disease is not seen until it is running its course, Kali Mur. should be given as the chief remedy, with Ferrum Phos. for the fever, except afternoon fever which calls for Kali Sulph. If bilious symptoms appear, with green, watery diarrhea, give a few doses of Natrum Sulph. When the patient wanders in mind, with low mutterings, or bubbles of saliva on the tongue, or great languor and weakness, give Natrum Mur. in alternation with Kali Phos. In cases of hemorrhage, which very rarely occur if the biochemic treatment is adhered to, Kali Phos., Ferrum Phos. and Natrum Mur. should be given, and also enemas of normal salt solution. If the blood is dark and clotted, Kali Mur. is indicated.

Nursing and diet are all-important in typhoid fever. As a rule, milk is the best food. It should be given fresh and unskimmed, not less than three pints in twenty-four hours. Give enough, but do not overfeed. Plain water, limewater or coffee may be added to the milk to modify its taste. Six-ounce feedings, day and night, are suggested. If curds or fat-globules show in the stools, it is evident that the milk is not being digested, and it should either be peptonized or replaced, wholly or in part, by buttermilk, koumys, albumen water, mutton or beef broth strained, clam broth, barley water, junket, gruels. If emaciation is rapid and extreme, give farinaceous gruels, well cooked.

During convalescence, also, the diet must be watched most carefully, as the intestinal tract is still in a very delicate condition, and should be irritated as little as possible. Broths, milk-toast, whipped cream, scraped beef, wine jelly, baked potato, mush and milk, etc., can be given, but no solid food until the temperature has been normal for a week. If at any time the temperature rises above 100° F., return at once to a liquid diet.

BIOCHEMIC TREATMENT

Ferrum Phos.—*In the initiatory stage,* chilliness, fever, etc. As an alternate remedy as long as inflammatory symptoms remain. Typhoid fever, with prostration and hemorrhage of bright red blood.

Kali Mur.—The *principal remedy* in this disease, in alternation with *Ferrum Phos.,* for the febrile symptoms. Typhoid fever, with gray or white fur on the tongue or looseness of the bowels. Light-yellow stools; abdominal swelling and tenderness. Hemorrhage of dark, clotted blood.

Kali Sulph.—Typhoid fever, with *evening aggravation, rise of temperature,* rapid pulse, etc. Typhoid fever, with very slow, labored pulse, indicating blood-poisoning (also *Kali Phos.*)

Kali Phos.—*Malignant symptoms* in typhoid fever, especially those which affect the brain, causing temporary insanity. Weakness and debility.. Putrid stools, sleeplessness, offensive breath or weak action of the heart, calls for this remedy. Sleeplessness, sordes on the teeth; *tongue coated like stale mustard,* very dry, cleaves to roof of mouth. Inarticulate speech from dryness of tongue. Hallucinations of the brain.

Natr. Mur.—Malignant symptoms in typhoid fever, with watery vomiting, dry tongue, twitching, stupor, drowsiness, hemorrhage, etc.

Natr. Sulph.—When there are distinct bilious symptoms present, watery bilious stools, etc.

Calc. Phos.—During decline of the disease, to promote rebuilding of tissue also intercurrently through the course of the disease.

Note: "In the treatment of typhoid fever, I should urge the use of copious injections of hot water, per rectum. When the fever is high and the pulse quick, when the disease goes from 'bad to worse,' an injection of hot water will give marvelous results. If the bowels are costive, an injection will do the work without fear of the results of a cathartic; if diarrhea is present, an injection will cleanse the unhealthy membranes and promote normal absorption. Patients treated in this manner, together with an intelligent use of the inorganic salts, will make rapid recovery and will escape the excessive emaciation so common in this disease."
(Dr. Chapman.)

CLINICAL CASES

Typhoid Fever:

Mr. G. H. P. Typhoid fever. Usual symptoms with the following treatment: *Ferrum Phos.* during the first week. *Kali Mur.* during the second week, and *Kali Sulph.* during the third week. The whole course of the disease, as well as the convalescence period was uneventful.
(Dr. G. A. Budd, Frankfort, Kentucky.)

Ferrum Phos. and Kali Mur. the most rational remedies in Typhoid:

The following report, from the pen of Dr. A. P. Davis, of Dallas, Texas, is of interest, since it illustrates the value of these remedies in this disease: "The most rational course to pursue is to supply deficiencies and to assist nature remove excesses. There is depression perceptible in all cases of typhoid fever; and as this depression is the result of molecular change, the molecules of several elements must receive our special attention. It is a conceded fact that the inflammation in the glands of Brunner and Peyer keeps up the fever, and the remedy that cures these glands cuts short the disease; and the remedies that I have found to do this most certainly are *Ferrum Phos.* and *Kali Mur.*, given in alternation, every hour during fever, where there is a white or grayish coating on the tongue. The *Ferrum Phos.* is the best fever remedy, and the *Kali Mur.* the best eliminator in such conditions. If the tongue should become brown, give *Kali Phos.*, and especially in those cases where the patient is delirious or nervous, and in the more malignant form of the disease. If the tongue assumes a yellow, shiny coating, then resort to *Magnes. Phos.*, and especially when there is pain in the bowels and a sensation of pressure in the stomach. If the tongue has a golden-yellow coating, creamy, moist, give *Natr. Phos.* Should the tongue have a dirty brownish-green coating, give *Natr. Sulph.* These remedies are especially indicated in this condition of the tongue. Last of all, when the patient begins to convalesce, finish up the treatment with *Calc. Phos.*, as a connective tissue and blood-cell constituent is needed. In all cases where these tissue remedies have been used by me, they have proved abundantly sufficient, and will cure, if given as indicated. They supply the inorganic elements that are disturbed or lacking in all diseased states, and if a strict observance is had in their selection, the physician will certainly cure any diseases that can be cured at all."

Kali Phos. rallied the patient:

Miss Nettie W., æt. 23; as called in consultation; found the patient apparently in last stage of the disease, with the symptoms usual in such cases. As other remedies had been tried and she seemed sinking, I advised *Kali Phos.* in solution. Under the use of this remedy she rallied, and it was continued some days, with the result that she ultimately recovered. (C. T. M.)

TYPHUS FEVER

(See Typhoid Fever.)

BIOCHEMIC TREATMENT

Ferrum Phos.—Initiatory stage, for febrile conditions. Alternate with *Kali Phos.*

Kali Phos.—*Chief remedy for the malignant conditions.* Putrid, camp, farm, or brain fever are met with this salt. Sleeplessness, stupor, delirium, etc. Tongue coated like stale mustard.

Kali Mur.—In typhus fever, for costiveness; light, ochre-colored stools. Alternate with *Kali Phos.*

Natr. Mur.—In alternation with *Kali Phos.*, when the stupor and sleeplessness is excessive; also for watery conditions.

ULCERS AND ULCERATIONS

(See Abscess and Exudations,)

BIOCHEMIC TREATMENT

Kali Mur.—*Ulcerations when there is a thick, white fibrinous discharge.* Ulceration of the neck of womb, with the above discharge. Secretions mild, non-irritating. Tongue is frequently coated white or grayish-white.

Ferrum Phos.—Ulcerations, *for the febrile conditions,* heat inflammation, pain, etc.

Silicea.—Ulcers of the extremities, deep-seated, *affecting the periosteum.* Ulcers secreting thin, foul, yellow matter. Fistulous ulcers. Hard swelling and suppuration of the glands requires this remedy in large doses. Use internally and also locally.

Calc. Sulph.—Ulcers, which continue to discharge after infiltration has ceased; after *Silicea. Ulcers of the glands* or extremities, when secreting sanious, yellow matter; *suppurations resulting from wounds,* bruises, burns, scalds, etc.

Calc. Fluor.—Ulceration of bone substance; *discharge of thick, yellow pus* and splinters of bone.

Calc. Phos.—Intercurrent remedy in ulcerations, especially of the bone.

Natr. Phos.—Ulceration of stomach or bowels, with *vomiting* of sour, acid fluids, or *of a dark substance like coffee-grounds.* Syphilitic ulcers, creamy yellow coating on the tongue.

CLINICAL CASES

Silicea in Chronic Ulcer:

Woman, age 28, single. Has had measles, mumps, and chickenpox. A lot of other data without hearing on the case was collected. History of present complaint is:

Born with talipes varus; operated upon when she was six years old. The foot was in fair position giving good service, but she had an ulcer on the outer side of the foot most of the time since then. Occasionally it healed and for a week or two would be free from the necessity of dressing her foot. She had used every salve she had ever heard of, and had been treated by physicians often, having some dead bone removed at one time about twelve years ago, but the abscess formation had continued. Examination showed simply the site of a sinus leading to the deep instep, little swelling, little redness, little pain.

I told her that there should be several radiographs made so that one could study the bones from different angles and make a careful, complete diagnosis of which bones were the seat of the chronic infection. She refused and said all she wanted was a salve. I told her she had been using that kind of treatment for twenty-two years and it hadn't advanced her far. I told her to keep on with any salve she wished and that I knew none of them would cure her; and in the meantime I would give her the only medicine I could think of that might clear up the trouble. I gave her *Silicea,* four times daily. I did not see her for about two months when she told me the foot had healed in about a week. I saw her again three months later, still healed. That has been four years ago now, and she has had no abscess formation since. I do not know what result I could have secured by radiographs and surgery.
(Dr. G. R. Reay, La Crosse, Wisconsin.)

Silicea and Calc. Phos.—Ulcers four years—cured in four weeks:

A girl came into my office, who had sores on both legs, running a thin, ichorous secretion, red, angry and painful, which had been bothering her for four years, breaking out, then scabbing over, partially healing, then taking on inflammation, so that sleep was disturbed; locomotion produced severe pains; in fact, the sores were seemingly very severe. I at once gave her *Silicea,* and *Calc. Phos.,* three doses each per day, bound up the limbs with flannel roller bandage, and in four weeks all the sores were healed up and the patient well, cheerful and happy.
(A. P. Davis, M. D.)

Calc. Fluor. in indolent Ulcers:

A. S., æt. 16; for three years had indolent ulcers on lower half of leg, which is red, very much swollen. Three fistulous ulcers secreting a thick, yellow pus, and which have thrown

off many splinters of bone. Pains principally at night. Emaciation; poor appetite. Frequent cough in morning, with thick, yellow expectoration and considerable weakness. Lungs normal. *Calc. Fluor.*, morning and evening for eight days, alternating with intervals of four days without medicine. Cured in five months. Externally, only glycerine. No enlargement of the limb was noticeable after six months.
(Dr. Husen, *Allg. Med. Zeit.*)

Natr. Phos. in syphilitic Ulcers:

In treating a chronic syphilitic ulcer, I observed a yellow coating on the surface of the ulcer, which had the appearance of half-dried cream. After *Natr. Phos.*, the coating disappeared within four days, and the patient was otherwise much improved.

Calc. Fluor. in tibial Ulcers:

A young lady had been treated by two physicians for several months, without being much or permanently benefited. She had a pricking pain near the shin-bone, and had irritated a raised spot like a pin-head, and ulceration set in. Her general health had been good, but being ordered to recline a great deal for relief, and even keep to bed, as she suffered pain and was lame on walking, her health began to give way. Mrs. G., her mother, applied for the new remedies, as the doctors seemed puzzled with the case. The appearance of the limb seemed quite normal, except the ulcer. This led me to give *Calc. Fluor.*—externally as a lotion on lint, and every two hours a dose internally. On very minute inquiry it turned out that she suffered from menstrual colic, with cramp in the legs; for the cramp *Magnes. Phos.* was taken, giving rapid relief, and special attention paid that none of her garments were tight. The sore, a varicose ulcer, healed in a very short time, and has not troubled her since a lapse of three years.

URINARY DISORDERS

(See Also Bright's Disease and Kidneys, Diseases of.)

ETIOLOGY

Urinary disorders arise in the kidneys or bladder and may have a variety of exciting causes resulting in a deficiency of one or more or several cell-salts. Nervous shock, exposure to cold and dampness, injudicious diet, overuse of stimulants, etc., will cause the cells of certain tissues in the kidneys and bladder to break down and lose their inorganic contents, the resulting symptoms varying according to the salt which is lacking. The most common trouble of the bladder is enuresis or inability to retain the urine, which arises from a deficiency of *Kali Phos.* In children this is largely due to habit and may be overcome to a large extent by preventing the child from sleeping upon its back. To do this, a spool or other hard article should be fastened at the child's back by a string tied to its waist.

It should be thoroughly understood that diseases of these excretory organs are extremely dangerous and should never be neglected. Treatment should begin as early as possible and the diet should be carefully restricted to foods that will not aggravate the condition.

The excessive use of intoxicating liquors is frequently the cause of most diseases of this region, the excretory organs being unable to cope with the constant presence of alcohol in the system. The use of alcoholic drinks should, therefore, be strictly abstained from by the patient whose kidneys or bladder have become diseased.

If Biochemic treatment is begun and a careful diet observed soon after the inception of the disease, a complete and early recovery may be anticipated. If, however, the disease has become chronic, improvement of the condition will necessarily be slow. For this reason it is obviously far better that treatment is begun as soon as possible.

Biochemistry does not conflict with any other recognized system of combating disease, and the Biochemic remedies will in no way interfere with the action of remedies that may be advised by a reputable physician. The Biochemic remedies supply the body's deficient cell-salts, and until those deficiencies are supplied the body cannot get well. Drugs may be taken to relieve pain or stimulate the resistive forces of the body; serums may be given to combat germs and bacilli; diet and proper nursing may overcome the exciting causes of the disease; but health cannot be restored until the deficiencies have been overcome and the tissue brought back to a normal condition.

BIOCHEMIC TREATMENT

Ferrum Phos.—This remedy is indicated *in all inflammatory conditions of the bladder and urethra,* when in the acute stage. First stage of cystitis, with pain, heat and fever. Wetting the bed, in children. Enuresis from weakness of the muscles; frequently noticed in women, when *coughing causes spurting of the urine.* Incontinence from weakness of the sphincter muscle. Retention of urine from inflammatory conditions. *Constant urging to urinate,* due often to retaining the urine too long, thereby setting up an inflammation. Excessive amount of urine.

Kali Mur.—Second stage of cystitis, with swelling. *Chronic cystitis, principal remedy.* Discharge of thick, white mucus in the urine, indicating secondary stage of inflammations. Dark-colored urine; deposit of uric acid, accompanied with torpor and inactivity of the liver; also *Natr. Sulph.*

Magnes. Phos.—*Retention of the urine, from spasm of the muscles.* "After use of catheter, a sensation as if the muscles did not contract. (Walker.) Gravel, for the excessive pain.

Kali Phos.—Cystitis in asthenic conditions, with prostration. *Frequent urination,* with excessive secretion of urine, from nervous weakness or paralytic conditions. *Paralysis of the muscles, with inability to retain the urine. Urine causing scalding of the parts where it touches. Passing of blood from the urethra* (also *Ferrum Phos.*). Wetting the bed from weakness of the muscles.

Natr. Sulph.—*Brick-dust-like sediment in the urine;* lithic deposit *clings to the bottom and sides of vessel.* High-colored urine, when associated with gout or bilious conditions. Sandy deposit in urine, indicating gravel.

Calc. Phos.—Gravel, calculous or phosphatic deposit; intercurrently with or after *Natr. Sulph.,* to check reformation of stone. Flocculent sediment. Passing of semen in urine (also *Natr. Phos.*). Enuresis in old people. Spasmodic retention of urine if *Magnes. Phos.* fails to give results.

Calc. Sulph.—Inflammation of the bladder, when pus is discharging.

Natr. Phos.—*Incontinence* of urine *in children,* with symptoms of acidity or worms. *Gravel in the kidneys.* Dark-red urine associated with rheumatism.

Natr. Mur.—Passing of large quantities of urine, providing other symptoms correspond. Enuresis, with corresponding symptoms of this remedy.

CLINICAL CASES

Ferrum Phos. in Cystitis:

Miss M., æt. 18; very nervous character; gave way to a violent fit of anger, which caused prolapsus of womb and acute cystitis. After suffering great pain for some time, the womb was replaced, but the cystitis still remained. A vaginal injection of hot water and internal treatment with *Ferrum Phos.* and *Kali Phos.* brought quick relief, and she made a rapid recovery. *Ferrum Phos.* reduced the inflammation, and *Kali Phos.* controlled the nervous symptoms.

(J. B. Chapman, M. D.)

Natr. Mur. in Enuresis:

Dr. Schuessler, in a private communication to Dr. Zoeppritz, mentions the case of a lad to whom he had given, without effect, *Ferrum Phos.* for enuresis. A pustular eruption near the corners of the mouth appeared, for which he prescribed *Natr. Mur.*, which cured both the eruption and the enuresis.

Calc. Phos. in spasmodic Retention of Urine:

Dr. Cornelius, Oldenburg, reports a case of spasmodic retention of the urine. No urine was at first excreted; even the catheter failed to bring any away. *Magnes. Phos.* was given, which relieved somewhat; some urine was passed. In five days, no permanent or decided results being obtained from this remedy, Schuessler's advice was followed and accordingly *Calc. Phos.* was given, which cured in one day. Some two months later another attack came on, which was likewise immediately cured by *Calc. Phos.*, for on the following day the patient was well.

Kali Phos. in Enuresis:

Ruth B., nine years old, had suffered from nocturnal enuresis for four years. Came to me, and I prescribed *Kali Phos.*, three tablets every three hours.

Improvement in two weeks.

Continued treatment with *Kali Phos.* and the report now is only an occasional accident at night.
(Dr. R. E. Titman, East Orange, N. J.)

UTERUS, DISEASES OF

(See also Dysmenorrhea; Menstruation; Leucorrhea; Metritis and Labor and Pregnancy.)

BIOCHEMIC TREATMENT

Ferrum Phos.—*All inflammatory conditions of the uterus*, in the first stage, for heat, pain, congestion, etc. Inflammation of the vagina, with pain from sexual intercourse. *Excessive* *dryness and sensitiveness of the vagina;* also inject a solution of the remedy in hot water.

Kali Mur.—*Second stage* of inflammatory processes, *when exudation has taken place. Ulceration of the os and cervix uteri, with characteristic* discharge of *thick, white, mild secretions* from the mucous membrane. Chronic congestion of the uterus. Enlargement of the uterus, when not of stony hardness.

Kali Phos.—*Uterine hemorrhage, with discharge of thin, deep-red or blackish-red blood.* Displacement of the uterus, for the nervous symptoms.

Calc. Fluor.—*Chief remedy in prolapsus* or displacement of the uterus, as a constitutional tonic to strengthen the relaxed muscles. Dragging pains in the region of uterus and thighs; also in small of back. Parts pulsate with voluptuous feelings, with feeling of weakness in sexual organs. Hypertrophy of the uterus, when of stony hardness (alternate *Kali Mur.*). Lacerations of the cervix.

Calc. Phos.—Prolapsus, with weak, sinking feelings. *Displacements, with rheumatic pains. Weakness and distress in uterine region.* Intercurrently in all womb troubles. Valuable as a constitutional remedy.

CLINICAL CASES

Magnes. Phos.—Ovaralgia:

Mrs. P., æt. 42, a washer-woman, strained herself turning a clothes-wringer, causing acute inflammation of left ovary. When I was called she had been suffering for several hours, and spasmodic symptoms had begun to appear. I prescribed *Ferrum Phos.* and *Magnes. Phos.* in alternation—frequent doses. In half an hour my patient was almost entirely free from pain, and made a rapid recovery. Hot applications, also, was used over the abdomen.
(J. B. Chapman.)

Kali Phos. in Anteflexion, with Neuroses:

Lady, about 40; anteflexion of uterus, with very peculiar nervous condition. Very solicitous about health; weak; exhausted with slight effort. Irritable and easily displeased, which was unnatural to her. Had suffered many annoyances. Hyperemia of the brain and hyperesthesia, which condition made her utterly miserable most of the time. *Kali Phos.* entirely cured.

(Sarah N. Smith, New York.)

Kali Phos. in Ovaralgia:

Miss B., æt. 20, had been suffering for the last two years with severe ovaralgia at the menstrual period. She had been under the treatment of several physicians, and the only relief that they were able to give her was by the use of *Morphine,* that being only temporary. Was called late one night to see her and found her suffering with severe pain in the left ovary, of a dull, dragging character, and but slightly intermittent. Patient hysterical and very excitable. Gave her *Kali Phos.* in water, every ten minutes for half an hour, when patient went to sleep, not waking until morning, when she was free from pain. Gave *Kali Phos.* once a day for a month, and now, after eighteen months, has had no more pain, and is feeling better every way.

(G. H. Martin, M. D.)

Calc. Fluor. in Papillomatous Erosion of Cervix:

Dr. Phil. Porter reports a cure of papillomatous erosion of the cervix with *Calc. Fluor.*, in which the local symptoms were accompanied by a dyscrasic condition, enlarged cervical glands, emaciation and weakness. His prescription was based upon the constitutional changes, the local conditons, the fissured appearance of the cervix, and an abundant yellowish leucorrhea.

VARICOSE ULCERS

(See Ulcers and Ulcerations.)

VEINS, DISEASES OF

BIOCHEMIC TREATMENT

Ferrum Phos.—A powerful vein remedy. Small aneurism, in the early stage; alternate with *Calc. Fluor.*, the chief remedy. For the pain in varicocele of the testicles.

Calc. Fluor.—*Chief remedy in dilation of the veins;* varicose veins of the extremities. Varicose ulcerations; also as a lotion on lint. A rubber bandage or elastic stocking should also be worn.

VERTIGO

BIOCHEMIC TREATMENT

Ferrum Phos.—Vertigo, or giddiness, from rush of blood to the head, with throbbing pain and flushed face, on arising from a stooping position.

Kali Phos.—*Dizziness, when from nervous causes or weakness.* Vertigo, with anemic conditions. *Vertigo worse from rising and looking upward.* Vertigo from exhaustion.

Natr. Sulph.—*Vertigo arising from bilious derangements,* yellow-coated tongue and bitter taste. Excess of bile.

Natr. Phos.—*Dizziness, with gastric derangements,* acid conditions, etc.

CLINICAL CASES

Natr. Phos. cured Vertigo with vomiting:

Dr. E. B. Rankin, of Washington, D. C., reports a case of vertigo of several weeks' standing, accompanied by vomiting of acid substances, cured by *Natr. Phos.* in one week.

Kali Phos. in Vertigo from rising:

A woman, æt. 64, came under my treatment, who had been for many years treated without success. She had taken baths

and quinine. She complained of a severe vertigo, felt mostly on rising from a sitting position and on looking upward. She was constantly in dread of falling, and did not venture to leave her room. I gave her all the usual remedies, without any benefit. At last I gave her, in May, two doses daily of *Kali Phos.* I had the pleasure of seeing a rapid and decided cure following this. The patient can attend to her domestic duties; she can go out alone, even to distances, and is almost completely cured of her painful sensation of giddiness.
(From Schuessler.)

VOMITING

BIOCHEMIC TREATMENT

Ferrum Phos.—Vomiting of undigested food, sometimes with sour fluids (*Natr. Phos., Natr. Mur.*). *Vomiting of bright-red blood,* which coagulates easily and quickly.

Kali Mur.—Vomiting of thick, white phlegm, or of dark, almost black blood, clotted and viscid.

Natr. Mur.—Vomiting or sour fluids. *Vomiting of watery, transparent mucus.* Water-brash, associated with constipation.

Kali Phos.—Vomiting of dark substances like coffee grounds.

Natr. Phos.—*Vomiting of sour* or *acid fluids,* or *curdy masses;* note also the coating on the back part of the tongue.

Natr. Sulph.—*Vomiting of bile* or bilious matter, with bitter taste in the mouth.

Calc. Phos.—Vomiting, from non-assimilation of the food, periodically at a certain hour of the night. Infants vomit often and easily from cold drinks.

Magnes. Phos.—Spasmodic vomiting, especially if accompanied with violent pains in stomach.

Calc. Fluor.—*Vomiting of undigested food,* if *Ferr. Phos.* does not give relief.

CLINICAL CASES

Ferrum Phos. in painless Vomiting:

F., æt. 54; had suffered for six months from vomiting of food. Some hours after dinner, unless it had consisted of milk foods, he would vomit it up painlessly and without exertion. The vomiting would be preceded by a shaking, as from a chill, and would occur with a gush. His appetite was good, and there was no other bad feeling. By moving about he could postpone the vomiting for about an hour. Immediately after vomiting he could eat more. On November 17, he received *Ferrum Phos.*, a dose morning and evening. On December 1st, he reported that he was entirely cured.

Calc. Phos. for morning Vomiting:

Mrs. W., æt. 35; vomited food every morning at 4 o'clock; no pains; hot water relieved. After trying a great many remedies, without any good results, I gave *Calc. Phos.*, five-grain dose before retiring; cured in one week.
(J. B. Chapman.)

Magnes. Phos. in persistent Vomiting:

W. J. Martin, M. D., in the Transactions Penn. Med. Society, reports a case of persistent vomiting, accompanied by pains in the abdomen, cured by *Magnes. Phos.*, after the ordinary remedies had failed.

Ferrum Phos. for painless Vomiting after meals:

A young girl, about 18, consulted me (so writes a student of medicine) for painless vomiting, which had existed for a long time, and occurred after almost every meal. The color of her face and the visible mucous membranes were pale. Menstruation was scanty and delayed. No other symptoms of importance; pregnancy was not present. I ordered *Ferrum Phos.* After a time I accidentally saw the patient again, and received the pleasing news that the vomiting had entirely disappeared from the commencement of the use of the remedy.

WHITLOW

(*See Abscess.*)

WHOOPING COUGH

This disease is caused by an accumulation of fibrin and other organic matter, in connective tissue adjoining the bronchial tubes and also the glottis, and a thickening of the epiglottis. The salts that are found in connection with this organic matter have fallen below the standard in amount. The principal deficiency is in the phosphate of magnesium which causes a contraction of muscular fibres and produces the spasmodic cough and "whoop." There is also a severe irritation of the mucous membranes of the bronchi, and a consequent heavy secretion of albuminous phlegm, denoting a molecular disturbance in the phosphate of lime.

BIOCHEMIC TREATMENT

Kali Mur.—*Principal remedy, if there is white-coated tongue or thick, white expectoration.* Also spasmodic cough similar to whooping-cough, but without the whoop.

Magnes. Phos.—Whooping cough, for the paroxysms of coughing ending in a whoop. A steady course of the remedy is necessary when the *fits of coughing are very acute;* dissolve the remedy in hot water. *Chronic whooping cough* (alternate with *Kali Mur.*).

Kali Phos.—An intercurrent remedy in whooping cough, for the symptoms of exhaustion, or in very nervous, sensitive subjects.

Ferrum Phos.—Whooping cough, for the febrile symptoms or vomiting of blood from excessive coughing.

Kali Sulph.—Whooping cough, with characteristic expectoration.

Natr. Mur.—The expectoration will guide in the selection of this remedy.

Calc. Phos.—Whooping cough, after *Magnes. Phos.*, or in obstinate cases, where the lime-salts are at fault.

CLINICAL CASES

The family doctor gave her up:

In the spring of last year, when there was an epidemic of whooping cough amongst the children here, a little child of ten months was given up by the family doctor. I heard this from the father of the child, who was in great grief. He mentioned that the spasms, which occurred about ten times in the course of a day, were so severe that the little face became quite livid, blue and swollen. I at once gave *Magnes. Phos.* One dose moderated the spasms so forcibly that they returned only occasionally, and the attacks were quite mild. Five days later I gave *Kali Phos.*, but without beneficial effect; then *Calc. Phos.*, and it had no effect. As the paroxysms grew only worse for want of *Magnes. Phos.*, I ordered it to be taken again, and in a very short time the spasms and whoop were gone, and the child recovered rapidly.
(From the *Rundschau.*)

Kali Sulph. in last stage of Whooping Cough:

Child, aged 18 months, in the last stage of whooping cough, with blistered lips and mouth; black, thin, offensive stools five times a day; hard and tympanitic abdomen; wasted to a shadow, and was given up to die by parents and another physician. I prescribed *Kali Sulph.* which effected complete cure in a short time.
(C. B. Knerr, M. D.)

WOMEN, DISEASES OF

(See Dysmenorrhea; Menstruation; Leucorrhea; Labor and Pregnancy; Metritis; Uterus, Diseases of.)

WORMS

BIOCHEMIC TREATMENT

Natr. Phos.—The *principal remedy* for all kinds of worms to destroy the excess of lactic acid upon which the worms live. Symptoms of acidity, in children, with pain in the bowels, picking of the nose, itching of the anus, restless sleep or grinding of the teeth are all signs of worms. A steady course of this remedy is necessary. For pin-worms, also an injection of a very strong solution of salt, in half a pint of warm water.

Calc. Fluor.—Itching at the anus, from piles; frequently mistaken for pin-worms.

Kali Mur.—Small, white thread-worms, with itching of anus, white tongue, etc. (alternate with *Natr. Phos.*).

Ferrum Phos.—*Intestinal worms, with passing of undigested food.* Febrile symptoms in worm troubles.

CLINICAL CASES

Natr. Phos. a worm remedy:

Dr. Schuessler recommends this drug as efficient in verminous affections. Dr. A. C. Kimball, of Barteville Station, Nebraska, reports a case in his practice with the following results: The patient, a boy aged 5 years, had spasms, and had been treated by several physicians, without benefit. After using *Natr. Phos.* for six weeks, three times a day, he passed four feet three inches of tape-worm, much to the astonishment of all interested. This is the first recorded case of *Natr. Phos.* producing such a result. It is believed that the entire worm was passed, there being no evidence of any remaining. *Natr. Phos.* is especially efficient in cases of pin-worms.

Natr. Phos. and Kali Phos. in Worms:

Case of a young girl, literally alive with pin worms. Vermifuge of different kinds had been administered by medical men for more than a year without results. *Natr. Phos.* given for four days, followed by a high enema of strong salt solution,

brought the worms by thousands. Worst case I ever saw. Continued the *Natr. Phos.* with *Kali Phos.* for 60 days, restricted candies and other sweets. Has never been troubled since.
(J. B. Chapman, M. D.)

Natr. Phos. in Worms:

Baby K., aged three years, has for a long time been troubled with worms and indigestion. On several occasions spasms came on as a result of the worms. Always has a coated tongue and an offensive breath. Child is cross and peevish, never satisfied, sleeps poorly. *Natr. Phos.*, a dose three times a day for three weeks, brought about such a change that all the neighbors were astonished. Child gained four pounds in flesh in these three weeks.
(Wm. Steinrauf, M. D.)

WOUNDS

(See Mechanical Injuries.)

PART IV.

Repertory of the Twelve Biochemic Remedies

Edited by

A. B. Hawes, M. D.

PART IV.

Repertory of the Twelve Biochemic Remedies

Edited by

A. B. Hawes, M. D.

GENERAL SYMPTOMS

Accumulation of serum or water in the areolar tissue: *Natr. Mur.*

Abscess, easily bleeding, after matter has been formed, to promote pus: *Silicea.*

Aggravation by motion: *Ferrum Phos.*

Aggravated in heated room or in the evening: *Kali Sulph.*

All ailments depending upon a deficiency or disturbance in the phosphate of lime molecules: *Calc. Phos.*

All inflammations where there is watery, yellow or greenish purulent secretions: *Kali. Sulph.*

All injuries to the soft tissues, strains, sprains, cuts, blows, or burns: *Ferrum Phos.*

All stomach and bowel troubles that are worse after eating fats: *Kali Mur.*

All symptoms that are worse in the morning and in damp, rainy weather, and better in dry, warm atmosphere: *Natr. Sulph.*

All symptoms of this remedy are relieved by heat, pressure, and rubbing: *Magnes. Phos.*

All symptoms of this remedy are worse from cold surroundings, cold air, draughts, etc.: *Magnes. Phos.*

Always better in the cool air: *Kali Sulph.*

Anguish, tremor and sweat during the pains: *Natr. Carb.*

Anemia: *Calc. Phos.*

Anemia, to build up the blood cells: *Ferrum Phos.*

Anemic conditions with characteristic symptoms of this remedy *Kali Phos.*

Anemic conditions with thin watery blood: *Natr. Mur.*

Anxious trembling with languor: *Calc. Phos.*

Atrophic conditions of old people; tissues dry, scaly, lack of vitality: *Kali Phos.*

Better by heat and in a warm room: *Silicea.*

Better from eating: *Kali Phos.*

Better from excitement: *Kali Phos.*

Better from motion: *Kali Phos.*

Better from pleasant company: *Kali Phos.*

Better from warm, dry atmosphere: *Calc. Sulph.*

Better in the evening: *Natr. Mur.*

Better in warm weather and in a warm room: *Calc. Phos.*

Bleeding from the nose in children, and anemic persons: *Ferrum Phos.*

Bones weak and friable, easily broken, will not unite; when new bone material is needed: *Calc. Phos.*

Bruises of the bones, with uneven, hard lumps: *Calc. Fluor.*

Burns of all degrees: *Kali Mur.*

Cachexia following ague, from excessive use of quinine: *Natr. Mur.*

Chlorosis: *Calc. Phos.*

Chlorotic conditions; chlorosis with torpid blood: *Natr. Mur.*

Chronic inflammation of lymphatic glands, watery secretions from some of the membranes: *Natr. Mur.*

Consumption, when the exudation is yellow, watery and green: *Natr. Sulph.*

Colic worse at night: *Calc. Phos.*

Congestive neuralgia, after catching cold, with inflammatory conditions: *Ferrum Phos.*

Convulsions: *Magnes. Phos., Calc. Phos.*

Chorea : *Magnes. Phos.*

Convulsions in teething children, young girls, and old people, when the lime salts are deficient : *Calc. Phos.*

Convulsions with fever in teething : *Ferrum Phos.*

Cramps worse at night : *Calc. Phos.*

Creeping paralysis : *Kali Phos.*

Convulsions worse at night : *Calc. Phos.*

Cuts and bruises if there is swelling and exudation : *Kali Mur.*

Defective development, with pale greenish white complexion : *Calc. Phos.*

Disease of the pancreas : *Calc. Phos.*

Digging pain down the back part of the thigh to the knee, accompanied by stiffness, great restlessness and pain : *Kali Phos.*

Drawing in the limbs : *Silicea.*

Dropsy arising from heart, liver, or kidney diseases, or from obstruction of the bile ducts, generally white coating on the tongue; whitish liquid on aspiration : *Kali Mur.*

Dropsy from heart disease : *Calc. Fluor.*

Dropsy in any part of the body : *Natr. Mur.*

Dropsy invading the areolar tissues of the body : *Natr. Mur.*

Dryness of some of the mucous membranes, with excess secretion in others : *Natr. Mur.*

Emaciation : *Calc. Phos., Natr. Mur.*

Emaciation : *Natr. Mur.*

Encysted tumors, swellings, and indurated enlargements, hardened glands, etc. : *Calc. Fluor.*

Epilepsy and spasms, occurring at night or from slight provocation, very obstinate cases : *Silicea.*

Epilepsy, chief remedy, with coated tongue, protruding appearance of the eyes : *Kali Mur.*

Epilepsy with sunken countenance, coldness and palpitation of the heart after the fit : *Kali Phos.*

Epilepsy from any cause : *Magnes. Phos.*

Epilepsy occurring with or after the suppression of eczema, or other eruptions : *Kali Mur.*

Epilepsy with rush of blood to the head and febrile conditions: *Ferrum Phos.*

Epithelial cancer with discharge; serious watery exudation from the membrane: *Kali Sulph.*

Exhaustion and weakness from any cause which has lowered the standard of the nervous system: *Kali Phos.*

Exuberant granulations: *Kali Mur.*

Exudation from any mucous membrane or flesh sore of a creamy-yellow or honey color which can be traced to a disturbance of the molecules of Sodium Phosphate in bone disease: *Natr. Phos.*

Exudation from the mucous lining which is corroding and chafing: *Kali Phos.*

Exudation mixed with blood: *Kali Phos.*

Face sore and sallow, when watery symptoms are present: *Natr. Mur.*

Facial paralysis: *Kali Phos.*

Feeling of weakness: *Natr. Mur.*

Fibrinous, thick, white, slimy exudations from any tissue, after inflammation or when not becoming absorbed it causes swelling or enlargement: *Kali Mur.*

Foul exudations: *Kali Phos.*

Gangrenous conditions in early stages of mortification: *Kali Phos.*

Glandular swellings: *Kali Mur.*

Hands and feet twitch during sleep: *Natr. Sulph.*

Hemorrhage from a small external vessel may be controlled by applying this remedy locally and binding on a compress tightly: *Ferrum Phos.*

Hemorrhage from any part of the body when the blood is bright red with tendency to coagulate rapidly: *Ferrum Phos.*

Hemorrhage from any part of the body when the blood is thin, dark, putrid, and not coagulating: *Kali Phos.*

Hemorrhage, hot applications will generally relieve, especially in hardened conditions: *Calc. Fluor.*

Hysteric attacks from sudden emotion, nervous fidgety feeling: *Kali Phos.*

Hysterical feeling worse in the morning or in cold weather: *Natr. Mur.*

Hysterical spasms and debility: *Natr. Mur.*

Ichorous exudations: *Kali Phos.*

In all cases of suppurations when the discharge continues too long: *Calc. Sulph.*

In anemia this remedy would be used intercurrently if skin affections are present: *Kali Mur.*

In bone diseases and fractures: *Ferrum Phos.*

In dropsy when the disease is caused by loss of blood: *Ferrum Phos.*

In epistaxis, locally in the nostrils: *Ferrum Phos.*

In ulceration of the tissues, to control fever and pain: *Ferrum Phos.*

Infantile paralysis: *Kali Phos.*

Infiltration: *Natr. Sulph.*

Involuntary shaking of the head: *Magnes. Phos.*

Lassitude, tired and weary feeling when accompanied by bilious symptoms: *Natr. Sulph.*

Inability to endure cold, occasioning coryza, colic and diarrhea: *Natr. Mur.*

Lock-jaw; frequent doses in hot water: *Magnes. Phos.*

Locomotor paralysis: *Kali Phos.*

Malignant, gangrenous inflammations: *Silicea.*

Mumps: *Natr. Mur.*

Neglected cases of injury, with suppuration: *Silicea.*

Nervous affections; patient irritable, impatient, dwells upon grievances, despondent, cries easily, makes mountains out of molehills; *Kali Phos.*

Nervous sensitiveness, feels pain very keenly; better when the attention is occupied by pleasant excitement: *Kali Phos.*

Nervousness, with trembling and palpitation of the heart and acid condition of the stomach: *Natr. Phos.*

Nervousness without any reasonable cause; hysteria: *Kali Phos.*

Neuralgia shooting pains along the nerve fibres, accompanied by flow of tears and saliva: *Natr. Mur.*

Neuralgias which are worse at night; colic, cramps, spasms: *Magnes. Phos.*

Neuralgic nerve pains with flow of saliva or tears, or when recurring periodically: *Natr. Mur.*

Neuralgic pains occurring in any organ, with depression, failure of strength, sensitiveness, noise, and light. Improved during pleasant excitement and gentle motion, but most felt when quiet and alone: *Kali Phos.*

Obstinate neuralgias occurring at night, when neither heat nor cold relieve: *Silicea.*

Offensive exudations: *Kali Phos.*

Pains all over the body like electric shocks, and at other times like trickling of cold water: *Calc. Phos.*

Pains are increased and aggravated by motion: *Kali Mur.*

Pains are severe at night with creeping sensation, also numbness and coldness: *Calc. Phos.*

Pains of a neuralgic nature, with tendency to shift from one place to another: *Kali Sulph.*

Pains worse from continued exercise: *Kali Phos.*

Paralysis agitans: *Magnes. Phos.*

Paralysis in which the vital powers are reduced, and stools have putrid odor; fetid breath; bad taste: *Kali Phos.*

Paralysis of any part of the body, and of all varieties: *Kali Phos.*

Paralysis when associated with rheumatism: *Calc. Phos.*

Patient is tired and weary: *Calc. Phos.*

Patient tired and exhausted: *Magnes. Phos.*

Patient suffering from suppressed sexual instinct or from excessive sexual indulgence: *Kali Phos.*

Polypi: *Calc. Phos.*

Poor nutrition through indigestion: *Calc. Phos.*

Proud flesh: *Kali Mur.*

Purulent discharge in gonorrhea, syphilis, bubo, leucorrhea, catarrh and consumption: *Calc. Sulph.*

Relaxed elastic tissue: *Calc. Fluor.*

Relieved by cold: *Ferrum Phos.*

Restlessness and twitching of the muscles: *Natr. Mur.*

Rheumatism with acid symptoms: *Natr. Phos.*

Rickets: *Calc. Phos.*

Rickets with offensive putrid stools: *Kali Phos.*

Rise of temperature in the evening, until midnight: *Kali Sulph.*

Sanious exudations: *Kali Phos.*

Sciatica: *Kali Phos.*

Scrofulous enlarged glands: *Silicea.*

Scurvy, gangrenous conditions: *Kali Phos.*

Scurvy with hard infiltrations: *Kali Mur.*

Sensation of numbness in parts affected, cannot bear to have spine touched; over-sensitive to pressure; paralytic pain in small of back: *Natr. Mur.*

Septic hemorrhages: *Kali Phos.*

Serous effusions, poor in albumen, slimy, like boiled starch: *Natr. Mur.*

Serous exudations: *Kali Phos.*

Slimy, frothy appearance of the tongue with watery secretions: *Natr. Mur.*

Smooth edematous swellings: *Natr. Sulph.*

Spasms and neuralgic pains in any tissue due to a deficiency or unequalization of the Magnesium Phosphate molecules: *Magnes. Phos.*

Spasms worse at night: *Calc. Phos.*

Spinal anemia from exhausting diseases: *Kali Phos.*

Sprains: *Kali Mur.*

Squinting, and grinding of the teeth with intestinal irritation; from worms: *Natr. Phos.*

Stunted growth: *Calc. Phos.*

Sudden or creeping paralysis of the vocal cords causing loss of voice: *Kali Phos.*

Suppurating glands with thick, yellow, offensive discharge of matter: *Silicea.*

Suppuration of bones and periosteum; ulcers, felons. etc.: *Calc. Fluor.*

Suppuration with offensive pus: *Kali Phos.*

Suppurations with ulcerations of the glands: *Calc. Sulph.*

Swelling of the glands: *Silicea.*

Symptoms aggravated by use of water in any form: *Natr Sulph.*

Symptoms are generally aggravated by noise, exertion, arising from sitting position: *Kali Phos.*

Symptoms are generally worse at night, in damp, cold weather, and change of weather, getting wet, etc.: *Calc. Phos.*

Symptoms are worse in the morning: *Natr. Mur.*

Tabes or atrophy of the muscles, organs or tissues: *Calc. Phos.*

Thick yellow or sanious discharge from any organ of the body: *Calc. Sulph.*

Trembling and involuntary motion of the hands: *Magnes. Phos.*

Ulceration and caries of bone: *Silicea.*

Ulceration of bone substance: *Calc. Phos.*

Ulcers of lower limbs, with characteristic discharge: *Calc. Sulph.*

Want of sensitiveness: *Magnes. Phos.*

Wasting diseases when putrid conditions are present: *Kali Phos.*

Wasting of spinal cord: *Kali Mur.*

Worse from getting wet: *Calc. Sulph.*

Worse in cold weather: *Natr. Mur.*

Worse in salty atmosphere: *Natr. Mur.*

Worse in the open air: *Silicea.*

Worse when alone: *Kali Phos.*

Writers cramp: *Magnes. Phos.*

Yellowish, watery secretions from any tissue: *Natr. Sulph.*

HEAD SYMPTOMS

All pains when heat relieves and cold aggravates: *Magnes. Phos.*

Asthenic conditions: *Kali Phos.*

Bald spots: *Calc. Phos.*

Blind headache: *Ferrum Phos.*

Blood tumors, on head: *Calc. Fluor.*

Brain, anemic conditions of: *Kali Phos.*

concussion of: *Kali Phos.*

to prevent dropsy of: *Calc. Phos.*

violent pains at base of: *Natr. Sulph.*

water on: *Calc. Phos.*

Cold applications relieve: *Ferrum Phos.*

Crawlings over head, with cold sensations: *Calc. Phos.*

Crusta lactea: *Calc. Sulph., Kali Mur., Kali Sulph.*

Crusts, yellow, on scalp: *Calc. Sulph.*

Dandruff: *Natr. Mur., Kali Sulph.*

Dilated pupils: *Kali Phos.*

Discharges of a sanious nature: *Calc. Sulph.*

Dizziness, from cerebral causes: *Kali Phos.*

Dropsy of brain, to prevent: *Calc. Phos.*

Dull stitching pain in the parietal bone: *Natr. Mur.*

Eruptions on scalp, with watery contents: *Natr. Mur.*

Eruption and nodules on the scalp with falling out of the hair: *Silicea.*

on the head with secretions of decidedly yellow, thin matter: *Kali Sulph.*

scalp with watery contents: *Natr. Mur.*

Fontanelles, closure of, delayed: *Calc. Phos.*

reopening of: *Calc. Phos.*

Giddiness, with gastric derangements: *Natr. Phos.*

Gone sensation at stomach: *Kali Phos.*

Hair, falling of: *Kali Phos., Silicea.*

loss of: *Calc. Phos.*

pulling causes pain: *Ferrum Phos.*

Hawking of thick, white mucus: *Kali Mur.*

Head, cold to touch: *Calc. Phos.*
inability to hold up: *Calc. Phos.*
involuntary shaking of: *Magnes. Phos., Kali Phos.*
rheumatic pains in: *Magnes. Phos.*
sore to touch: *Ferrum Phos.*
suppurations of: *Calc. Sulph.*
sweat on, of children: *Calc. Phos., Silicea.*
trembling of: *Magnes. Phos., Kali Phos.*
tumors on, in new-born infants: *Calc. Fluor.*
ulceration on bony surface of: *Calc. Fluor.*
ulcers on top of: *Calc. Phos.*
Headache, bruising, throbbing, beating: *Ferrum Phos.*
accompanied by:
chills up and down spine: *Magnes. Phos.*
cold feeling on head: *Calc. Phos.*
confusion: *Kali Phos.*
constipation: *Natr. Mur., Kali Mur.*
drowsiness: *Natr. Mur.*
dull, heavy, hammering: *Natr. Mur., Ferrum Phos.*
feeling as if skull were too full: *Natr. Phos.*
frothy coating on tongue: *Natr. Mur.*
hammering, throbbing: *Ferrum Phos.*
hysteria: *Kali Phos.*
inability for thought: *Kali Phos.*
intermittent and spasmodic pains: *Magnes. Phos.*
loss of strength: *Kali Phos., Calc. Phos.*
nodules, on head: *Silicea.*
pain in temples: *Ferrum Phos., Natr Phos.*
over eye: *Ferrum Phos.*
in stomach: *Natr. Phos.*
on top of head: *Ferrum Phos., Natr. Sulph.*
profusion of tears: *Natr. Mur.*
prostrated feeling: *Kali Phos.*

Headache, accompanied by restlessness and nervousness at puberty: *Calc. Phos.*
rush of blood to head: *Ferrum Phos.*
sharp, shooting pains: *Magnes. Phos.*
suffused eyes: *Ferrum Phos.*
tearful mood: *Kali Phos.*
thick white coating on the tongue: *Kali Mur.*
unrefreshing sleep: *Natr. Mur.*
vomiting of frothy phlegm: *Natr. Mur.*
weariness: *Kali Phos.*
yawning and stretching: *Kali Phos.*
after taking thick sour milk: *Natr. Phos.*
aggravated by mental work: *Calc. Phos., Kali Phos.*
in evening: *Kali Sulph.*
heated room: *Kali Sulph.*
near sutures: *Calc. Phos.*
when alone: *Kali Phos.*
from loss of sleep: *Kali Phos.*
mental work: *Kali Phos.*
in nervous subjects: *Kali Phos.*
Neuralgic: *Kali Phos., Magnes. Phos.*
with humming in the ears: *Kali Phos., Ferrum Phos.*
of girls at puberty: *Natr. Mur., Calc. Phos.*
nervous character, with illusions of light: *Magnes. Phos.*
on awakening in the morning: *Natr. Phos.*
crown of head: *Natr. Phos.*
top of head, with pressure: *Natr. Phos.*
with heat: *Natr. Phos.*
relieved by cheerful excitement: *Kali Phos.*
cool air: *Kali Sulph.*
rheumatic, evening aggravations: *Kali Sulph.*
sick, from sluggish action of liver: *Kali Mur.*
with bitter taste in mouth: *Natr. Sulph.*

Headache, accompanied by vomiting of acid sour fluids: *Natr. Phos.*
undigested food: *Natr. Phos., Ferrum Phos*
Heaviness from the nape of the neck to the vertex: *Silicea.*
of the head in the morning after waking, with giddiness and dullness: *Natr. Mur.*
Inability to hold up the head: *Calc. Phos.*
Inflammatory condition of the scalp: *Ferrum Phos.*
Mouth, bitter taste in: *Natr. Sulph.*
Neck, sharp pain in nape of: *Magnes. Phos.*
Neuralgia of head when pain is sharp: *Magnes. Phos.*
Neuralgic headache with humming in the ears, better under cheerful excitement, worse alone, tearful mood: *Kali Phos.*
Noises in head when falling asleep: *Kali Phos.*
Nose-bleed relieves: *Ferrum Phos.*
Pain in the nape of the neck of a sharp character: *Magnes. Phos.*
Painful pustules, suppurating wounds, with characteristic thick, yellow discharge of pus: *Silicea.*
Pain and weight in the back part of the head, with weariness and exhaustion: *Kali Phos.*
Pain, aggravated by cold: *Magnes. Phos.*
relieved by cheerful excitement: *Kali Phos.*
gentle motion: *Kali Phos.*
heat: *Magnes. Phos.*
Parietal bone, dull stitching pain in the: *Natr. Mur.*
Scalp, eruption on: *Silicea.*
inflammatory conditions of: *Ferrum Phos.*
nodules on: *Silicea.*
painful, pustules on: *Silicea.*
sensitive: *Silicea.*
sore to touch: *Silicea., Ferrum Phos.*
suppurations of, discharge yellow and purulent: *Calc. Sulph.*
tight sensations of: *Calc. Phos.*
white scales on: *Natr. Mur., Kali Mur., Kali Sulph.*

Sick headache arising from sluggish action of the liver, want of bile frequently accompanied by constipation: *Kali Mur.*

when the material vomited is undigested food: *Ferrum Phos.*

with bitter taste in the mouth; vomiting of bile or bilious diarrhea: *Natr. Sulph.*

vomiting of sour fluids: *Natr. Phos.*

Skull, thin and soft: *Calc. Phos.*

Sleeplessness: *Kali Phos.*

Spasmodic symptoms and delirium: *Ferrum Phos.*

Spinal meningitis, with determination of blood to the head; spasmodic symptoms and delirium: *Natr. Sulph.*

Secondary remedy: *Kali Mur.*

Spirits, hopeless, dejected: *Natr. Sulph.*

Stitches in the head: *Natr. Mur.*

Sun-stroke: *Natr. Mur.*

Suppuration of the head or scalp, when the discharge is yellow, purulent matter, or when forming crusts of the same matter: *Calc. Sulph.*

Tic Douloureux: *Calc. Phos., Ferrum Phos. Magnes. Phos.*

Tongue, dirty coating on: *Natr. Sulph.*

greenish-brown coating on back part of: *Natr. Sulph.*

greenish-gray coating on: *Natr. Sulph.*

Trembling and involuntary shaking of the head: *Magnes Phos.*

Tumors on the head of new born infants, blood tumors: *Calc. Fluor.*

Ulceration of bone surface: *Calc. Fluor.*

Ulcers on top of the head: *Calc. Phos.*

Vertigo: *Calc. Phos.*

cold applications relieve pain and momentarily contracting the excessively congested tissues: *Ferrum Phos.*

Vertigo: giddiness from excessive secretions of bile, tongue ha a dirty greenish or gray or greenish brown coating at the back part, bitter taste in the mouth: *Natr. Sulph.*

from exhaustion and weakness: *Kali Phos.*

Very severe headache on top of the head with intense pressure and heat: *Natr. Sulph.*

Violent pains at the base of the brain: *Natr. Sulph.*

Vomiting of white phlegm: *Kali Mur.*

Water on the brain: *Kali Phos.*

White scales on the scalp: *Natr. Mur.*

Wounds, suppurating, with thick yellow discharge: *Silicea.*

MENTAL SYMPTOMS

Anxious about future: *Calc. Phos.*

Backwardness: *Kali Phos.*

Brain, congestion of, from any cause: *Ferrum Phos.*

Brain, rush of blood to, causing delirium: *Ferrum Phos.*

softening of: *Kali Phos.*

Brain-fag, from overwork: *Kali Phos.*

Cerebritis: *Ferrum Phos.*

Children, crossness of: *Kali Phos.*

crying and screaming: *Kali Phos.*

ill-tempered: *Kali Phos.*

peevish and fretful: *Calc. Phos.*

screaming of, at night, during sleep: *Kali Phos. Natr. Phos.*

somnambulism in: *Kali Phos.*

Delirium, accompanied by frothy appearing tongue: *Natr. Mur.*

muttering and wandering: *Natr. Mur.*

during febrile diseases: *Kali Phos., Ferrum Phos., Natr. Mur.*

low in typhoid fever: *Natr. Mur.*

typhus fever: *Natr. Mur.*

tremens: *Natr. Mur., Ferrum Phos., Kali Phos.*

Depressed spirits: *Kali Phos., Calc. Phos., Natr. Mur.*
Desires solitude: *Calc. Phos.*
Despondent moods: *Natr. Mur., Natr. Sulph., Silicea.*
Discouraged, feels: *Natr. Sulph.*
Dizziness: *Ferrum Phos., Kali Phos.*
Fainting of nervous sensitive persons: *Kali Phos.*
    tendency to: *Kali Phos.*
Fits of crying: *Kali Phos.*
    laughing: *Kali Phos.*
Grasping at imaginary objects: *Kali Phos.*
Home-sickness: *Kali Phos.*
Hopeless, with dejected spirits: *Natr. Mur.*
Hyperemia: *Ferrum Phos.*
Illusions, mental: *Magnes. Phos., Kali Phos.*
Impatience and nervousness: *Kali Phos.*
Insanity: *Kali Phos.*
Irritable: *Kali Phos.*
Irritation, due to biliousness: *Natr. Sulph.*
Life, disgusted with: *Silicea.*
    looks on the dark side of: *Kali Phos.*
Melancholy: *Natr. Mur., Kali Phos.*
Memory, poor: *Calc. Phos., Kali Phos., Magnes. Phos.*
Mental abstraction: *Silicea.*
Mental disorders, in general: *Kali Phos.*
Mind, wanders from one subject to another: *Calc. Phos.*
Moods, anxious: *Kali Phos.*
    gloomy: *Kali Phos.*
    maniacal: *Ferrum Phos.*
Overstrain, from mental employment: *Kali Phos.*
Puerperal mania: *Kali Phos.*
Self-abuse, mind weak in those practicing: *Calc. Phos.*
Sensitiveness: *Kali Phos.*
Shyness: *Kali Phos.*
Sleeplessness: *Natr. Mur., Kali Phos.*
Stupor: *Natr. Mur.*

Suicide, tendency to: *Natr. Sulph.*
with wildness and irritability: *Natr. Sulph.*
Thought, cannot concentrate: *Calc. Phos.*
difficulty of: *Silicea.*
Visions, haunted by, of the past: *Kali Phos.*
Weeps easily: *Natr. Mur.*
Worse after disappointment: *Calc. Phos.*
grief: *Calc. Phos.*
in damp weather: *Natr. Sulph.*
morning *Natr. Sulph.*

EYE SYMPTOMS

Abscess of the cornea: *Ferrum Phos.*
Acrid tears in the eyes: *Natr. Mur.*
Acute inflammation of eyes: *Ferrum Phos.*
pain in eyes, worse from motion: *Ferrum Phos.*
use: *Ferrum Phos.*
Agglutination at night with smarting of the lids: *Silicea*
Agglutination of lids in morning: *Natr. Phos.*
All eye affections with flow of tears; *Natr. Mur.*
Asthenopia, muscular: *Natr. Mur., Magnes. Phos.*
Blisters on the cornea: *Natrum Mur.*
Blurred vision, after straining eye: *Calc. Fluor.*
Boils around eyelids: *Silicea.*
Burning of edges of lids: *Natr. Sulph.*
Cataract of eye: *Calc. Fluor.*
after eruptions: *Silicea.*
dimness of crystalline lens: *Kali Sulph., Natr. Mur.*
Colors before eyes: *Magnes. Phos.*
Conjunctivitis, chronic, with blister-like granulation on lids: *Natr. Sulph.*
with lachrymation: *Natr. Mur.*
mucous secretions: *Natr. Mur.*
Conjunctiva, yellow: *Natr. Sulph.*

Contracted pupils: *Magnes. Phos.*
Cornea, abscess of the, for pain: *Ferrum Phos., Calc. Sulph.*
blisters on: *Natr. Mur.*
crusts on eyelids, yellow: *Kali Sulph.*
inflammation of, with thick yellow discharges: *Calc. Sulph.*
Dimness of sight from weakness of the optic nerve: *Kali Phos.*
Diplopia: *Magnes. Phos.*
Discharge, golden-yellow creamy: *Natr. Phos.*
thick white mucus: *Kali Mur.*
yellow: *Calc. Sulph.*
greenish, serous: *Kali Sulph.*
slimy secretions: *Kali Sulph.*
Drooping of lids: *Kali Phos., Magnes. Phos.*
Dry inflammation of eyes: *Ferrum Phos. Natr. Mur.*
Excited appearance of eye: *Kali Phos.*
Eyes, blood-shot: *Ferrum Phos.*
glued together in the morning, with a creamy discharge: *Natr. Phos.*
Eye-bails, ache: *Calc. Phos.*
pain in the, relieved by resting eyes: *Calc. Fluor.*
Eyelids, specks of matter on: *Kali Mur.*
yellow, mattery scabs on: *Kali Mur.*
Flow of tears from the eyes when associated with colds in the head: *Kali Mur.*
Granulations on eyelids: *Ferrum Phos., Kali Mur.*
Feeling in the lids: *Calc. Phos.*
Hypopyum: *Calc. Sulph.*
Illusion ot sense of sight: *Magnes. Phos.*
Indurations around eyelids: *Silicea.*
Inflammation of the conjunctiva with characteristic discharge: *Kali Sulph.*
or cornea with characteristic discharge: *Calc. Sulph.*
Inflammation of the eye in measles, with great intolerance of light: *Ferrum Phos.*

Inflammation of the eyes with characteristic discharge, especially in scrofulous subjects: *Calc. Phos.*
when pus is discharging: *Calc. Sulph.*
secreting a golden yellow, creamy matter: *Natr. Phos.*
with discharge of thick yellow matter: *Silicea.*

Injuries of the eye, neglected cases, with subsequent suppuration of thick yellow matter: *Silicea.*

Lachrymal-ducts, disease of: *Silicea.*
fistula of: *Silicea.*
occlusion of, from cold: *Natr. Mur.*

Lachrymation, from weakness: *Natr. Mur.*
on going into open air: *Natr. Mur.*
when wind strikes eye: *Natr. Mur.*

Lachrymation, with fresh colds: *Natr. Mur.*
neuralgic pains in eye: *Natr. Mur. Magnes. Phos.*

Lids, hot feeling of: *Calc. Phos.*

Light, great intolerance of: *Ferrum Phos., Calc. Phos.*
sensitive to artificial: *Calc. Phos., Magnes. Phos.*

Muscular asthenopia: *Natr. Mur.*

Neuralgic pains in eyes: *Calc. Phos., Magnes. Phos.*

Neuralgic pain in the eyes with flow of tears: *Natr. Mur.*

Optic nerve, dullness of sight, from weakness of: *Kali Phos., Magnes. Phos.*

Pain as from excoriation in the eyes: *Natr. Mur.*
in the eyes with tears; recurring daily at certain times: *Natr. Mur.*

Paralysis of the retina causing dimness and loss of sight: *Calc. Phos.*

Pupils, contracted: *Magnes. Phos.*
dilated during disease: *Kali Phos.*

Redness and inflammation of the whites of the eyes with sensation as if the eyeballs were too large: *Natr. Mur.*

Retinitis, in first stages of: *Ferrum Phos.*
third stages of: *Calc. Sulph.*
with exudation: *Kali Mur.*

Retina, paralysis of: *Kali Phos., Calc. Phos.*

Scrofulous condition of eyes: *Natr. Mur., Silicea.*
subjects, inflammation of eyes in: *Calc. Phos.*

Sensitive to artificial light: *Calc. Phos.*
light; diplopia: *Magnes. Phos.*

Smarting secretions, with tears: *Natr. Mur.*

Sparks before eyes: *Magnes. Phos.*

Sore eyes with specks of matter on the lids or yellow mattery scabs: *Kali Mur.*

Spasms of eyelids: *Calc. Phos., Magnes. Phos.*

Spasmodic twitching of lids: *Magnes. Phos., Calc. Phos.*

Stoppage of tear ducts from cold: *Natr. Mur.*

Superficial flat ulcer, arising from a vesicle: *Kali Mur.*

Squinting: *Calc. Phos., Magnes. Phos.*
after diphtheria: *Kali Phos.*
caused by irritation, from worms: *Natr. Phos.*

Staring appearance of eyes: *Kali Phos.*

Sty on lids: *Silicea.*

Ulcers, deep-seated, of the cornea: *Calc. Sulph.*
superficial, flat, arising from a vesicle: *Kali Mur.*

Weak eyes with tears when going into the cold air or when wind strikes the eyes: *Natr. Mur.*

Yellow crusts on the eyelids: *Kali Sulph.*

Yellow-green matter in the eye: *Kali Sulph.*

Yellowness of the conjunctiva: *Kali Sulph.*

EAR SYMPTOMS

Aching pain and swelling of the glands of the face and neck: *Calc. Phos.*

After inflammation of the ear when the secretion is thin, bright, and yellow, or greenish: *Kali Sulph.*

Beating in the ears: *Silicea.*
Boils around external ear: *Silicea.*
Catarrh of ear, causing deafness: *Kali Sulph.*
involving eustachian tubes: *Kali Sulph.*
middle ear: *Ferrum Phos., Kali Mur.*
Cracking noises in ear on blowing nose: *Kali Mur.*
swallowing: *Kali Mur.*
Cutting pain under ears: *Kali Sulph.*
Cystic tumors around ear: *Silicea.*
Deafness, accompanied by evening aggravation: *Kali Sulph.*
exhaustion of nervous system: *Kali Phos.*
thick yellow discharge: *Calc. Sulph.*
from inflammatory action: *Ferrum Phos.*
swelling of eustachian tubes: *Natr. Mur.*
Kali Mur., Silicea, Kali Sulph.
external ear: *Kali Sulph.*
thickening of drum membrane: *Kali Mur.*
want of nervous perception: *Kali Phos.*
Discharges, foul, ichorous, offensive: *Kali Phos.*
mixed with blood: *Kali Phos.*
sanious: *Kali Phos*
thick, yellow, bloody: *Calc. Sulph.*
Dullness of hearing from disease of the auditory nerve fibre: *Magnes. Phos.*
throat affections or swelling of the middle ear: *Kali Mur.*
with noise in the ear: *Kali Phos.*
swelling and catarrh of the eustachian and tympanic cavity: *Kali Mur.*
Ear affections, involving bones: *Calc. Fluor.*
periosteum: *Calc. Fluor.*
with excessive secretions of saliva: *Natr. Mur.*
Ears, swollen, burning, itching: *Calc. Phos.*
Earache, accompanied by albuminous discharge: *Calc. Phos.*
beating, throbbing pain: *Ferrum Phos.*
excoriating discharge: *Calc. Phos.*

Earache, gray or white-furred tongue: *Kali Mur.*
lightning-like pain through ears: *Natr. Sulph.*

Earache, accompanied by swelling of eustachian tube: *Kali Mur.*
glands: *Kali Mur.*
tonsils: *Kali Mur.*
yellow, mattery discharge: *Kali Sulph.*
aggravated by cold: *Magnes. Phos.*
damp weather: *Natr. Sulph.*
of nervous character: *Magnes. Phos.*
spasmodic character: *Magnes, Phos.*
relieved by heat: *Magnes. Phos.*

External meatus swollen: *Silicea.*

Exudations from ear, thick, white and moist: *Kali Mur.*

Glands around the ear swollen; noises in the ear; snapping and cracking from unequalization of air in the eustachian tubes: *Kali Mur.*

Glandular swelling of scrofulous persons: *Calc. Phos.*

Granulations moist, gray or thick white exudation from the ear: *Kali Mur.*

Hard hearing: *Natr. Mur.*

Heat and burning of the ears with gastric symptoms: *Natr. Phos.*

Humming in the ears: *Natr. Mur.*

Inflammation of the ears, first stage for the fever and pain: *Ferrum Phos.*
external ear with beefy redness and burning: *Ferrum Phos.*
meatus: *Silicea.*

Noises in ears and head, with confusion: *Kali Phos.*
like running water: *Ferrum Phos.*

Otitis, for fever and pain: *Ferrum Phos.*
with thick yellow discharge: *Silicea.*
thin bright-yellow, organic secretions: *Kali Sulph.*

Otorrhea, with caries of mastoid: *Silicea.*

Outer ear sore and scabby: *Natr. Phos.*
with creamy discharge: *Natr. Phos.*
Scabs, with creamy, yellow appearance: *Natr. Phos.*
Scrofulous persons, swollen glands: *Calc. Phos.*
Sharp pain under ears: *Kali Sulph.*
Singing or tingling in the ears: *Natr. Mur.*
Stitches in the ears: *Natr. Mur.*
Swelling of the parotid gland with stitching pain: *Silicea.*
Suppurative otitis, when discharge is thick yellow matter: *Silicea.*
Tympanitis: *Ferrum Phos.*
Ulceration of the ear when the discharge is foul, ichorous, offensive, sanious, or mixed with blood: *Kali Phos.*
Whizzing and ringing in the ears with diminution of hearing: *Magnes. Phos.*

NOSE SYMPTOMS

Albuminous discharge, thick and tough, dropping from the posterior nares, causing constant hawking and spitting, worse out of doors: *Calc. Phos.*
Bleeding from the nose: *Ferrum Phos.*
in delicate constitutions, when the blood is thin, blackish or coagulating; predisposition to bleeding: *Kali Phos.*
anemic persons, the blood is thin and watery: *Natr. Mur.*
Boils on edges of nostrils: *Silicea.*
Burning in nose: *Natr. Sulph.*
Caries of nasal bones: *Silicea.*
Catarrh, accompanied by fever: *Ferrum Phos.*
acute or chronic, with shiny yellow, greenish discharges: *Ferrum Phos. Kali Phos.*

Catarrh, aggravated in evening: *Kali Sulph.*
warm room: *Kali Sulph.*
chronic, with purulent discharges from anterior or posterior nares: *Kali Sulph., Silicea.*
of anemic persons: *Natr. Mur.*
with fetid discharges: *Kali Phos.*
salty mucus: *Natr. Mur.*
with stuffy sensation: *Kali Mur.*
white, not transparent phlegm: *Kali Mur.*
Cold in the head with yellow creamy discharge from the nose; itching of the nose: *Natr. Phos.*
in the third stage of resolution, when the discharge is thick, yellow, purulent, and sometimes tinged with blood; Calc. *Sulph.*
with dry, harsh skin; to produce perspiration: *Kali Sulph.*
Coryza, initiatory stage: *Ferrum Phos.*
stage of resolution: *Calc. Sulph.*
with albuminous discharge: *Calc. Phos.*
dry, harsh skin: *Kali Sulph.*
mattery, slimy discharge: *Natr. Mur.*
Crusts in the vault of the pharynx: *Kali Mur.*
Discharge, albuminous: *Calc. Phos.*
clear, watery, transparent mucus: *Natr. Mur.*
fetid: *Kali Phos.*
slimy, yellow, watery, greenish: *Kali Sulph.*
thick and white: *Kali Mur.*
yellow, fetid: *Silicea.*
lumpy, green: *Calc. Fluor.*
purulent, bloody: *Calc. Sulph.*
yellow, creamy: *Natr. Phos.*
Diseases of nose affecting bones: *Calc. Fluor., Silicea.*
Disposition to take cold in anemic persons: *Calc. Phos.*
Dropping of watery, salty secretions from the posterior nares: *Natr. Mur.*
Dry catarrh with stuffy sensation: *Kali Mur.*

Dry coryza: *Natr. Mur.*
Dryness and burning in the nose: *Natr. Sulph.*
Dryness of nose, with scabbing: *Natr. Mur., Silicea.*
  in nose: *Natr. Sulph.*
Edges of nostrils itch: *Silicea.*
First or inflammatory stage of colds: *Ferrum Phos.*
Fluent coryza: *Natr. Mur.*
Frequent sneezing: *Silicea.*
Fresh cold and discharge of clear, watery transparent mucus, and sneezing: *Natr. Mur.*
Hawking and spitting, constant: *Calc. Phos.*
Hay fever: *Natr. Mur.*
Head, cold in, with yellow, creamy discharge: *Natr. Phos.*
Influenza, with sneezing: *Natr. Mur.*
  watery discharge from eyes and nose: *Natr. Mur.*
Itching of tip of nose: *Silicea.*
  the nose: *Natr. Phos.*
Large pedunculated nasal tumor: *Calc. Phos.*
Loss of smell or perversion of the sense of smell, under certain conditions not connected with the cold: *Magnes. Phos.*
  with dryness and rawness of the pharynx: *Natr. Mur.*
Nasal catarrh: *Natr. Sulph.*
  polypi, large and pedunculated: *Calc. Phos.*
Nose, inflamed at edges of nostrils: *Silicea*
  swollen: *Calc. Phos.*
Ozena, affecting periosteum: *Silicea.*
  submucous connective tissues: *Silicea.*
  syphilitica: *Natr. Sulph.*
  worse in damp weather: *Natr. Sulph.*
  with offensive lumpy discharges: *Calc. Fluor., Kali Phos., Silicea*
  foul odor: *Silicea, Kali Phos.*
Perversion of sense of smell, not from cold: *Magnes. Phos.*
Pharynx, dryness and rawness of: *Natr. Mur.*

Picks at nose: *Natr. Phos.*

Posterior nares, dropping of watery salty secretions from: *Natr. Mur., Calc. Phos.*

tough, albuminous mucus from: *Calc. Phos.*

Pus changes to green when exposed to light: *Natr Sulph.*

Sneezing: *Natr. Mur.*

Stuffy cold in head, with yellow, lumpy, green discharges: *Calc. Fluor.*

with collection of greenish mucus: *Kali Sulph., Silicea.*

Takes cold easily: *Ferrum Phos., Calc. Phos.*

Tips of nose red: *Silicea.*

Tongue coated white or gray: *Kali Mur.*

FACE SYMPTOMS

Anemic face: *Calc. Phos.*

Beard, tender pimples under: *Calc. Sulph.*

with bloody secretions: *Calc. Sulph.*

Blotches on face, come and go suddenly: *Natr. Phos.*

Cancer of face: *Kali Sulph.*

Caries and necrosis of bones of the jaw: *Silicea.*

Cellular tissues, indurations of, after boils: *Silicea.*

Chaps of lips: *Calc. Fluor.*

Cheek swollen and painful: *Kali Mur.*

Chlorosis: *Natr. Mur.*

Chlorotic face: *Calc. Phos.*

Cracks and rhagades of the corners of the mouth: *Calc. Phos*

Creeping pains in face: *Calc. Phos.*

Dirty-looking face: *Calc. Phos.*

Eruption on the face from any cause, with discharge: *Silicea.*

Erysipelas, for inflammation and pain: *Ferrum Phos., Natr. Sulph.*

smooth, red, shiny, swelling: *Natr. Sulph.*

Face, bloated, without fever: *Natr. Phos.*
flushed, cold sensation at nape of neck: *Ferrum Phos.*
livid: *Kali Phos.*
pale, sickly, sallow: *Kali Phos., Calc. Phos.*
pallid and pale: *Ferrum Phos., Calc. Phos.*
red, without fever: *Natr. Phos.*
Faceache, accompanied by constipation: *Natr. Mur.*
flow of tears: *Natr. Mur.*
rheumatic pains: *Magnes. Phos.*
small lumps on face: *Silicea.*
vomiting of clear mucus: *Natr. Mur.*
from swelling of cheek: *Kali Mur.*
gums: *Kali Mur.*
Feeling of coldness of face: *Calc. Phos.*
numbness of face: *Calc. Phos.*
Feverish complexion: *Ferrum Phos.*
Florid complexion: *Ferrum Phos.*
Freckles: *Calc. Phos.*
Frothy bubbles at edge of tongue: *Natr. Mur.*
Grinding pains in face: *Magnes. Phos., Calc. Phos.*
Growths on cheek-bones: *Calc. Fluor.*
Hard swelling on cheeks, with toothache: *Calc. Fluor.*
Headache, with flushed burning face: *Ferrum Phos.*
Heat in face: *Calc. Phos.*
Inflammatory neuralgia of the face: *Ferrum Phos.*
Jaundiced face: *Natr. Sulph.*
Lightning-like pains in face: *Magnes. Phos.*
Lupus: *Calc. Phos.*
discharge of thick matter: *Silicea.*
Necrosis of bones of jaw: *Silicea.*
Neuralgia, accompanied by flow of tears: *Natr. Mur.*
shifting pains: *Magnes. Phos. Kali Sulph.*
shooting pains: *Magnes. Phos.*
spasmodic pains: *Magnes. Phos.*
aggravated by being in heated room: *Kali Sulph.*
Cold: *Magnes. Phos.*

Neuralgia, in the evening: *Kali Sulph.*
touch: *Magnes. Phos.*
from exhaustion of nervous system: *Kali Phos.*
relieved by being in cool air: *Kali Sulph.*
hot applications: *Magnes. Phos.*
Nodules on face: *Calc. Sulph.*
Nose cold: *Calc. Fluor.*
Osseous lumps on jaw: *Calc. Fluor.*
Pains and heat in face: *Ferrum Phos.*
cold applications soothe: *Ferrum Phos.*
Pale face in children when teething is difficult: *Calc. Phos.*
pallid face from a lack of red blood corpuscles: *Ferrum Phos.*
Pimples on face, mattery: *Calc. Sulph.*
at age of puberty: *Calc. Sulph., Calc. Phos.*
Rheumatism of face: *Calc. Phos.*
worse at night: *Calc. Phos.*
Skin cold and clammy: *Calc. Phos.*
Swellings on face: *Calc. Sulph.*
Sycosis: *Natr. Mur.*
Tearing pain in face: *Magnes. Phos. Calc. Phos.*
Tongue, covered with clear mucus: *Natr. Mur.*
cream-colored: *Natr. Phos.*
Whiskers fall out: *Natr. Mur.*
White about mouth and nose: *Natr. Phos.*
Yellow, sallow, or jaundiced face due to biliousness: *Natr. Sulph.*

MOUTH SYMPTOMS

Acid taste in mouth: *Natr. Phos.*
Aphthae, with flow of saliva: *Natr. Mur.*
Bad taste in mouth: *Natr. Sulph., Kali Phos.*
in morning *Calc. Phos.*

Begins speaking with teeth closed: *Magnes. Phos.*
Bitter taste in mouth: *Natr. Sulph.*
Blisters like pimples on the tip of the tongue: *Calc. Phos.*
Canker of lips: *Kali Mur.*
mouth: *Kali Mur.*
Catarrh of mouth and pharynx, with watery discharges: *Natr. Mur.*
Chronic swelling of the tongue: *Calc. Fluor.*
Clean tongue showing an inflammatory condition: *Ferrum Phos.*
Coating on the tongue white and slimy: *Kali Mur.*
yellow, sometimes with whitish edge: *Kali Sulph.*
Constant hawking of foul, slimy mucus from the mouth to the trachea, oesophagus and stomach: *Natr. Sulph.*
Constant spitting of frothy mucus: *Natr. Mur.*
Cracked lips: *Calc. Fluor.*
Creamy, golden-yellow exudation from tonsils and pharynx: *Natr. Phos.*
Creamy, yellow coating at back part of roof of mouth: *Natr. Phos.*
Dirty greenish gray or greenish brown coating on the root of the tongue with saliva: *Natr. Mur.*
Disease of the mouth if accompanied with purulent secretion: *Calc. Phos.*
Dryness of the lower lips; skin pulls off in large flakes: *Kali Phos.*
tongue in low fevers with watery discharge from the bowels: *Natr. Mur.*
Epithelial cancer of lips: *Kali Sulph.*
Gangrenous canker of mouth: *Kali Phos.*
Glands and gums swollen: *Kali Mur.*
swelling of, under tongue: *Natr. Mur.*
Gums hot, swollen and inflamed: *Ferrum Phos.*
Hard swelling on jaw-bones: *Calc. Fluor.*
Hawking, constant, of foul, slimy mucus from trachea and stomach: *Natr. Sulph.*

Inflammation of salivary glands, when secreting excessive amount of saliva: *Natr. Mur.*

Inflammation of the tongue when suppurating: *Calc. Sulph.*
with excessive dryness: *Kali Phos*

Lock-jaw: *Magnes. Phos.*

Mouth full of thick, greenish-white, tenacious slime: *Natr. Sulph.*

Purulent secretions in diseases of mouth: *Calc. Sulph.*

Ranula: *Natr. Mur.*

Rawness of mouth: *Kali Mur.*

Saliva, excess of, during disease: *Natr. Mur.*

Salivation: *Natr. Mur.*

Skin peels off in large flakes: *Kali Sulph.*

Sour taste in mouth: *Natr. Phos.*

Spasms, stammering: *Magnes. Phos.*

Speaks slowly: *Magnes. Phos.*

Stomatitis: *Ferrum Phos.*
accompanied by bad taste in mouth: *Kali Phos.*
fetid, offensive breath: *Kali Phos.*

Swelling of glands under 'he tongue: *Natr. Mur.*

Tetanic spasms: *Magnes. Phos.*

Thrush in children: *Kali Mur.*
with much saliva: *Natr. Mur.*

Tongue has a cracked appearance, tongue becoming indurated after inflammation: *Calc. Fluor.*
is coated like slate, brownish liquid mustard: *Kali Phos.*
dark red and inflamed with swelling: *Ferrum Phos.*
has clear, watery coating, with small frothy bubbles: *Natr. Mur.*
stiff and numb: *Calc. Phos.*
swollen: *Calc. Phos.*
very dry in the morning; feels as if it clung to the roof of the mouth: *Kali Phos.*

Twitching, spasmodic, of lips: *Magnes. Phos.*
mouth: *Magnes. Phos.*

Ulcers on tongue: *Silicea.*
Very offensive breath: *Kali Phos.*
Vesicles on the tongue: *Natr. Mur.*
Water canker: *Kali Phos.*

TONGUE

Bitter taste in mouth: *Natr. Sulph.*
Blisters on tip of tongue: *Natr. Mur., Calc. Phos.*
Breath, offensive: *Kali Phos.*
Chronic swelling of: *Calc. Fluor.*
Clean and red: *Ferrum Phos.*
Cling to roof of mouth, feels as if it would: *Kali Phos.*
Coating, clear, slimy, watery, on: *Natr. Mur.*
  dirty, greenish-gray, on root of: *Natr. Sulph.*
  golden-yellow, on back part of: *Natr. Phos.*
  grayish-white, of: *Kali Mur.*
  like stale brownish liquid mustard, on: *Kali Phos.*
  moist, creamy, on back part of: *Natr. Phos.*
  yellow and slimy, on: *Kali Sulph.*
Cracked appearance of: *Calc. Fluor.*
Dark red and inflamed: *Ferrum Phos.*
Dry in the morning: *Kali Phos.*
Dryish or slimy: *Kali Mur.*
Dryness of, in low fevers, with watery discharges from bowels: *Natr. Mur.*
Frothy bubbles on edges of: *Natr. mur.*
Hardening of: *Silicea.*
Induration of, after inflammations: *Silicea, Calc. Fluor.*
Inflammation of, for swelling: *Ferrum Phos., Kali Mur.*
  with exhaustion: *Kali Phos.*
  when suppurating: *Silicea, Calc. Sulph.*
Numbness of: *Calc. Phos.*
Pimples on tip of: *Calc. Phos.*

Swollen: *Kali Mur., Calc. Phos.*
Stiffness of: *Calc. Phos.*
Ulcers on: *Silicea.*

TEETH

Children grind teeth during sleep: *Natr. Phos.*
Convulsions during dentition: *Magnes. Phos.*
Cramps during dentition: *Magnes. Phos.*
Decay of teeth as soon as they appear: *Calc.* ***Phos.***
Enamel, brittle: *Calc. Fluor.*
 rough and thin: *Calc. Fluor.*
Gastric derangements during teething: *Natr. Phos.*
Gums bleed easily: *Kali Phos.*
 pale: *Calc. Phos.*
 predisposition of, to bleed: *Kali Phos.*
Gum-boil on jaw: *Silicea.*
 before pus begins to form: *Kali Mur.*
Infants, teething of, with drooling: *Natr. Mur.*
Nervous chattering of teeth: *Kali Phos.*
Neuralgia of teeth: *Natr. Mur.*
Rapid decay of teeth: *Calc. Fluor.*
Retarded dentition: *Calc. Phos.*
Seam, bright-red, on gums: *Kali Phos.*
Sockets, teeth loose in: *Calc. Fluor.*
Teeth sensitive to cold air: *Magnes. Phos.*
 touch: *Magnes. Phos.*
 tender, due to looseness: *Calc. Fluor.*
Toothache, accompanied by deep-seated pain in periosteum: *Silicea.*
 excessive flow of tears: *Natr. Mur.*
 saliva: *Natr. Mur.*
 neuralgia of face: *Magnes. Phos.*
 rheumatic pains: *Magnes. Phos.*
 sharp, shooting pains: *Magnes. Phos.*

Toothache, spasmodic pains: *Magnes. Phos.*
swelling of gums or cheeks: *Kali Mur., Ferrum Phos.*
ulceration: *Silicea.*
after exhaustion: *Kali Phos.*
mental labor: *Kali Phos.*
aggravated by being in warm room: *Kali Sulph.*
hot liquids: *Ferrum Phos.*
in evening: *Kali Sulph.*
motion: *Ferrum Phos.*
from chilling feet: *Silicea.*
from loss of sleep: *Kali Phos.*
in nervous subjects: *Magnes. Phos., Kali Phos.*
relieved by being in open air: *Kali Sulph.*
cold applications: *Ferrum Phos.*
liquids: *Ferrum Phos.*
gentle motion: *Kali Sulph.*
hot applications: *Magnes. Phos.*
Ulceration of roots of teeth: *Calc. Sulph.*
with swelling gums and cheeks: *Calc. Sulph.*

THROAT SYMPTOMS

After-effects of diphtheria, weakness of sight, partial paralysis: *Kali Phos.*
All throat ailments in the third stage of the inflammation or when discharging mattery secretion: *Calc. Sulph.*
Burning sensation in the pharynx and cases of chronic catarrh, when there is considerable dropping from the posterior nares: *Calc. Phos.*
Catarrh, chronic dropping of mucus from posterior nares to throat: *Calc. Phos., Natr. Mur.*
of pharynx: *Natr. Sulph.*
Choking on attempting to swallow: *Magnes. Phos.*

Chronic enlargement of the tonsils: *Calc. Phos.*
Constricted feeling of: *Magnes. Phos.*
Closing of larynx by spasms or cramp: *Magnes. Phos.*
Constant hoarseness: *Calc. Phos.*
Croup in the last stage, for syncope, nervous prostration, pale or livid countenance: *Kali Phos., Kali Mur.*
Deglutition, painful: *Calc. Phos.*
Diphtheria: *Kali Mur.*
after-effects of: *Kali Phos.*
with weakness of sight: *Kali Phos.*
partial paralysis: *Kali Phos.*
face puffy and pale: *Natr. Mur.*
flow of saliva: *Natr. Mur.*
in first stage: *Ferrum Phos.*
involving trachea: *Calc. Fluor.*
vomiting of clear water: *Natr. Mur.*
greenish water: *Natr. Sulph.*
with drowsiness: *Natr. Mur.*
Dry, red and inflamed: *Ferrum Phos.*
Elongation of the uvulae, causing tickling cough, by dropping into the throat: *Calc. Fluor.*
Enlargement of the: *Calc. Fluor., Natr. Mur.*
False diphtheria with creamy coating of the palate and back part of the tongue: *Natr. Phos.*
First stage of all throat diseases, when there is pain, heat and redness: *Ferrum Phos.*
Gangrenous condition of: *Kali Phos.*
Glands painful, aching: *Calc. Phos.*
Goitre: *Silicea, Calc. Phos., Natr. Phos.*
with mattery symptoms: *Calc. Phos., Natr. Mur.*
Hoarseness, constant: *Calc. Phos., Ferrum Phos.*
Inflammation of the mucous lining of the throat with characteristic watery secretions: *Natr. Mur.*
tonsils: *Ferrum Phos.*
with swelling and grayish white patches: *Kali Mur.*

Larynx, burning and soreness in: *Calc. Phos.*
closing of, by spasm: *Magnes. Phos.*
Loss of voice: *Kali Mur.*
from strain: *Ferrum Phos.*
Lump in, on swallowing: *Natr. Sulph.*
Mumps, when watery symptoms are present: *Natr. Mur.*
with swelling of testicles: *Kali Mur.*
Neck, thin, with chlorotic condition: *Natr. Mur.*
Nervous prostration, in disease of: *Kali Phos.*
Pharynx, burning and soreness in: *Calc. Phos.*
Quinsy, acute and chronic: *Ferrum Phos., Kali Mur.*
Raw feeling in: *Natr. Phos.*
Redness and inflammation: *Ferrum Phos.*
Relaxed condition of: *Calc. Fluor.*
Relaxation of blood-vessels of: *Calc. Fluor.*
Scraping of, when talking: *Calc. Phos.*
Sticking pain in, on swallowing: *Calc. Phos.*
Shrill voice, coming on suddenly while speaking: *Magnes. Phos., Kali Phos.*
Sore, raw feeling in the throat; tonsils and throat inflamed.
with creamy, yellow, moist coating: *Natr. Phos.*
throat as if a plug had lodged in the throat: *Natr. Mur.*
of singers and speakers: *Ferrum Phos.*
quinsy and tonsillitis when suppurating, or before matter has formed to prevent its formation: *Calc. Sulph.*
with excessive dryness or too much secretion: *Natr. Mur.*
Speech, slow, indicating paralysis: *Kali Phos.*
Spasms of the throat: *Magnes. Phos.*
Spasmodic cough: *Magnes. Phos.*
Stinging sore throat, only when swallowing, the neck being painful to touch: *Silicea.*
Suppuration of throat: *Calc. Sulph.*
to prevent: *Calc. Sulph.*
Thirst, with dry mouth: *Calc. Phos.*
tongue: *Calc. Phos.*

Tonsils, chronic enlargement of: *Calc. Phos.*
creamy, yellow, moist coating on: *Natr. Phos.*
gray-white patches on: *Kali Mur.*
inflamed: *Natr. Phos., Ferrum Phos.*
Tonsilitis, after pus has begun to form: *Silicea.*
Ulcerations, with thick yellow discharges: *Silicea.*
Ulcerated throat, with fever and pain: *Ferrum Phos.*
white or gray patches: *Kali Mur.*
Uvula, elongated, causing tickling cough: *Calc. Fluor., Natr. Phos.*
relaxed, with much saliva in: *Natr. Mur., Calc. Fluor.*
Vocal cords, paralysis of: *Kali Phos.*
Windpipe, spasmodic closing of: *Magnes. Phos.*

GASTRIC SYMPTOMS

Abnormal appetite, but food causes distress: *Calc. Phos.*
Acid drinks aggravate: *Magnes. Phos.*
All conditions and diseases of the stomach when excess of saliva and watery vomiting present; tongue has a clear, frothy, transparent coating: *Natr. Mur.*
of the stomach when there are sour acid risings, or the tongue has a moist, creamy yellow coating: *Natr. Phos.*
Appetite not satisfied: *Kali Phos.*
Belching brings back taste of food: *Ferrum Phos.*
wind relieves: *Calc. Phos.*
Bilious colic: *Natr. Sulph.*
Biliousness from too much bile: *Natr. Sulph.*
Bitter taste in mouth: *Natr. Sulph.*
Bloated, stomach feels: *Calc. Phos.*
Blood, vomit of dark, clotted: *Kali Mur.*
bright-red: *Ferrum Phos.*

Burning in stomach: *Calc. Phos., Kali Mur., Ferrum Phos.*
Catarrh of the stomach with yellow, slimy tongue: *Kali Sulph.*
Clear, frothy, transparent coating on tongue: *Natr. Mur.*
Coffee-ground vomit: *Natr. Phos.*
Cold drinks relieve: *Ferrum Phos.*
aggravate: *Calc. Phos., Magnes. Phos.*
Constant desire to nurse: *Calc. Sulph.*
Constipation, with water-brash: *Natr. Mur.*
Cough, with pain in left hypochondriac region: *Natr. Sulph.*
Craving for salt or salty food: *Natr. Mur.*
Distress about heart: *Kali Phos.*
Dizziness: *Natr. Sulph.*
Dread of hot drinks: *Kali Sulph.*
Dyspepsia with acid risings: *Kali Phos.*
characteristic coating on tongue: *Kali Sulph.*
flushed face and throbbing pain in the stomach *Ferrum Phos.*
pain after eating, if watery symptoms are present: *Natr. Mur.*
white gray coating on the tongue, heavy pain under the right shoulder blade, eyes look large and protruding: *Kali Mur.*
Eating, pain after: *Natr. Phos.*
Enlargement of the liver, worse lying on the left side: *Natr Mur.*
Eructations: *Silicea.*
Evacuations, bilious, green: *Natr. Sulph.*
Excess of saliva: *Natr. Mur.*
Eyeballs, yellow: *Natr. Sulph.*
Eyes, large and protruding: *Kali Mur.*
Faint, sick feeling in the region of the stomach: *Calc. Phos.*
Fatty food disagrees: *Kali Mur.*
Flatulence, with distress about heart: *Kali Phos.*
Flatulence with sluggishness of the liver: *Kali Mur.*
Food aggravates: *Calc. Phos.*
causes pain: *Natr. Phos.*

Food distresses: *Calc. Phos.*
persistent vomiting of: *Ferrum Phos.*
Fullness at pit of stomach: *Kali Sulph.*
Gastric abrasions, superficial ulcerations, pain after eating, calls for this remedy if the accompanying acid conditions are present: *Natr. Phos.*
Gastric derangements causing flatulence: *Natr. Phos.*
giddiness: *Natr. Phos.*
Gastric fever: *Ferrum Phos.*
with rise of temperature in the evening: *Kali Sulph.*
Gastritis, accompanied by abrasions: *Natr. Phos.*
catarrh, with yellow, slimy-coated tongue: *Kali Sulph.*
Gastritis, accompanied by gone sensation in stomach: *Kali Phos., Calc. Phos.*
gray or white-coated tongue: *Kali Mur.*
greenish-brown coating on tongue: *Natr. Sulph.*
nervous prostration: *Kali Phos.*
weakness and debility: *Kali Phos.*
caused by hot drinks: *Kali Mur.*
first stage: *Ferrum Phos.*
greasy food disagrees: *Kali Mur.*
second stage: *Kali Mur.*
Great thirst: *Natr. Mur.*
Headache: *Natr. Sulph.*
with vomiting of food: *Ferrum Phos.*
Heartburn: *Silicea, Ferr Phos., Calc. Phos., Natr. Phos.*
Heaviness in stomach: *Calc. Phos.*
Hiccough: *Magnes. Phos.*
hot applications relieve: *Ferrum Phos., Calc. Phos., Magnes. Phos.*
water relieves: *Magnes. Phos.*
Hungry feeling after eating: *Kali Phos.*
Indigestion, accompanied by griping pains: *Magnes. Phos.*

Indigestion with pain in the stomach and watery gathering in the mouth, or sour taste in the mouth: *Natr. Mur.*
pressure and fullness at the pit of the stomach: *Kali. Sulph.*
vomiting of greasy, white opaque mucus: *Kali Mur.*
watery vomiting and salty taste in the mouth: *Natr. Mur.*

Induration of the polypi; *Silicea.*

Infants vomit sour curdled milk: *Calc. Phos.*

Inflammation of the stomach when it comes too late under treatment, with weakness, debility, and nervous prostration: *Kali Phos.*

Irritable liver: *Natr. Sulph.*

Jaundice, from vexation: *Natr. Sulph.*
with watery symptoms: *Natr. Mur.*

Lead colic: *Natr. Sulph.*

Liver, cutting pain in region of: *Natr. Sulph.*
enlargement of: *Natr. Sulph.*
worse lying on left side: *Natr. Sulph.*

Lump, food lies in a: *Calc. Phos.*

Milk, infants vomit curdled: *Calc Phos., Natr. Phos.*

Moist, creamy, yellow coating on tongue: *Natr. Phos.*

Morning sickness: *Natr. Phos.*

Mouth full of slime: *Natr. Sulph.*

Nausea, with sour risings: *Natr. Phos.*

Nausea immediately after a meal: *Natr. Mur.*
with gone sensation in the stomach: *Kali Phos.*

Neuralgia of stomach: *Magnes. Phos.*
relieved by heat or pressure: *Magnes. Phos.*

Nurse, constant desire to: *Calc. Phos.*

Nurses, child vomits as soon as it: *Calc. Phos., Ferrum Phos., Silicea.*

Pain after eating: *Natr. Mur., Calc. Phos., Natr. Phos.*

Pain after eating: *Calc. Phos.*
in the left hypochondriac region, frequently accompanied by a cough: *Natr. Sulph.*
is remittent and spasmodic: *Magnes. Phos.*
sometimes relieved by belching wind: *Calc. Phos.*
worse from eating even the smallest amount of food: *Calc. Phos.*

Pastry disagrees: *Kali Mur.*

Pressure at pit of stomach: *Kali Sulph.*

Pylorus, induration of: *Silicea.*

Remittent pain: *Magnes. Phos.*

Right shoulder-blade, pain under: *Kali Mur.*

Salty taste in mouth: *Natr. Mur.*

Sick headache from gastric derangements: *Natr. Sulph.*

Skin dry and hot: *Kali Sulph.*
sallow: *Natr. Sulph.*

Sour, acid risings: *Natr. Phos*

Spasmodic pain: *Magnes. Phos.*

Spasms of stomach, with griping: *Magnes. Phos.*

Stomach sore to touch: *Calc. Phos.*
tender to touch: *Ferrum Phos.*

Stomachache, accompanied by constipation: *Kali Mur.*
depression: *Kali Phos.*

Stomachache, accompanied by exhaustion: *Kali Phos.*
loose evacuations: *Ferrum Phos.*
after febrile diseases: *Kali Phos.*
from acidity of the stomach: *Natr. Phos.*
chill: *Ferrum Phos.*
worms: *Natr. Phos.*

Temperature, rise of, in evening: *Kali Sulph.*

Thirst, great: *Natr. Mur.*

Thirstlessness: *Kali Phos.*

Tongue, clean: *Magnes. Phos.*
slimy yellow coated: *Kali Sulph.*

Ulceration of the stomach when the least amount of food causes pain and the tongue and palate have the characteristic creamy yellow coating: *Natr. Phos.*
with vomiting of sour acid fluids or substance like coffee grounds: *Natr. Phos.*

Vomiting, after cold drinks: *Calc. Phos.*
bile: *Natr. Sulph.*
bright-red blood: *Ferrum Phos.*

Vomiting, dark, clotted blood: *Kali Mur., Ferrum Phos.*
fluids like coffee-grounds: *Natr. Phos.*
from stomachache: *Magnes. Phos.*
greenish water: *Natr. Sulph.*
sour acid fluids: *Natr. Phos.*
thick white phlegm: *Kali Mur.*
undigested food: *Ferrum Phos., Calc. Fluor.*
watery: *Natr. Mur.*

Water-brash, with constipation: *Natr. Mur.*

Water gathers in mouth: *Natr. Mur.*

APPETITE AND TASTE

Acidity in the stomach: *Silicea*

Bitter taste in the morning: *Silicea.*

Bitterness in the mouth: *Natr. Mur.*

Eructations and acidity: *Silicea.*

Excessive appetite: *Natr. Mur.*
but food causes distress: *Calc. Phos.*

Great thirst and loss of appetite: *Silicea.*

Putrid taste: *Natr. Mur.*

Sour taste: *Natr. Mur.*

Thirst without appetite: *Kali Mur.*

ABDOMEN

Abdomen, bloated: *Kali Sulph., Magnes. Phos.*
cold to touch: *Kali Sulph.*
cutting pains in: *Natr. Sulph., Magnes. Phos. Ferrum Phos.*
distended: *Magnes. Phos.*
sunken: *Calc. Phos.*
swollen: *Kali Phos., Kali Mur.*
tender to touch: *Kali Mur.*
Acidity of stomach: *Natr. Phos.*
Anus, itching at: *Natr Phos., Calc. Fluor.*
cracks and fissures of the: *Calc. Phos.*
Anus, pain in: *Kali Mur.*
Appendicitis, second stage: *Kali Mur.*
Back, pain in: *Calc. Fluor.*
Belching of wind: *Magnes. Phos.*
Bilious evacuations: *Natr. Sulph.*
Bowels, loose, in old people: *Natr. Sulph.*
sore and tender: *Ferrum Phos.*
Burning in the bowels: *Silicea.*
sore pain in the pit of the stomach: *Ferrum Phos.*
Burning pain in rectum: *Natr. Mur.*
Cholera, rice-water stool: *Kali Phos.*
Colic from sudden changes: *Kali Sulph.*
of infants: *Magnes. Phos.*
with constipation: *Silicea.*
Constant urging to stool: *Kali Mur.*
Constipation, accompanied by drowsiness: *Natr. Mur.*
dull, heavy headache: *Natr. Mur.*
profusion of tears: *Natr. Mur.*
Constipation, accompanied by vomit of frothy mucus: *Natr. Mur.*
during consumption: *Calc. Sulph.*
light-colored stools: *Kali Mur.*
of old people and infants: *Calc. Phos.*

Crest of ileum, pain above: *Kali Sulph.*
Delirious: *Kali Phos.*
Depression of nerves: *Kali Phos.*
Diarrhea after fatty foods: *Kali Mur.*
alternated with constipation: *Natr. Mur.*
causes soreness and smarting: *Natr. Mur.*
from eating green fruit: *Calc. Phos.*
in teething children: *Calc. Phos.*
of children: *Natr. Phos.*
school-girls: *Calc. Phos.*
pus-like, slimy: *Calc. Sulph.*
putrid, foul evacuations: *Kali Phos.*
stool frothy mucus: *Natr. Mur.*
watery: *Magnes. Phos., Natr. Mur.*
with dark, greenish stools: *Natr. Sulph.*
straining: *Natr. Phos.*
watery stools: *Natr. Mur.*
worse in cold, wet weather: *Natr. Sulph.*
Discharge of matter, or blood and matter from the bowels: *Calc. Sulph.*
Distended abdomen: *Magnes. Phos.*
Dryness of tongue: *Kali Phos., Natr. Mur.*
Duodenum, catarrh of the: *Kali Mur.*
Dysentery, accompanied by sanious, purulent discharges: *Kali Mur.*
sharp, griping pains: *Magnes. Phos.*
Dyspepsia with flushed face and throbbing pain in the stomach: *Ferrum Phos.*
Enteric fever, first stage: *Ferrum Phos.*
Enteritis, second stage: *Kali Mur.*
Eyeballs protrude: *Kali Mur.*
Face pale and anxious: *Calc. Phos.*
Feces, inability to expel: *Calc. Fluor.*
Fissures of anus: *Calc. Phos., Calc. Fluor.*
Fistulae, without pain: *Calc. Phos.*
Flatulence, with pains in left side: *Kali Phos.*

Flatulent colic: *Natr. Phos., Natr. Sulph.*
Flatulent distention of the abdomen: *Natr. Mur.*
Flatus, passing of much: *Magnes. Phos.*
Food, child craves, it should not eat: *Calc. Phos.*
Frequent calls to stool, no passage: *Calc. Phos., Kali Phos., Magnes. Phos.*
Fretful children: *Calc. Phos.*
Gnawing in bowels: *Magnes. Phos.*
Head, sweating of, in children: *Silicea.*
Headache with vomiting of food: *Ferrum Phos.*
Heart, distress about: *Kali Phos.*
Heartburn: *Ferrum Phos.*
Heat in lower bowels: *Natr. Sulph., Ferrum Phos.*
Hemorrhoids, accompanied by albuminous discharges: *Calc. Phos.*
constipation: *Natr. Mur.*
cutting pains: *Magnes. Phos.*
dark, thick blood: *Kali Mur.*
flow of bright-red blood: *Ferrum Phos.*
in anemic persons: *Calc. Phos.*
Inflammation of bowels, first stage: *Ferrum Phos.*
Infant cries when it nurses: *Calc. Phos.*
Inflammation of the inguinal glands: *Silicea.*
Jaundice when caused by a chill resulting in catarrh of the duodenum, white coated tongue, and white colored stools: *Kali Mur.*
Jelly-like masses of mucus: *Natr. Phos.*
Legs, drawing up of: *Magnes. Phos.*
Liver, abscess of: *Silicea.*
with purulent discharge: *Calc. Sulph.*
congestion of: *Natr. Sulph., Ferrum Phos.*
induration of: *Silicea.*
irritable, after mental strain: *Natr. Sulph., Kali Phos.*
Liver, pains in region of: *Kali Mur.*
sensitive: *Natr. Sulph.*
sharp, shooting pains in: *Natr. Sulph.*

Liver, sluggish: *Kali Mur.*
sore to touch: *Natr. Sulph.*
Marasmus: *Calc. Phos.*
Navel, pain near: *Calc. Phos.*
Neuralgia of bowels: *Magnes. Phos.*
rectum: *Calc. Phos.*
Offensive stools: *Calc. Phos., Kali Phos.*
Orchitis, first stage, when there is fever, pain and throbbing: *Ferrum Phos.*
Pain in the abdomen, just above the crest of the ilium on a line of the umbilicus deep within beside the right hip: *Kali Sulph.*
near the navel: *Calc. Phos.*
rectum and abdomen: *Natr. Mur.*
of a colicky nature caused by sudden change from hot to cold: *Kali Sulph.*
Pains, relieved by pressure: *Magnes. Phos.*
rubbing: *Magnes. Phos.*
warmth: *Magnes. Phos.*
Peritonitis, first stage: *Ferrum Phos.*
second stage: *Kali Mur.*
with chilliness: *Ferrum Phos.*
Piles, accompanied by bleeding, bright-red blood: *Ferrum Phos*
itching: *Calc. Phos., Calc. Fluor., Ferrum Phos.*
pain and soreness: *Calc. Fluor.*
rush of blood to head: *Calc. Fluor., Ferrum Phos*
stinging pains: *Natr. Mur.*
thick, yellow, mattery discharges: *Silicea.*
yellow, slimy coating on tongue: *Kali Sulph.*
protruding: *Calc. Phos., Calc. Fluor., Ferrum Phos.*
Prolapsus recti: *Kali Phos., Calc. Fluor.*
Rectum, pain in: *Magnes. Phos.*
Remittent pains: *Magnes. Phos.*
Right shoulder-blade, pains under: *Kali Mur.*
Second stage of peritonitis: *Kali Mur.*
Sleep, restless: *Natr. Phos.*

Sluggish action of the liver, with pale yellow evacuations; pain in region of liver or under the right shoulder blade: *Kali. Mur.*

constipation, with furred tongue and protruding eyeballs: *Kali Mur.*

Sore crack near end of bowel: *Calc. Fluor.*

Spasmodic pains: *Magnes. Phos.*

Sulphurous odor of gas from bowels: *Kali Sulph.*

Summer complaint: *Calc. Phos.*

Swelling of abdomen: *Kali Mur.*

Tabes mesenterica: *Calc. Phos.*

Tongue, white-furred: *Kali Mur.*

yellow and slimy, sometimes with whitish edge: *Kali Sulph.*

Torn feeling after stool: *Natr. Mur.*

To prevent formation of gall stones: *Calc. Phos.*

To reduce inflammation: *Ferrum Phos.*

Typhlitis to assist to reduce inflammation: *Ferrum Phos., Natr. Sulph.*

Typhoid, enteric or typhus fevers with evening aggravation and rise of temperature: *Kali Sulph.*

Ulceration of bowels: *Natr. Phos., Calc. Sulph.*

Vomiting ot bile: *Natr. Sulph.*

curdled masses: *Natr. Phos.*

Weakness of bowels: *Natr. Mur.*

muscles of abdomen: *Natr. Mur.*

Worms of all kinds with accompanying symptoms of picking at the nose, itching at the anus, pain in the abdomen, acidity of the stomach, restless sleep: *Natr. Phos.*

Worse after change of weather: *Calc. Phos., Silicea.*

at night: *Calc. Phos.*

STOOLS

Bowels discharging mattery substances or very constipated in later stages of consumption: *Calc. Sulph.*

Cholera infantum, the child craves food it should not eat: *Calc. Phos.*

when the stools are profuse and have the appearance of rice water: *Kali Phos.*

Constipation from dryness of the mucous membrane with watery secretions in other parts: *Natr. Mur*

in typhus fever: *Kali Mur.*

light colored stool, showing want of bile: sluggish action of the liver: *Kali Mur.*

with drowsiness and watery symptoms from the eyes or mouth: *Natr. Mur.*

dull, heavy headache, profusion of tears or vomiting of frothy mucus: *Natr. Mur.*

Diarrhea after eating greasy food: *Kali Mur.*

fruit, abdomen sunken: *Calc. Phos.*

alternating with constipation: *Natr. Mur.*

especially of children, with green, sour smelling stools caused by an acid condition: *Natr. Phos.*

in teething children; stools slimy, green, undigested, with colic: *Calc. Phos.*

like water: *Natr. Mur.*

with sanious discharge from the bowels: *Calc. Sulph.*

of school girls, accompanied by headache: *Calc. Phos.*

stools frothy, slimy, causing soreness and smarting: *Natr. Phos.*

when there is much straining at stool or constant urging to stool with passing of jelly-like mucus indicating acidity: *Natr. Phos.*

with greenish, bilious stools or vomiting of bile: *Natr. Sulph.*

pale, yellow, clay-colored stool, swelling of the abdomen, slimy stools: *Kali Mur.*

Diarrhea, putrid, foul evacuations, depression and exhaustion of the nerves: *Kali Phos.*

yellow, slimy, purulent matter: *Kali Sulph.*

Dysentery, purging with slimy, sanious evacuations, pain in the abdomen, constant urging to stool; straining with great pain in the anus extorting cries: *Kali Mur.*

when accompanied by sharp grinding pains in the abdomen which are relieved by warmth, rubbing or pressure: *Magnes. Phos.*

the stools consist of pure blood, abdomen swollen, patient becomes delirious, stools have a foul, putrid odor, dryness of the tongue: *Kali Phos.*

with sanious discharge from the bowels: *Calc. Sulph.*

Flatulent colic with green sour smelling stools, or vomiting of curdled masses: *Natr. Phos.*

Frequent call for stool, but passes nothing: *Calc. Phos.*

Griping pain in the abdomen with watery diarrhea, stools expelled with force; *Natr. Mur.*

Loose morning stool, worse in cold, wet weather: *Natr. Sulph*

Looseness of the bowels in old people: *Natr. Sulph.*

with watery stools: *Natr. Mur.*

Offensive stools: *Calc. Phos.*

Retention of stool: *Natr. Mur.*

Stool is hot, often noisy and offensive: *Calc. Phos.*

Stools are dry and often produce fissures in the rectum: *Natr. Mur.*

Summer complaint caused by inability to properly digest the food: *Calc. Phos.*

Typhoid or enteric fever, white coated tongue and looseness of the bowels, stools pale color: *Kali Mur.*

Varices of the anus: *Natr. Mur.*

URINARY ORGANS

After febrile diseases for the characteristic discharge of pus and mucus in the urine: *Silicea.*

Albuminous urine: *Kali Phos., Calc. Phos.*

Bladder, catarrh of, when secreting watery, transparent fluid: *Natr. Mur.*

chronic inflammation of: *Kali Mur., Ferrum Phos., Calc. Sulph.*

Blood passing from urethra: *Kali Phos.*

Brickdust sediment in urine: *Natr. Sulph.*

Bright's disease: *Kali Phos., Calc. Phos.*

Bright's disease, with fever and congestion: *Ferrum Phos.*

Burning after urinating: *Natr. Mur., Ferrum Phos.*

pain over kidneys: *Ferrum Phos.*

Catarrh of the bladder when secreting transparent watery fluid: *Natr. Mur.*

Chronic inflammation of the bladder when passing sanious or bloody matter: *Calc. Fluor.*

Constant urging to urinate, if not chronic: *Ferrum Phos.*

Cutting and burning after urinating: *Natr. Mur.*

Cystitis, chronic: *Kali Mur.*

discharge or yellow, slimy matter from urethra· *Kali Sulph.*

thick, white, slimy mucus *Kali Mur.*

first stage *Ferrum Pho*

second stage, with swelling and discharge of thick, white, slimy mucus: *Kali Mur.*

third stage of inflammation: *Kali Sulph.*

for prostration: *Kali Phos.*

Constant urging to urinate: *Ferrum Phos.*

Cutting after urinating: *Natr. Mur.*

pains at neck of bladder: *Calc. Phos.*

Dark red urine with rheumatism: *Natr. Phos.*

Desire to urinate with scanty emission: *Silicea.*

Diabetes insipidus: *Natr. Mur.*
mellitus: *Calc. Phos., Natr. Sulph.*
with feverishness and congestion: *Ferrum Phos.*

Enuresis of children: *Kali Phos., Natr. Phos., Ferrum Phos.*
if from worms: *Natr. Phos.*

Excessive flow of watery urine: *Natr. Mur., Ferrum Phos.*
secretion of urine when diabetic: *Natr. Sulph.*

First stage of inflammation of the bladder causing retention of urine with pain and smarting when urination: *Ferrum Phos.*

Febrile diseases, after, when mucus and pus in urine: *Silicea.*

Frequent micturition at night, also unsuccessful desire to urinate: *Natr. Mur.*
urging to urinate with sharp shooting pains, cutting at the neck of the bladder and along the urethra: *Calc. Phos.*
urination with inability to retain the urine with corresponding symptoms of acidity; more frequently seen in children: *Natr. Phos.*
passing of much water, sometimes scalding: *Kali. Phos.*

Gravel in bilious persons: *Natr. Sulph.*
pain while passing: *Natr. Sulph., Magnes Phos.*
sediment in urine: *Natr. Sulph., Calc. Phos.*
with gouty symptoms: *Natr. Sulph.*

Great quantity of urine: *Ferrum Phos.*

Great thirst, with excessive flow of watery urine: *Natr. Mur.*

Highly-colored urine: *Calc. Phos., Ferrum Phos.*
with fever: *Natr. Phos., Ferrum Phos.*

Hunger, voracious: *Kali Phos.*

Inability to retain urine, from nervous debility: *Kali Phos.*

Incontinence from paralysis of sphincter: *Kali Phos.*
weakness of sphincter: *Ferrum Phos.*

Increase in quantity of urine: *Calc. Phos.*

Increased quantity of urine when traced to a relaxed condition of the muscle fibres of the urinary organs: *Calc. Fluor.*

Inflammation of the kidneys: *Ferrum Phos.*
second stage: *Kali Mur.*
Involuntary emission of urine while walking: *Natr. Mur.*
Lithia deposit in urine: *Natr. Sulph.*
Micturition almost every night: *Silicea.*
Nephritis, first stage: *Ferrum Phos.*
second stage: *Kali Mur.*
third stage: *Silicea.*
Pain when passing gravel: *Magnes. Phos.*
Passing of blood from the urethra: *Kali Phos.*
Phosphatic deposits in urine: *Calc. Phos.*
Polyuria: *Natr. Mur.*
Rheumatism, with dark-red urine: *Ferrum Phos.*
Sandy deposits in urine: *Natr. Sulph.*
Sediment clings to side of vessel: *Natr. Sulph.*
Sharp shooting pains at neck of bladder: *Calc. Phos.*
Sleeplessness: *Kali Phos.*
Smarting on urinating: *Ferrum Phos.*
Sore pain over kidneys: *Ferrum Phos.*
Spasmodic retention of urine: *Magnes. Phos.*
Spasms of bladder, with painful straining: *Magnes Phos., Ferrum Phos., Kali Phos.*
urethra, with painful straining: *Magnes. Phos. Ferrum Phos., Kali Phos.*
Stone, to prevent reformation of: *Calc. Phos.*
Urine frequently scalding: *Kali Phos.*
suppression of, through heat: *Ferrum Phos.*
dark colored, deposits of uric acid when there is torpidity and inactivity of the liver: *Kali Mur.*
high colored: *Calc. Phos.*
feverish smell: *Ferrum Phos.*
Wetting the bed from weakness of the muscles of the neck of the bladder, if from worms: *Ferrum Phos.*

MALE GENITAL ORGANS

Albuminous discharge from urethra: *Calc. Phos.*

Bubo, first stage, when there is fever, pain, and throbbing: *Ferrum Phos.*

for soft swelling: *Kali Mur.*

syphilitic or gonorrheal in the suppurative stage, with sanious purulent discharge: *Calc. Sulph.*

Condylomata, of syphilitic origin: *Natr. Sulph.*

Discharge of prostatic fluid: *Natr. Mur.*

Dropsy of testicles: *Calc. Fluor., Calc. Phos.*

Evening aggravation of syphilis, gleet when yellow and slimy: *Kali Sulph.*

Excessive sexual desire: *Natr. Mur.*

Gleet, yellow, slimy discharge: *Kali Sulph.*

Gonorrhea: *Kali Mur.*

chronic, thick, yellow discharge: *Silicea.*

with transparent watery, scalding, slimy discharge: *Natr. Mur.*

for inflammation, first stage: *Ferrum Phos.*

with discharge of blood: *Kali Phos.*

sanious, purulent discharge: *Calc. Sulph.*

slimy, yellow or greenish discharge: *Kali Sulph.*

Hardening of testicle: *Calc. Fluor.*

Hydrocele: *Calc. Phos., Natr. Mur., Natr. Phos., Silicea.*

Inflammation of prostate gland: *Ferrum Phos.*

Inflammatory swelling of the testicles from suppressed gonorrhea: *Kali Mur.*

Inguinal hernia: *Calc. Phos., Calc. Fluor.*

Irregularity of the sexual desires, either gone or increased when there are other indications of acid conditions of the system: *Natr. Phos.*

Irritation of prostate gland: *Ferrum Phos.*

Itching and humid spots in the scrotum: *Silicea.*

in the scrotum with much sweat: *Silicea.*

Masturbation: *Calc. Phos.*

Orchitis: *Ferrum Phos., Calc. Phos.*
from suppressed gonorrhea: *Kali Mur., Calc. Phos*
Phagedenic chancres: *Kali Phos.*
Preputial edema: *Natr. Sulph., Natr. Mur.*
Prostate gland, suppurative abscess of: *Calc. Sulph.*
Prostatitis, when suppuration has commenced: *Silicea.*
Scrotum itches: *Calc. Phos., Silicea.*
relaxed: *Calc. Phos.*
soreness of: *Calc. Phos.*
sweating of: *Calc. Phos., Silicea.*
Seminal emissions, without dreams: *Natr. Phos.*
Sexual desire is very much excited: *Silicea.*
Sexual desires, irregularity of: *Natr. Phos.*
Suppurating abscess of the prostate gland: *Calc. Sulph.*
Sweating and soreness of the scrotum: *Calc. Phos.*
Swelling of the testicles: *Calc. Phos.*
Syphilis in the suppurating stage: *Calc. Sulph.*
Syphilis, chronic, with hardening and suppuration of tissues: *Silicea.*
serous discharge: *Natr. Mur.*
white discharges: *Kali Mur.*
evening aggravation: *Kali Sulph.*
Varicocele: *Ferrum Phos.*

FEMALE GENITAL DISORDERS

Abdominal spasms followed by leucorrhea: *Magnes. Phos.*
Abscess of labia: *Silicea.*
Aching in the intestines: *Calc. Phos.*
Aching in uterus: *Calc. Phos.*
Acid leucorrhea, worse after menstruating, or with sexual excitement: *Calc. Phos.*
Acrid pain during leucorrhea, with yellowness of the face: *Natr. Mur.*

After confinement when the pelvic muscles are relaxed: *Calc. Fluor.*
All displacements of the uterus: *Calc. Fluor.*
Amenorrhea, with depression: *Kali Phos.*
Anteversion: *Calc. Fluor.*
Ball rising in throat: *Kali Phos.*
Colic in nervous, lachrymose women: *Kali Phos., Magnes. Phos.*
Congestion of the uterus, chronic or second stage, menstrual periods too frequent; lasting too long: *Kali Mur.*
Discharge, deep-red or blackish-red: *Kali Phos.*
scalding, smarting: *Natr. Mur.*
sickening: *Natr. Phos.*
sour-smelling: *Natr. Phos.*
thick, white, bland: *Kali Mur.*
Discharge, thin, with offensive odor: *Kali Phos.*
Displacement of uterus: *Calc. Fluor., Calc. Phos., Kali Phos.*
Dragging in groin: *Calc. Fluor.*
small of back: *Calc. Fluor.*
Dryness of vagina: *Natr. Mur.*
Dysmenorrhea: *Magnes. Phos.*
labor-like pains during: *Magnes. Phos.*
to prevent: *Ferrum Phos.*
Dysmenorrhea with congestion: *Ferrum Phos.*
vomiting of undigested food: *Ferrum Phos.*
First stage of gonorrhea: *Ferrum Phos.*
Flexions of the womb: *Calc. Fluor.*
Gonorrhea: *Kali Mur., Ferrum Phos., Calc. Sulph., Kali Sulph.*
Hypertrophy, second stage, to reduce the swelling, if very bad: *Kali Mur.*
Hysteric fits of crying: *Kali Phos.*
Increased menses: *Silicea.*
sexual desire, especially before menstruation: *Calc. Phos.*
Inflammation of uterus: *Ferrum Phos.*
vagina: *Ferrum Phos.*

Leucorrhea, accompanied by albuminous discharge: *Calc. Phos.*
milky-white, non-irritating discharge: *Kali Mur.*
rawness and itching of parts: *Natr. Phos.*
scalding, acrid discharge: *Natr. Mur., Kali Phos.*
thick, yellow, bloody discharge: *Calc. Sulph.*
watery, slimy, excoriating discharge: *Natr. Mur.*
yellow, creamy discharge: *Natr. Phos.*
slimy, greenish discharge: *Kali Sulph.*

Listlessness: *Calc. Phos., Kali Phos.*

Menstruation, accompanied by acrid leucorrhea: *Calc. Phos. Natr. Phos.*
bearing-down pains: *Calc. Fluor.*
cold extremities: *Calc. Phos., Ferrum Phos.*
colic: *Natr. Sulph., Kali Phos., Magnes. Phos.*
constipation: *Silicea, Natr. Sulph.*
excitableness: *Kali Phos.*
fetid sweating of feet: *Silicea.*
flushed face: *Ferrum Phos., Calc. Phos.*
by frontal headache: *Natr. Phos.*
fullness in abdomen: *Kali Sulph.*
headache: *Natr. Mur., Ferrum Phos. Kali Phos.*
hysteria: *Kali Phos.*
icy coldness of body: *Silicea.*
increased sexual desire: *Calc. Phos.*

Menstruation, accompanied by labor-like pains: *Calc. Phos., Magnes. Phos.*
leucorrhea: *Natr. Mur.*
morning diarrhea: *Natr. Sulph.*
nervousness: *Kali Phos.*
pains in back: *Calc. Phos.*
sadness: *Natr. Mur.*
weeping: *Natr. Mur.*
weight in abdomen: *Kali Sulph.*

Menstruation, delayed, in young girls: *Natr. Mur.*
repressed: *Kali Mur.*
retarded: *Kali Mur.*
thin, watery blood: *Natr. Mur., Kali Phos.*
too frequent: *Calc. Phos.*
late: *Natr. Mur., Kali Sulph., Kali Phos.*
profuse: *Kali Mur., Calc. Fluor., Kali Phos.*
Menstrual flow bright-red blood: *Ferrum Phos.*
dark, clotted, black blood: *Kali Mur.*
stringy and fibrous: *Magnes. Phos.*
Menstruations of pale, nervous, sensitive women: *Kali Phos.*
Metritis: *Ferrum Phos., Kali Mur.*
Metrorrhagia from standing in water: *Silicea.*
Neuralgia of the ovaries: *Magnes. Phos.*
Ovaralgia: *Magnes. Phos.*
Pains precede monthly flow: *Magnes. Phos.*
Pudenda, burning and itching of: *Silicea.*
Retroversion: *Calc. Fluor.*
Sexual desire increased: *Calc. Phos.*
intercourse painful: *Natr. Mur., Ferrum Phos.*
Spasms of the vagina with excessive dryness: *Ferrum Phos.*
Spasmodic pain in the hypogastrium: *Natr. Mur.*
Sterility due to acid secretions: *Natr. Phos.*
Sticking pains in vagina: *Natr. Mur.*
Thighs, pain extends to: *Calc. Fluor.*
Ulceration of cervix uteri: *Kali Mur.*
os: *Kali Mur.*
Uterine secretions, acid: *Natr. Phos.*
creamy, yellow: *Natr. Phos.*
watery: *Natr. Phos., Natr. Mur.*
weakness: *Calc. Phos., Calc. Fluor., Kali Phos.*
Uterus hard, like stone: *Calc. Fluor.*
relaxed and flabby: *Calc. Fluor.*
Vagina, weakness of, after urinating: *Natr. Mur.*
smarting of, after urinating: *Natr. Mur.*

Vaginal secretions, acid: *Natr. Phos.*
watery, creamy, yellow: *Natr. Phos.*
Vaginismus: *Ferrum Phos., Magnes. Phos.*
with dryness: *Natr. Mur., Ferrum Phos.*
Vulva, itching of: *Natr. Mur., Calc., Phos.*
Weakness in the uterine region from prolapsus uteri and other uterine displacements: *Calc. Phos.*

PREGNANCY

Aching in limbs during: *Calc. Phos.*
After-pains: *Ferrum Phos.*
when too weak: *Calc. Fluor.*
Bitter taste in mouth: *Natr. Sulph.*
Brain function perverted: *Kali Phos., Kali Mur.*
Contract, uterus does not: *Calc. Fluor.*
Convulsions: *Magnes. Phos.*
Expulsive efforts, excessive: *Magnes. Phos.*
Fistulous ulcers of breast: *Silicea.*
Hard knots in breast: *Calc. Fluor., Kali Mur., Silicea.*
Hemorrhage: *Calc. Fluor., Ferrum Phos.*
Labor pains, feeble: *Kali Phos.*
ineffectual: *Kali Phos.*
spasmodic: *Magnes. Phos.*
spurious: *Kali Phos.*
with cramps in legs: *Magnes. Phos.*
spasmodic twitchings: *Magnes. Phos.*
tedious, from weakness: *Kali Phos.*
Lacerations, to aid in healing: *Ferrum Phos.*
Mania: *Kali Mur., Kali Phos.*
Mastitis, first stage, for fever: *Ferrum Phos.*
for swelling, before pus forms: *Kali Mur.*
to control suppuration: *Silicea.*
with brown, dirty, offensive discharge: *Kali Phos.*
suppurations: *Calc. Sulph., Silicea.*

Milk, salty: *Natr. Mur.*
watery: *Natr. Mur., Calc. Phos.*
Miscarriage in weak subjects: *Kali Phos.*
Morning sickness: *Kali Mur.*
accompanied by sour, acid vomiting: *Natr. Phos.*
vomiting of bilious fluids: *Natr. Sulph.*
food: *Ferrum Phos.*
Nausea, with sour risings: *Natr. Phos.*
Nipples, sore: *Calc. Phos., Ferrum Phos.*
Nurse, child refuses to: *Calc. Phos.*
Nursing, debility from long: *Calc. Phos.*
Puerperal fever: *Kali Phos., Kali Mur., Ferrum Phos.*
Septic poisons: *Kali Mur., Kali Phos.*
Vomiting, frothy phlegm: *Natr. Mur.*
sour, curdled milk: *Calc. Phos.*
watery phlegm: *Natr. Mur.*
white phlegm: *Kali Mur.*

RESPIRATORY ORGANS

Abscess of lungs: *Silicea.*
Absence of expectoration: *Magnes. Phos.*
Aching in chest: *Calc. Phos.*
Acute inflammation of the windpipe with expectoration of frothy, watery mucus, constant frothy expectoration: *Natr. Mur.*
edema of the lungs, spasmodic cough, threatening suppuration: *Kali Phos.*
Acute, painful, short, irritating cough: *Ferrum Phos.*
All inflammatory conditions of the respiratory tract, in the first stage: *Ferrum Phos.*
All symptoms worse in damp weather, also rainy weather: *Natr. Sulph.*

Anemia: *Ferrum Phos., Calc. Phos.*

Aneurism: *Ferrum Phos.*

Arteritis in the congestive stage: *Ferrum Phos.*

Asthma, accompanied by belching of gas: *Magnes. Phos.*
constrictive cough: *Magnes. Phos.*
difficult expectoration: *Calc. Fluor.*
expectoration of frothy, watery mucus: *Natr. Mur.*
tiny, yellow lumps: *Kali Phos., Calc. Fluor.*
gastric derangements: *Kali Mur.*
greenish, purulent expectoration: *Natr. Sulph.*
by labored breathing: *Kali Phos.*
loose evacuations in morning: *Natr. Sulph.*
pain in chest: *Magnes. Phos.*
by soreness in chest: *Ferrum Phos.*

Blood thin and watery; will not coagulate: *Natr. Mur.*

Breath, short of, from asthma: *Kali Phos.*
worse from motion: *Kali Phos.*

Breathing, hurried, at beginning of disease: *Ferrum Phos.*

Bronchial asthma: *Kali Sulph.*
when expectoration is fetid: *Kali Phos.*
with yellow expectoration: *Kali Sulph.*
catarrh: *Natr. Sulph., Natr. Mur.*

Bronchitis, first stage: *Ferrum Phos.*
last stage: *Calc. Sulph.*
mucus frothy, watery: *Natr. Mur.*

Carditis in the congestive stage: *Ferrum Phos.*

Catch in breath: *Ferrum Phos.*

Children, cough of teething: *Calc. Phos.*

Chronic coughs: *Calc. Phos.*

Chronic whooping cough: *Calc. Phos.*

Cold in chest: *Ferrum Phos.*

Constant spitting of frothy water: *Natr. Mur.*

Constriction of chest: *Magnes. Phos.*

Consumption, bloody, mattery expectoration: *Calc. Sulph.*
chronic, cough of: *Natr. Mur.*
dryness of throat in: *Calc. Phos.*
expectoration causes rawness of mouth: *Natr. Phos.*
soreness of lips: *Natr. Phos.*
heavy cough: *Kali Mur.*
incipient: *Calc. Phos*
purulent expectoration: *Calc. Sulph.*
soreness of throat in: *Calc. Phos.*
Convulsive fits of coughing: *Magnes. Phos.*
Cough, better in cool open air: *Kali Sulph.*
hard, dry: *Ferrum Phos.*
irritating, painful: *Ferrum Phos.*
pain in chest from: *Natr. Mur., Ferrum Phos.*
with headache: *Natr. Mur.*
with hectic fever: *Calc. Sulph.*
lachrymation: *Natr. Mur.*
mattery sputa: *Calc. Sulph.*
Cough, worse in evening: *Kali Sulph.*
warm room: *Kali Sulph.*
Countenance, pale, livid: *Kali Phos.*
Croup, first stage, for febrile symptoms: *Ferrum Phos.*
for exudation: *Kali Mur.*
last stage: *Kali Phos., Calc. Sulph.*
Croupy hoarseness: *Kali Mur., Kali Sulph.*
Debility: *Silicea, Calc. Phos., Natr. Mur.*
Deficiency of red blood corpuscles: *Ferrum Phos.*
Dilatation of the blood vessels, the elastic fibres of the walls of the blood vessels have been relaxed: *Calc. Fluor.*
heart or of the blood vessels: *Ferrum Phos.*
Edema of the lungs with watery expectoration: *Natr. Mur., Kali Phos.*
Embolism, for the condition of the blood which favors the formation of clots which act as plugs: *Kali Mur.*

Endocarditis in the congestive stage: *Ferrum Phos.*

Exhaustion: *Kali Phos.*

Expectoration, albuminous: *Calc. Phos.*
difficult: *Natr. Mur., Kali Mur.*
salty: *Natr. Mur.*
slips back: *Kali Sulph.*
streaked with blood: *Ferrum Phos.*
thick, yellow, green pus: *Silicea.*
tiny yellow lumps: *Calc. Fluor., Silicea.*
watery: *Natr. Mur.*
yellow, green, slimy: *Kali Sulph.*

Extreme weakness: *Kali Phos.*

Eyes, protruded appearance of: *Kali Mur.*

Fainting from fright, fatigue or weak heart action; pulse low and hardly perceptible: *Kali Phos.*

First stage of aneurism: *Calc. Phos.*

Flow of tears: *Natr. Mur.*

Full, rapid, quick pulse in fevers: *Ferrum Phos.*

Glottis, spasm of: *Magnes Phos.*

Gurgling of mucus in chest: *Kali Sulph.*

Harsh breathing: *Natr. Sulph.*

Hawking, to clear throat: *Calc. Phos.*

Hay asthma, for depression: *Kali Phos.*

Hectic fever: *Silicea.*

Hemorrhage, bright-red, from lungs: *Ferrum Phos.*

Hoarseness from cold: *Kali Mur.*
overexertion of voice: *Calc. Phos.*
of speakers: *Ferrum Phos.*

Hypertrophy or enlargement of the heart: *Calc. Fluor.*

In asthma when the expectoration is difficult and consists of small yellow lumps: *Calc. Fluor.*

In consumption when expectoration causes soreness of the lips or rawness of the tongue and mouth: *Natr. Phos.*

In the beginning of all colds: *Ferrum Phos.*

In whooping cough for the yellow, slimy expectoration: *Kali. Sulph.*
frothy, watery expectoration: *Natr. Mur.*
Incipient consumption: *Calc. Phos.*
Inflammation of the blood vessels: *Ferrum Phos.*
respiratory tract when tissue destruction has gone to that stage in which there is copious expectoration of thick yellow or greenish-yellow pus accompanied with hectic fever, profuse night sweats, and great debility: *Silicea.*
Inflammatory condition of the respiratory tract when the expectoration is decidedly yellowish, greenish and slimy: *Kali Sulph.*
Involuntary sighing: *Calc. Phos.*
sighing or moaning during sleep: *Kali Phos.*
Irregularities of the heart action, when due to prolapsus of the uterus and other relaxing diseases: *Calc. Phos.*
Intercurrently in most cases of heart troubles with characteristic symptoms: *Calc. Phos.*
Intermittent irregular pulse: *Kali Phos.*
action of the heart after violent excitement, grief or care: *Kali Phos.*
Involuntary sighing: *Calc. Phos., Kali Phos.*
Last stage of consumption when the expectoration is purulent, watery, and sometimes bloody: *Calc. Sulph.*
croup, pneumonia or bronchitis: *Calc. Sulph.*
Leuchemia (excess of white blood corpuscles): *Calc. Phos.*
Loss of voice: *Kali Mur.*
Loss of voice from paralysis of the vocal cords: *Kali Phos.*
Loud, noisy cough: *Kali Mur.*
Milky sputa: *Kali Mur.*
Moaning during sleep: *Kali Phos.*

Must go in open air for relief: *Kali Sulph.*
sit up, in asthma: *Magnes. Phos.*
Naevi; varicose veins: *Ferrum Phos.*
Neuralgic spasms of the breast: *Magnes. Phos.*
Nervous depression: *Kali Phos.*
Night-sweats about head: *Calc. Phos., Silicea, Natr. Mur.*
profuse: *Silicea.*
Oppression: *Ferrum Phos.*
Pain in side: *Ferrum Phos.*
Pain in the chest: *Natr. Mur.*
Painful hoarseness and huskiness of speakers and singers when due to irritating bronchi: *Ferrum Phos.*
Paralysis of vocal cords: *Kali Phos.*
Pleurisy in the inflammatory stage, and as long as the pain lasts: *Ferrum Phos.*
second stage, with thick, white, viscid expectoration: *Kali Mur.*
when serous effusion has taken place: *Kali Mur., Natr. Mur.*
Pneumonia, first stage: *Ferrum Phos.*
second stage: *Kali Mur.*
last stage: *Calc. Sulph.*
watery, frothy expectoration: *Natr. Mur.*
yellow, slimy expectoration: *Kali Sulph.*
Prostration: *Calc. Fluor., Kali Phos.*
Pus forms in cavity of lungs: *Calc. Sulph.*
spreads out: *Calc. Sulph., Silicea.*
Râles in chest: *Kali Mur.*
Rattling in chest: *Kali Mur., Natr. Mur.*
Rheumatic pains in lungs: *Calc. Phos.*
Rise of temperature in evening in consumption: *Kali Sulph.*
Second stage of all inflammatory conditions of the respiratory tract, with thick white phlegm or milky sputa: *Kali Mur.*
Sensation of weariness to pressure, speaking is fatiguing: *Kali Sulph.*
Sharp pains in chest: *Magnes. Phos.*

Short spasmodic cough like whooping cough: *Kali Mur.*

Shortness of breath from asthma or with exhaustion or want of proper nerve power; worse from motion or exertion: *Kali Phos.*

Sighing during sleep: *Kali Phos.*

Soreness of chest: *Ferrum Phos.*

Spasms of glottis: *Magnes. Phos.*

Spasmodic cough: *Magnes Phos., Kali Phos., Kali Mur.*
 at night: *Magnes. Phos.*
 worse lying down: *Magnes. Phos.*

Speaking fatigues: *Kali Sulph.*

Spurting of urine: *Natr. Mur., Ferrum Phos.*

Sputa, thick, much and pus-like: *Silicea.*

Sudden, shrill voice: *Magnes. Phos.*

Suffocates in heated room: *Kali Sulph.*

Stomach cough: *Kali Mur.*

Thick, tenacious, white phlegm: *Kali Mur.*

Threatened suffocation: *Kali Phos.*

Tickling in throat: *Calc. Fluor.*

Tongue coated white: *Kali Mur.*

Uvula, elongated: *Calc. Fluor.*

Vessel, pus falls to bottom of: *Calc. Sulph.*

Want of breath: *Calc. Phos.*

Weakness and prostration: *Calc. Phos.*

Weariness in pharynx: *Kali Sulph.*

Whooping-cough, chronic cases: *Calc. Phos.*
 febrile symptoms: *Ferrum Phos.*
 watery, frothy expectoration: *Natr. Mur.*
 white expectoration: *Kali Mur.*
 with depression: *Kali Phos.*
 yellow, slimy expectoration: *Kali Sulph.*

Winter Cough: *Natr. Mur.*

CIRCULATORY ORGANS

Anemia: *Ferrum Phos., Calc. Phos.*
palpitation in: *Natr. Mur.*
Aneurism: *Ferrum Phos., Calc. Fluor.*
Angina pectoris: *Magnes. Phos.*
Arteritis, in congestive stage: *Ferrum Phos.*
Blood, thin, watery: *Natr. Mur.*
Blood-vessels, dilatation of: *Ferrum Phos., Calc. Fluor.*
inflammation of: *Ferrum Phos.*
Carditis: *Ferrum Phos.*
Circulation, poor: *Kali Phos., Calc. Phos.*
Dilatation of heart: *Ferrum Phos.*
Dizziness: *Kali Phos.*
Embolism: *Kali Mur.*
Endocarditis: *Ferrum Phos.*
Face, pallid: *Kali Sulph.*
Fainting: *Kali Phos.*
from fright, grief: *Kali Phos.*
Hands and feet cold: *Calc. Phos., Natr. Mur.*
Hyperemia: *Ferrum Phos.*
Hypertrophy: *Calc. Fluor., Kali Mur.*
Ileum, throbbing, boring pain over: *Kali Sulph.*
Irregularity of heart from prolapsus uteri: *Calc. Fluor.*
Leuchemia: *Ferrum Phos.*
Naevi: *Ferrum Phos.*
Palpitation, accompanied by anxiety: *Kali Phos.*
melancholia: *Kali Phos.*
nervousness: *Kali Phos.*
restlessness: *Kali Phos.*
sleeplessness: *Kali Phos.*
after violent emotion: *Kali Phos.*
followed by weakness: *Calc. Phos., Kali Phos.*
from indigestion: *Natr. Phos.*
inflammations: *Ferrum Phos.*
on ascending stairs: *Kali Phos.*

Pericarditis, first stage: *Ferrum Phos.*
second stage: *Kali Mur.*
Phlebitis: *Ferrum Phos.*
Pressure about heart: *Natr. Sulph., Kali Phos.*
Pulse felt all over body: *Natr. Mur.*
full, rapid, quick: *Ferrum Phos.*
intermittent: *Kali Phos., Natr. Mur.*
irregular: *Kali Phos.*
sluggish: *Kali Phos., Kali Sulph.*
subnormal: *Kali Phos.*
Shortness of breath: *Kali Phos.*
Skin hot and dry, harsh: *Kali Sulph.*
Temperature rises toward evening: *Kali Sulph.*
Trembling about heart: *Natr. Phos.*
worse after eating: *Natr. Phos.*
Uneasiness about heart: *Natr. Sulph.*
Varicose veins: *Ferrum Phos., Calc. Fluor.*
Veins seem as if they would burst: *Calc. Fluor.*
Vertigo, with giddiness: *Natr. Sulph.*

BACK AND EXTREMITIES

Acid, sour smelling perspiration: *Natr. Phos.*
diathesis: *Natr. Phos.*
Acute and chronic rheumatism, very painful, parts feel stiff, severe morning, after rest, or when rising from a sitting position; worse from exertion or fatigue, relieved by gentle movement: *Kali Phos.*
Abscess, deep-seated, on bones: *Calc. Phos., Kali Phos.*
Aggravations in morning after rest: *Kali Phos.*
Arthritis: *Ferrum Phos., Natr. Sulph.*
Articular rheumatism: *Natr. Phos., Ferrum Phos.*
spinal irritation: *Calc. Phos.*
when rising from sitting posture: *Calc. Phos.*

Back, feeling of coldness in: *Natr. Mur.*
pains in: *Natr. Mur., Ferrum Phos.*
Backache, relieved by lying on something hard: *Natr. Mur.*
Blisters on hands, containing water: *Natr. Mur.*
Bones soft and friable: *Calc. Phos.*
ulcerations of: *Silicea, Calc. Sulph., Calc. Phos.*
Burning of soles of feet in consumption: *Calc. Sulph.*
pains in sacrum: *Calc. Fluor.*
Cannot sit still: *Natr. Mur.*
Carbuncles, on back, suppuration: *Calc. Sulph.*
to hasten suppuration: *Silicea.*
Caries of bones, with fistulous openings: *Silicea.*
Chilblains on hands and feet: *Kali Phos., Kali Mur.*
Chronic swelling of feet and legs: *Kali Mur.*
Coccyx, injuries of: *Calc. Phos.*
Coldness, feeling of, in back: *Natr. Mur.*
of limbs: *Calc. Phos.*
Cold water being poured over limbs, sensation as of: *Calc Phos.*
Convulsions, with clenched fingers: *Magnes. Phos., Calc. Phos*
stiffening of limbs: *Magnes. Phos*
Cracking of joints: *Natr. Phos.*
Creaking of muscles at back of wrist: *Kali Mur.*
Curvature of spine: *Calc. Phos.*
Cysts: *Calc. Phos.*
Discharges, bony fragments: *Silicea, Calc. Fluor.*
Dislocations, easy: *Calc. Fluor.*
Drowsy: *Natr. Mur.*
Electric shocks in limbs: *Magnes. Phos.*
Enlargement of joints: *Calc. Fluor.*
Excrescences on bones: *Calc. Fluor.*
Feeling of coldness in the back: *Natr. Mur.*
Fidgets: *Natr. Mur.*
Fingers painful or inflamed through rheumatism or other causes: *Ferrum Phos.*
Fetid perspiration of feet: *Silicea.*
Fungoid inflammation of joints: *Kali Sulph.*

Glands of neck swollen: *Kali Mur.*
Gout: *Natr. Phos., Natr. Sulph.*
Gouty enlargement of the joints: *Calc. Fluor.*
Head, determination of blood to: *Natr. Sulph.*
pain in back of: *Natr. Sulph.*
Hip-joint disease, before pus forms: *Kali Mur.*
first stages: *Ferrum Phos.*
to control suppuration: *Silicea*
Hydroma patellae: *Calc. Phos.*
Hydrops: *Calc. Phos.*
Idiospinal softening of the spinal cord with gradual moleculai deadening of the nervous centres: *Kali Phos.*
Inflammatory pains over kidneys: *Ferrum Phos.*
through loins: *Ferrum Phos.*
Injuries to the coccyx: *Calc. Phos.*
Involuntary movement of legs: *Natr. Mur.*
Jerking of limbs during sleep: *Natr. Phos., Natr. Mur.*
Lameness: *Natr. Phos.*
Languid: *Natr. Mur.*
Limbs, asleep: *Calc. Phos.*
feel better by moving: *Calc. Phos.*
Lumbago: *Calc. Phos., Ferrum Phos.*
with dragging pain: *Calc. Fluor.*
Neck, muscles stiff: *Ferrum Phos.*
Neuralgic pains, as if on bone: *Calc. Phos.*
better in cool air: *Kali Sulph.*
in thin children: *Calc. Phos.*
commencing at night: *Calc. Phos.*
in back: *Kali Sulph., Natr. Phos.*
limbs: *Magnes. Phos., Natr. Phos.*
worse in evening: *Kali Sulph.*
warm room: *Kali Sulph.*
Numbness, feeling of: *Calc. Phos., Kali Phos.*
Pains during rest: *Kali Phos.*
in damp weather: *Calc. Phos.*
worse at night: *Calc. Phos.*

Paralysis of limbs: *Kali Phos.*
Parts feel bruised: *Kali Phos.*
stiff: *Kali Phos.*
Periodic rheumatic gout: *Natr. Mur.*
Periostitis of syphilitic origin: *Calc. Phos.*
Pott's disease: *Silicea.*
Power of motion deficient: *Magnes. Phos.*
Psoas abscess: *Silicea.*
Rheumatism, acute, articular: *Magnes. Phos.*
bilious: *Natr. Sulph.*
between shoulders: *Calc. Phos.*
for inflammation and fever: *Ferrum Phos.*
from catching cold: *Ferrum Phos.*
gouty: *Natr. Sulph.*
of joints: *Natr. Mur., Calc. Phos., Natr. Phos*
relieved by gentle motion: *Kali Phos.*
sciatic: *Magnes. Phos.*
with swelling: *Kali Mur.*
worse from violent exertion: *Kali Phos.*
Rickets: *Calc. Phos.*
Sciatic rheumatism with violent pains: *Magnes. Phos.*
Shins, pain in: *Calc. Phos.*
Slow learning to walk: *Calc. Phos.*
Soreness of joints: *Natr. Phos.*
Spasms in back: *Natr. Sulph., Magnes. Phos.*
Spinal cord, idiopathic softening of: *Kali Phos.*
meningitis: *Natr. Sulph.*
Sprains: *Ferrum Phos.*
Stiff back: *Ferrum Phos.*
worse from motion: *Ferrum Phos.*
Stiffness: *Kali Phos.*
Strains: *Ferrum Phos.*
Suppuration, first remedy: *Ferrum Phos.*
of joints: *Silicea, Calc. Sulph.*
Swellings, hard · *Calc. Fluor.*
Threatened suppuration: *Silicea.*

Ulcers, deep-seated, on bones: *Calc. Phos.*
on extremities: *Kali Mur.*
Varicose ulcerations of veins of limbs: *Calc. Fluor.*
Wandering rheumatic pains: *Kali Sulph.*
Weakness: *Natr. Mur.*
Whitton: *Calc. Fluor., Silicea, Calc. Sulph.*

NERVOUS SYMPTOMS

Chorea: *Magnes. Phos., Calc. Phos.*
Coldness: *Calc. Phos.*
after fit: *Kali Phos.*
Cold water, pains like trickling of: *Calc. Phos.*
Colic, worse at night: *Calc. Phos.*
Convulsions in old people: *Calc. Phos.*
young people: *Calc. Phos.*
of teething children: *Ferrum Phos., Calc. Phos. Magnes. Phos.*
Cramps in limbs: *Magnes. Phos.*
worse at night: *Calc. Phos.*
Creeping numbness: *Calc. Phos.*
Cries easily: *Kali Phos.*
Despondent: *Kali Phos.*
Dwells upon grievances: *Kali Phos.*
Epilepsy, accompanied by bulging of eyeballs: *Kali Mur.*
eczema: *Kali Mur.*
rush of blood to head: *Ferrum Phos.*
white-coated tongue: *Kali Mur.*
after suppressed eruptions: *Kali Mur.*
from slight provocation:
Silicea, Magnes. Phos., Calc. Phos., Kali Mur.
in general: *Magnes. Phos.*
Electrical shocks, pains like: *Calc. Phos.*
Feels pain keenly: *Kali Phos.*
Feet twitch during sleep: *Natr. Sulph.*

Grinding of teeth, from worms: *Natr. Phos.*

Hands twitch during sleep: *Natr. Sulph.*

Head, involuntary shaking of: *Magnes. Phos.*

Heart, palpitation of: *Natr. Phos.*
    trembling of: *Natr. Phos.*

Hemiplegia: *Kali Phos.*

Hysteria: *Natr. Mur., Kali Phos.*

Impatient: *Kali Phos.*

Involuntary motion of hands: *Magnes. Phos.*

Irritable: *Kali Phos.*

Lassitude: *Natr. Sulph.*

Lock-jaw: *Magnes. Phos.*

Makes mountains out of mole hills: *Kali Phos.*

Nervous sensitiveness: *Kali Phos.*

Neuralgia, accompanied by congestion, after taking cold: *Ferrum Phos.*
        depression: *Kali Phos.*
        failure of strength: *Kali Phos.*
        flow of saliva: *Natr. Mur.*
            tears: *Natr. Mur.*
        shifting pains: *Kali Sulph.*
    in any organ: *Kali Phos.*
    obstinate, heat or cold gives no relief: *Silicea.*
        occurring at night: *Silicea, Calc. Phos.*
    periodic: *Magnes. Phos., Natr. Mur.*
    relieved by gentle motion: *Kali Phos.*
        pleasant excitement: *Kali Phos.*
    sensitive to light: *Kali Phos.*
    noise: *Kali Phos.*
    worse at night: *Kali Phos.*
        in cold weather: *Natr. Mur.*
            the morning: *Natr. Mur.*
        when alone: *Kali Phos.*

Palpitation after fits: *Kali Phos.*

Paralysis, accompanied by fetid breath: *Kali Phos.*
fetid odor of stools: *Kali Phos.*
rheumatism: *Calc. Phos.*
agitans: *Kali Phos., Magnes. Phos.*
creeping: *Kali Phos.*
facial: *Kali Phos.*
infantile: *Kali Phos.*
in general: *Kali Phos.*
locomotor: *Kali Phos.*
partial: *Kali Phos.*
Sensibility, want of: *Magnes. Phos.*
Spasms occurring at night: *Silicea, Magnes. Phos., Calc. Phos.*
Spinal anemia from exhausting diseases: *Kali Phos.*
Tired, weary and exhausted: *Calc. Phos., Magnes. Phos., Kali Phos.*
Tired, weary, with biliousness: *Natr. Sulph.*
Trembling hands: *Magnes. Phos.*
Vocal cords, paralysis of: *Kali Phos.*
Writer's cramp: *Magnes. Phos.*

SKIN SYMPTOMS

Abscess, for heat and pain: *Ferrum Phos.*
Acne rosacea: *Calc. Phos.*
Acne, with thick white contents: *Kali Mur.*
Albuminous discharge: *Calc. Phos.*
Anus, fissures of: *Calc. Fluor.*
Blebs, with sanious, watery contents: *Kali Phos.*
Blisters, with sanious, water contents: *Kali Phos.*
watery contents: *Natr. Mur.*
Boils, for the swelling before pus forms: *Kali Mur.*
if deep seated and discharge thick, heavy yellow pus: *Silicea.*
inflammatory stage, to relieve heat, pain and throbbing: *Ferrum Phos.*
to abort them: *Calc. Sulph.*

Burns, when suppurating: *Calc. Sulph.*

Burning, as from nettles: *Calc. Phos.*

Carbuncles, for swelling before pus forms: *Kali Mur.*
if deep seated, and discharging a heavy, thick, yellow pus: *Silicea.*
inflammatory stage to relieve heat, pain, and throbbing: *Ferrum Phos.*

Chafed skin of infants: *Natr. Sulph., Natr. Phos., Natr. Mur.*

Chapped hands from cold: *Ferrum Phos., Calc. Fluor.*

Chicken-pox, for fever: *Ferrum Phos.*

Chilblains: *Kali Phos., Kali Mur.*

Colorless, watery vesicles: *Natr. Mur.*

Cracks in palms of hands: *Calc. Fluor.*

Crusta lactea: *Calc. Sulph., Natr. Phos.*

Dandruff: *Kali Sulph., Natr. Mur., Kali Mur.*

Desquamation: *Kali Sulph.*

Discharge, albuminous: *Calc. Phos.*
blood and pus: *Calc. Sulph.*

Discharge, fetid: *Kali Phos.*
thick, yellow pus: *Silicea.*

Dry skin: *Calc. Phos., Kali Sulph.*

Eczema, accompanied by nervous irritation: *Kali Phos.*
oversensitiveness: *Kali Phos.*
acid, creamy, yellow secretion: *Natr. Phos.*
from deranged uterine functions: *Kali Mur.*
eating too much salt: *Natr. Mur.*
when eruption is suddenly suppressed: *Kali Sulph.*
white scales: *Natr. Mur., Kali Mur.*
yellow crusts: *Calc. Phos.*
white exudations: *Kali Mur.*

Epithelial cancer, thin, purulent discharge: *Kali Sulph.*

Eruptions from bad vaccine: *Kali Mur.*
with watery contents: *Natr. Mur.*
thick, white contents: *Kali Mur.*

Erysipelas, for the febrile symptoms of the first stage: *Ferrum Phos.*
smooth, red, shiny, tingling, or painful swelling of the skin: *Natr. Sulph.*
Erythema, for swelling and white coated tongue: *Kali Mur.*
rose rash: *Natr. Phos.*
Excessive dryness of skin: *Natr. Mur.*
Exudations, when white and fibrinous indicate a deficiency in: *Kali Mur.*
albuminous: *Calc. Phos.*
yellow with small, tough lumps: *Calc. Fluor.*
like gold: *Natr. Phos.*
yellowish and slimy or watery: *Kali Sulph.*
greenish, thin: *Kali Sulph.*
clear, transparent, thin like water: *Natr. Mur.*
mattery, or streaked with blood: *Calc. Sulph.*
pus is thick, yellow: *Silicea.*
very offensive smelling: *Kali Phos.*
causing soreness and chafing: *Natr. Mur., Kali Phos.*
Face full of pimples: *Calc. Phos.*
Felons, if deep seated, and discharging thick, yellow, heavy pus: *Silicea.*
inflammatory stage, to relieve heat, pain and throbbing: *Ferrum Phos.*
or any other skin disease, when the matter discharging becomes fetid: *Kali Phos.*
Festers easily: *Calc. Sulph., Silicea.*
Fevers, with skin dry and hot: *Kali Sulph.*
Fistulous abscess of long standing: *Natr. Sulph.*
surrounded by a blue border: *Natr. Sulph.*
Freckles: *Calc. Phos.*
Glands, swollen: *Kali Mur.*

Greasy scales on skin: *Kali Phos.*
Hard, callous skin: *Calc. Fluor.*
Heals slowly: *Silicea.*
Herpes, in bend of knees: *Natr. Mur.*
Herpetic eruptions: *Natr. Mur.*
Hives: *Natr. Phos.*
Horny skin: *Calc. Fluor.*
Inflammation of skin, for fever and heat: *Ferrum Phos.*
with yellow, watery exudations: *Natr. Sulph.*
Ingrowing toe-nail: *Kali Mur., Silicea.*
Intertrigo between the thighs and scrotum, and acrid excoriating discharge: *Natr. Mur.*
Irritating secretions: *Kali Phos.*
Irritation of the skin similar to chillblains: *Kali Mur.*
Itching, as from nettles: *Calc. Phos.*
of skin, with crawling: *Kali Phos., Calc. Phos.*
while undressing: *Natr. Sulph.*
without eruptions. *Calc. Phos.*
Leprosy, copper-colored spots: *Silicea.*
nasal ulcerations: *Silicea.*
nodes: *Silicea.*
Lupus: *Calc. Phos., Kali Mur.*
Malignant pustules: *Kali Phos.*
Mattery scabs on heads of pimples: *Calc. Sulph.*
Measles, hoarse cough, glandular swellings, white furred tongue: *Kali Mur.*
skin dry and hot, with suppressed rash: *Kali Sulph.*
when the rash has been suppressed: *Kali Sulph.*
Moist scabs on skin: *Natr. Sulph.*
Nails, diseased: *Kali Sulph., Silicea.*
interrupted in growth: *Kali Sulph., Silicea.*
Nettle-rash, after becoming overheated: *Natr. Mur.*
with violent itching: *Natr. Mur.*
Pemphigus malignus: *Kali Phos.*
yellow, watery exudation: *Natr. Sulph.*

Perspiration, lack of: *Kali Sulph.*
on hands, from spinal weakness: *Calc. Phos.*
to promote: *Kali Sulph.*
Pimples all over body, like flea-bites: *Natr. Phos.*
with itching: *Calc. Phos.*
under beard: *Calc. Sulph.*
Pruritus of vagina: *Calc. Phos.*
with or without albuminous leucorrhea: *Calc. Phos.*
Pustules on face: *Silicea, Kali Mur.*
painful: *Silicea.*
Rawness of skin in little children: *Natr. Phos.*
Rupia, blisters, with watery contents: *Natr. Mur.*
Scalds, when suppurating: *Calc. Sulph.*
Scales freely on sticky base: *Kali Sulph.*
Scaling eruptions on skin: *Calc. Phos.*
Scarlet fever: *Kali Mur., Natr. Mur.*
for fever: *Ferrum Phos.*
twitchings: *Natr. Mur.*
Scarlet fever, watery vomit: *Natr. Mur.*
when rash has been suppressed: *Kali Sulph.*
Scrofulous eruptions: *Silicea, Calc. Phos.*
Secretions irritate: *Kali Phos.*
Shingles: *Natr. Mur., Kali Mur.*
Skin affections with vesicular eruptions containing yellowish water: *Natr. Sulph.*
yellow scabs: *Calc. Sulph.*
diseases which arise from using bad vaccine lymph: *Kali Mur.*
festers easily: *Calc. Sulph.*
hard and horny: *Calc. Fluor.*
heals slowly and suppurates easily after injuries: *Silicea.*
dry, hot, and burning, lack of perspiration: *Kali Sulph.*
itching and burning; as from nettles: *Calc. Phos.*
scales freely on a sticky base: *Kali Sulph.*
withered and wrinkled: *Kali Phos.*

Small-pox, heat and fever: *Ferrum Phos.*
pustules discharging: *Calc. Sulph.*
putrid conditions: *Kali Phos.*
when rash has been suppressed: *Kali Sulph.*
with drowsiness: *Natr. Mur.*
flow of saliva: *Natr. Mur.*
Stings of insects: *Natr. Mur.*
Suppurates easily: *Silicea.*
Sycosis: *Kali Mur.*
To aid desquamation in eruptive diseases: *Kali Sulph.*
To assist in the formation of new skin: *Kali Sulph.*
Tongue coated white: *Kali Mur.*
Ulcers around nails: *Silicea.*
fistulous, thick, yellow pus: *Silicea. Calc. Fluor. Calc. Sulph.*
Unhealthy-looking skin: *Silicea.*
Vesicular erysipelas: *Kali Mur.*
eruptions containing yellow, watery pus: *Natr. Sulph.*
Yellow scabs: *Calc. Sulph.*
scales on skin: *Natr. Sulph.*
Warts: *Kali Mur.*
in palms of hands: *Natr. Mur.*
Withered skin: *Kali Phos.*
Wounds do not heal readily: *Calc. Sulph.*
neglected, discharge pus: *Calc. Sulph.*
Wrinkled skin: *Kali Phos.*

TISSUES

Abscess bleeds easily after pus forms: *Silicea.*
Anemia: *Calc. Phos., Ferrum Phos.*
Anemia, with skin affections: *Kali Mur.*
Ameliorates pain of cancer: *Kali Phos.*
Atrophic condition of old people: *Kali Phos.*

Bleeding from nose in anemic persons: *Ferrum Phos.*
Calc. Phos.
children: *Ferrum Phos.*
Blood coagulates rapidly: *Ferrum Phos.*
Bones, diseased, soft parts inflamed: *Ferrum Phos.*
easily broken: *Calc. Phos.*
friable: *Calc. Phos.*
weak: *Calc. Phos.*
will not unite: *Calc. Phos.*
Bruises: *Ferrum Phos.*
on bones: *Calc. Fluor.*
Burns: *Kali Mur.*
Cancer, offensive discharge: *Kali Phos.*
epithelial: *Kali Sulph.*
Caries of bone: *Silicea.*
Catarrh, purulent discharge in: *Calc. Sulph.*
Chlorosis: *Calc. Phos., Natr. Mur.*
Complexion, pale, greenish or white: *Calc. Phos., Natr. Mur.*
Consumption, purulent discharge in: *Calc. Sulph.*
Debility: *Kali Phos.*
Development, defective: *Calc. Phos.*
Discharge continues too long: *Calc. Sulph.*
thick, yellow, sanious: *Calc. Sulph.*
Dropsy: *Natr. Sulph., Natr. Mur.*
from heart disease: *Calc. Fluor.*
kidney diseases: *Kali Mur.*
loss of blood: *Ferrum Phos.*
obstruction of bileducts: *Kali Mur.*
invading areolar tissues: *Natr. Sulph.*
Dropsy, of extremities, with hard, glistening appearance: *Kali Mur.*
Effusions, slimy, serous: *Natr. Mur.*
Elastic tissues relaxed: *Calc. Fluor.*
Emaciations: *Calc. Phos.*
of neck: *Natr. Mur.*
Encysted tumors: *Calc. Fluor.*

Energy: lack of: *Kali Phos.*
Epithelial cancer: *Kali Sulph.*
Exhaustion: *Kali Phos.*
Exuberant granulations: *Kali Mur.*
Exudations, creamy yellow: *Natr. Phos.*
fibrinous, slimy, thick, yellow: *Kali Mur.*
mucous, corroding: *Kali Phos.*
sanious, mixed with blood: *Kali Phos.*
serous, ichorous, offensive: *Kali Phos.*
Face pale and sallow: *Natr. Mur.*
Fibrinous exudation becomes hard: *Calc. Fluor.*
Gangrenous conditions: *Kali Phos.*
inflammations: *Silicea.*
Glands, enlargement of, from scrofula: *Kali Mur.*
suppuration of, yellow, thick, offensive discharge: *Silicea.*
swelling of: *Silicea, Kali Mur.*
Gonorrhea, purulent discharge in: *Calc. Sulph.*
Hardened glands: *Calc. Fluor., Silicea, Kali Mur.*
Hemorrhage, bright-red blood: *Ferrum Phos.*
does not coagulate: *Kali Phos.*
thin, dark, putrid: *Kali Phos.*
Indurated enlargements: *Calc. Fluor.*
Infiltration: *Natr. Sulph.*
Injury, neglected cases of, with suppuration: *Silicea.*
Leucorrhea, purulent discharge: *Calc. Sulph.*
Lymphatic glands, chronic inflammation of: *Natr. Mur.*
Malignant inflammations: *Silicea.*
Mucous membrane, dry: *Natr. Mur.*
excess of secretion: *Natr. Mur.*
Mumps: *Ferrum Phos., Kali Mur., Natr. Mur.*
Neuralgic pains in any tissue: *Magnes. Phos.*
Nutrition, through indigestion, poor: *Calc. Phos.*
Pancreas, diseases of: *Calc. Phos.*

Periosteum, suppuration of: *Calc. Fluor.*
Polypi: *Calc. Phos.*
Proud flesh: *Kali Mur.*
Rheumatism, with acid symptoms: *Natr. Phos.*
Rickets: *Calc. Phos.*
putrid stools: *Kali Phos.*
Scrofulous enlargement of glands: *Silicea, Calc. Phos.*
Scurvy, gangrenous conditions: *Kali Phos.*
hard infiltrations: *Kali Mur.*
Secretions yellow, watery, purulent: *Kali Sulph.*
Serum in areolar tissues: *Natr. Mur.*
Smooth, edematous swelling: *Natr. Sulph.*
Soft tissues, all injuries to: *Ferrum Phos.*
Sores, unhealthy: *Calc. Sulph.*
Spasms in any tissue: *Magnes. Phos.*
Sprains: *Ferrum Phos.*
Strains: *Ferrum Phos.*
Stunted growth: *Calc. Phos.*
Suppuration of glands: *Calc. Sulph.*
Syphilis, with purulent discharges: *Calc. Sulph.*
Tabes: *Calc. Phos.*
Thin, watery blood: *Natr. Mur.*
Tissues dry scabby: *Kali Phos.*
Tongue coated white: *Kali Mur.*
slimy, frothy: *Natr. Mur.*
Ulceration of bone: *Calc. Phos., Silicea.*
glands: *Calc. Sulph.*
lower limbs: *Calc. Sulph.*
for fever: *Ferrum Phos.*
Uneven, hard lumps: *Calc. Phos.*
Urine, white, sediment of mucus in: *Kali Mur.*
Vitality, lack of: *Kali Phos.*
Wasting disease: *Kali Phos.*
Yellow, white, greenish secretions: *Natr. Sulph.*

FEBRILE SYMPTOMS

Acid symptoms during febrile diseases: *Natr. Phos.*

After typhoid and other fevers as the disease declines, to promote the deposit of new molecules in place of those destroyed: *Calc. Phos.*

All febrile conditions with grayish white, dry or slimy coating on the tongue: *Kali Mur.*

All febrile diseases with low malignant, putrid symptoms: *Kali Phos.*

All kinds of fevers when there are malignant symptoms, such as stupor, drowsiness, watery vomiting, twitchings, etc.: *Natr. Mur.*

Bilious fevers: *Natr. Sulph.*

Blood-poisoning threatens: *Kali Sulph.*

Brain fever, low muttering of: *Kali Phos.*

Catarrhal fever, chilly sensations: *Ferrum Phos.*

quickened pulse: *Ferrum Phos.*

Chicken-pox, for heat and congestion: *Ferrum Phos.*

Chill commencing in the morning about 10 o'clock and continuing till noon, preceded by intense heat, increased headache and thirst, sweat, weakening, more backache and headache; great languor, emaciation, sallow complexion and blisters on the lips: *Natr. Mur.*

Chilliness at beginning of fevers: *Ferrum Phos.*

in back: *Natr. Mur.*

Chills run up and down spine: *Magnes. Phos.*

Clammy sweat on body: *Calc. Phos.*

Cold sweat on face: *Calc. Phos.*

Copious night sweat with prostration, in phthisis: *Silicea.*

Delirium: *Kali Phos.*

Desquamation, to aid: *Kali Sulph.*

Diarrhea, with sanious, bloody discharge: *Calc. Sulph.*

Drowsiness: *Natr. Mur.*

Dull, heavy headache: *Natr. Mur.*

Dysentery, with sanious, bloody discharge: *Calc. Sulph.*

Enteric fever, first stage: *Ferrum Phos.*
second stage, to restore the integrity of the tissues: *Kali Mur.*
when the temperature rises in the evening: *Kali Sulph*

Excessive exhausting perspiration or sweating, while eating, with weakness at the stomach: *Kali Phos.*

Feeling of chilliness especially in the back; watery saliva; full heavy headache, increased heat: *Natr. Mur.*

Fevers, during suppurative processes: *Silicea.*
from relaxed conditions: *Calc. Fluor.*
vomit of sour fluids during: *Natr. Phos.*
with chills and cramps: *Magnes. Phos., Ferrum Phos.*
gastric, typhoid, scarlet, enteric, when the temperature rises in the evening: *Kali Sulph.*

First stage of chicken pox for the heat and congestion: *Ferrum Phos.*
enteric fever for the heat and congestion: *Ferrum Phos.*
gastric fever for the heat and congestion: *Ferrum Phos.*
measles for the heat and congestion: *Ferrum Phos.*
rheumatic fever for the heat and congestion: *Ferrum Phos.*
scarlet fever for the heat and congestion: *Ferrum Phos.*
smallpox for the heat and congestion: *Ferrum Phos.*
typhoid fever for the heat and congestion: *Ferrum Phos.*
typhus for the heat and congestion: *Ferrum Phos.*

Flashes of heat from indigestion: *Natr. Phos.*

Frontal headache from flashes of heat: *Natr. Phos.*

Gastric fever, first stage: *Ferrum Phos.*
secondary remedy to restore integrity of the tissues: *Kali Mur.*
when the temperature runs in the evening: *Kali Sulph.*

Hectic fever: *Calc. Sulph.*
with burning of soles of feet: *Silicea.*

Increased thirst: *Natr. Mur.*

Inflammations, first stage: *Ferrum Phos.*
second stage: *Kali Mur.*

In fevers when blood poison threatens: *Kali Sulph.*

In eruptive fevers to aid desquamation: *Kali Sulph.*

Intermittent fever after the abuse of quinine: *Natr. Mur.*
fetid, profuse, debilitating perspiration: *Kali Phos.*
the chief remedy in all stages: *Natr. Sulph.*
with cramps in the calves of the legs: *Magnes. Phos.*
vomiting of food, continual fever, with quickened pulse and chilly sensation: *Ferrum Phos.*

Living in damp regions or in newly turned ground: *Natr. Mur.*
with malignant symptoms and low muttering: *Kali Phos.*

Malignant conditions of typhoid fever: *Kali Phos.*
symptoms: *Kali Phos.*

Measles, for heat and congestion: *Ferrum Phos.*

Much sweat in the daytime: *Natr. Mur.*

Nervous chills, with chattering of teeth: *Magnes. Phos.*
Kali Phos.
fever, low muttering in: *Kali Phos.*

Nervous fever with malignant symptoms and low muttering: *Kali Phos.*

Night sweats: *Silicea.*
in phthisis: *Calc. Phos.*

Offensive foot-sweats: *Silicea.*

Perspiration, excessive: *Calc. Phos., Kali Phos.*
sour-smelling: *Natr. Phos.*
Profuse night-sweats: *Natr. Mur., Silicea, Calc. Phos.*
Prostration in phthisis: *Silicea.*
Puerperal fever: *Kali Mur., Kali Phos.*
Pulse, subnormal: *Kali Phos.*
Rheumatic fever, for exudation: *Kali Mur.*
heat and congestion: *Ferrum Phos.*
Saliva clear, watery: *Natr. Mur.*
Scarlet fever, for heat and congestion: *Ferrum Phos.*
for the putrid, malignant conditions: *Kali Phos.*
when the temperature rises in the evening: *Kali Sulph.*
with stupor, drowsiness, watery vomiting and twitchings: *Natr. Mur.*
Second stage of inflammations and congestions of any organ: *Kali Mur.*
Shivering at beginning of fever: *Calc. Phos., Ferrum Phos.*
Sleeplessness: *Kali Phos.*
Small-pox, for heat and congestion: *Ferrum Phos.*
Stupor: *Natr. Mur., Kali Phos.*
Sweat of head in children: *Silicea.*
while eating: *Kali Phos.*
To assist in promoting perspiration: *Kali Sulph.*
Tongue coated dirty, greenish-brown: *Natr. Sulph.*
grayish-white, slimy: *Kali Mur.*
Twitching: *Natr. Mur.*
Typhoid fever, first stage: *Ferrum Phos.*
when the temperature rises in the morning: *Kali Sulph.*
for the putrid malignant condition: *Kali Phos.*
with sanious, bloody discharges from the bowels: *Calc. Sulph.*
second remedy, to restore integrity to the tissues: *Kali Mur.*
with stupor, drowsiness, watery vomiting and twitchings: *Natr. Mur.*

Typhus fever, for the constipation: *Kali Mur.*
with malignant symptoms, with low fever, muttering: *Kali Phos.*
sanious discharge: *Calc. Sulph.*
stupor, drowsiness, watery vomiting and twitchings: *Natr. Mur.*

Vomit of bile: *Natr. Sulph.*
bitter fluids: *Natr. Sulph.*
brown or black fluids: *Natr. Sulph.*

Watery vomit: *Natr. Mur.*

Yellow fever, black vomit of: *Natr. Sulph.*
of remittent type: *Natr. Sulph.*

SLEEP

Better in evening: *Natr. Sulph.*
Congestion of blood to the head at night: *Silicea.*
Constant desire to sleep in morning: *Natr. Mur.*
Drawing pain in the back at night during sleep: *Natr. Mur.*
Dreams much: *Natr. Sulph.*
Drowsiness, with bilious symptoms: *Natr. Sulph.*
Drowsy: *Natr. Mur., Magnes. Phos., Calc. Phos.*
Dull: *Natr. Mur.*
Emptiness in stomach: *Kali Phos.*
Excessive sleep, from an excess of moisture in brain: *Natr. Mur.*
Frequent dreams and exclamations during sleep: *Silicea.*
Great drowsiness: *Silicea.*
Grits teeth: *Natr. Phos.*
Hard to wake in morning: *Calc. Phos.*
Heavy, anxious dreams: *Natr. Sulph.*
Hysterical yawning: *Kali Phos.*
Jerking of limbs during sleep: *Silicea. Natr. Sulph.*
Lethargy, with hectic fever: *Calc. Sulph.*
Much yawning: *Silicea.*

Nightmare, with bilious symptoms: *Natr. Mur., Natr. Sulph. Kali Sulph.*

Picks nose: *Natr. Phos.*

Restless sleep, from worms: *Calc. Phos., Natr. Phos.*

Screams in sleep: *Natr. Phos.*

Sleep does not refresh: *Natr. Mur.*

Sleepiness, with hectic fever: *Calc. Sulph.*

Sleeplessness, after excitement: *Ferrum Phos., Natr. Phos.*
worry: *Ferrum Phos., Kali Phos.*
from nervous causes: *Kali Phos.*
orgasm of blood: *Silicea.*

Sleepy in morning: *Natr. Sulph.*

Somnambulism: *Kali Phos.*

Stretching, from nervous causes: *Kali Phos.*

Stupid: *Natr. Mur.*

Tired in morning: *Natr. Mur., Natr. Sulph.*

Vivid dreams: *Calc. Phos.*

Wakefulness: *Kali Phos., Ferrum Phos.*

Wakefulness in old people with phthisis: *Silicea.*

Weariness, from nervous causes: *Kali Phos.*
with bilious symptoms: *Natr. Sulph.*

Yawning, from nervous causes: *Kali Phos.*
with spasmodic straining of lower jaw: *Natr. Phos.*

MODALITIES

Complaints after free use of poisonous things: *Natr. Mur.*
periodic: *Natr. Mur.*

Rise in temperature in evening till midnight: *Kali Sulph.*

Stomach symptoms worse after eating fats, pastry or rich food: *Kali Mur.*

Pains, aggravated by continued exercise: *Kali Phos.*
motion: *Kali Mur., Ferrum Phos.*
rest: *Kali Phos.*

Pains, ameliorated by gentle motion: *Kali Phos.*
heat: *Magnes. Phos.*
pressure: *Magnes. Phos.*
rubbing: *Magnes. Phos.*

Symptoms, aggravated:
arising from sitting position: *Kali Phos.*
at night: *Silicea, Calc. Phos.*
change of weather: *Calc. Phos.*
chilling feet: *Silicea.*

Symptoms, aggravated:
cold: *Natr. Mur., Calc. Phos., Magnes. Phos.*
cold air: *Magnes. Phos., Kali Sulph.*
damp weather: *Calc. Phos., Natr. Sulph.*
draughts: *Magnes. Phos.*
eating water plants: *Natr. Sulph.*
exertions: *Kali Phos.*
eating fish: *Natr. Sulph.*
getting wet: *Calc. Phos., Calc. Sulph.*
heated atmosphere: *Kali Sulph.*
in the morning: *Natr. Sulph., Natr. Mur.*
evening: *Silicea, Calc. Phos., Kali Sulph.*
open air: *Silicea.*
motion: *Ferrum Phos.*
noise: *Kali Phos.*
rainy weather: *Natr. Sulph.*
salty atmosphere: *Natr. Mur.*
water: *Natr. Sulph.*

ameliorated:
cold: *Ferrum Phos.*
eating: *Kali Phos.*
evening: *Natr. Mur.*
excitement: *Kali Phos.*
gentle motion: *Kali Phos.*
heat: *Magnes. Phos., Calc. Fluor.*
pleasant excitement: *Kali Phos.*
pressure: *Magnes. Phos.*
rubbing: *Magnes. Phos.*
warm room: *Calc. Phos.*
weather: *Calc. Phos. Calc. Sulph.*

THE INORGANIC SALTS

Copied from "A Text-Book of Physiology."

By William H. Howell, Ph.D., M.D., Sc.D., LL.D.,
Professor of Physiology in The Johns Hopkins University, Baltimore.

"The body contains in its tissues and liquids a considerable amount of inorganic material. When any organ is incinerated this material remains as the ash. If we include the bones, which are rich in mineral matter, the average amount of ash in the body amounts to about 4.3 to 4.4 per cent of its weight. The bones, however, in the adult contain most of this ash (five-sixths). In the soft tissues, like the muscle, the ash constitutes about 0.6 to 0.8 per cent of the moist weight. The ash consists of chlorids, phosphates, sulphates, carbonates, fluorids, or silicates of potassium, sodium, calcium, magnesium, and iron; iodin occurs also, especially in the thyroid tissues.

In the liquids of the body the main salts are sodium chlorid, sodium carbonate, sodium phosphate, potassium and calcium chlorid or phosphate. In considering the organic foodstuffs weight was laid upon their value as sources of energy, as well as upon their function in constructing tissue. The salts have no importance from the former standpoint. Whatever chemical changes they undergo are not attended by any liberation of heat energy—none at least of sufficient importance to be considered.

They have, however, most important functions. They maintain a normal composition and osmotic pressure in the liquids and tissues of the body, and by virtue of their osmotic pressure they play an important part in controlling the flow of water to and from the tissues. Moreover, the salts constitute an essential part of the composition of living matter. In some way they are bound up in the structure of the living molecule and are necessary to its normal reactions or irritability. Even the proteins of the body liquids contain definite amounts of ash, and if this ash is removed their properties are seriously altered, as is shown by the fact that ash-free native proteins lose their property of coagulation by heat. The globulins are precipitated from their solutions when the salts are removed.

The special importance of the calcium salts in the coagulation of blood and the curdling of milk has been referred to, as also the peculiar part played by the calcium, potassium, and sodium salts in the rhythmical contractions of heart muscle, the irritability of muscular and nervous tissues, and the permeability of the capillary walls and other membranes. The special importance of the iron salts for the production of hemoglobin is also evident without comment.

There can be no doubt, in fact, that each one of the salts of the body has a special nutritive value and a special metabolic history. The time will doubtless come when the special importance of the potassium, sodium, calcium, and magnesium will be understood as well, at least, as we now understand the significance of iron, and quite possibly this knowledge will find a direct therapeutic application as in the case of iron."

INDEX